Silent Myocardial Ischemia and Infarction

FUNDAMENTAL AND CLINICAL CARDIOLOGY

Editor-in-Chief

Samuel Z. Goldhaber, M.D.

*Harvard Medical School
and Brigham and Women's Hospital
Boston, Massachusetts*

Associate Editor, Europe

Henri Bounameaux, M.D.

*University Hospital of Geneva
Geneva, Switzerland*

38. *Cardiac Rehabilitation: A Guide to Practice in the 21st Century,* edited by Nanette K. Wenger, L. Kent Smith, Erika Sivarajan Froelicher, and Patricia McCall Comoss
39. *Heparin-Induced Thrombocytopenia,* edited by Theodore E. Warkentin and Andreas Greinacher
40. *Silent Myocardial Ischemia and Infarction, Fourth Edition,* by Peter F. Cohn

ADDITIONAL VOLUMES IN PREPARATION

Cardiac Arrhythmias, edited by Peter M. Spooner and Michael R. Rosen

Silent Myocardial Ischemia and Infarction

Fourth Edition

Peter F. Cohn

*Professor of Medicine
and Chief, Cardiology Division
State University of New York
Health Sciences Center at Stony Brook
Stony Brook, New York*

MARCEL DEKKER, INC.   NEW YORK · BASEL

ISBN: 0-8247-0354-5

This book is printed on acid-free paper.

Headquarters
Marcel Dekker, Inc.
270 Madison Avenue, New York, NY 10016
tel: 212-696-9000; fax: 212-685-4540

Eastern Hemisphere Distribution
Marcel Dekker AG
Hutgasse 4, Postfach 812, CH-4001 Basel, Switzerland
tel: 41-61-261-8482; fax: 41-61-261-8896

World Wide Web
http://www.dekker.com

The publisher offers discounts on this book when ordered in bulk quantities. For more information, write to Special Sales/Professional Marketing at the headquarters address above.

Series Introduction

Marcel Dekker, Inc., has focused on the development of various series of beautifully produced books in different branches of medicine. These series have facilitated the integration of rapidly advancing information for both the clinical specialist and the researcher.

My goal as editor-in-chief of the Fundamental and Clinical Cardiology series is to assemble the talents of world-renowned authorities to discuss virtually every area of cardiovascular medicine. In this fourth edition of *Silent Myocardial Ischemia and Infarction*, Peter F. Cohn has fully revised this much-needed and timely book. Future contributions to this series will include books on molecular biology, interventional cardiology, and clinical management of such problems as coronary artery disease and ventricular arrhythmias.

Samuel Z. Goldhaber

Preface to the Fourth Edition

Since the third edition of this book was published in 1993, there has been an important change in the way silent coronary artery disease is perceived by physicians: it is now regarded not as an esoteric phenomenon but as a key component of the ischemic spectrum. If 1970–1979 was the decade for defining this syndrome and understanding its pathophysiology, and 1980–1989 was a time for documenting its impact on prognosis and the effectiveness of anti-ischemic treatment, then 1990–1999 was the decade for tying these diverse strands together and assessing the impact of therapy on prognosis. With the new millennium upon us, it is now time to sum up what we know.

For this edition, I thank Ms. Carol Pascale for her excellent secretarial assistance.

Peter F. Cohn

Preface to the First Edition

The purpose of this monograph is to discuss what is known—and what is not known—about asymptomatic coronary artery disease and its two major components: silent myocardial ischemia and silent myocardial infarction. These disorders afflict millions of persons, yet little is written about their mechanisms, prognosis, and other characteristics mainly because physicians—and the lay public—traditionally associate myocardial ischemia and infarction with chest pain (or its equivalents). That this is not necessarily so is becoming more and more evident. Symptomatic episodes may represent only the tip of the iceberg of myocardial ischemia.

To evaluate the subject in a systematic way, this book has been organized into five major parts: pathophysiology, prevalence, detection, prognosis, and management of asymptomatic coronary artery disease.

Many of the studies discussed in the following chapters were performed with the assistance of my colleagues at Harvard Medical School and the Brigham and Women's Hospital in Boston, and the State University of New

York Health Sciences Center at Stony Brook. Their contributions are greatly appreciated, as is the expert secretarial assistance of Mrs. Marlene Landesman.

Peter F. Cohn

Contents

Silent Myocardial Ischemia and Infarction

Introduction

Where have we been? Where are we going? These themes are necessary for summing up, but especially so as we end the twentieth century. In the case of silent coronary artery disease, these are especially pertinent questions since the realization that not all manifestations of coronary artery disease must be symptomatic is not new but, until the 1970s, did not receive the attention it deserved.

The history of asymptomatic coronary artery disease is basically a history of its two major syndromes—silent myocardial ischemia and silent myocardial infarction. *Silent (painless, asymptomatic) myocardial ischemia is* best defined as objective evidence of transient ischemia (on ECG, radionuclide studies, etc.) in the absence of angina or its usual equivalents. *Silent (unrecognized) myocardial infarction is* essentially an ECG diagnosis. Autopsy reports of extensive coronary disease in persons apparently free of symptoms were the first important clues to the existence of this syndrome [1]. The next important—although indirect—milestones were studies of unexpected sudden death in which large numbers of previously asymptomatic persons were involved. But it was not until patients with coronary artery disease were actually observed to be free of pain during episodes of transient myocardial ischemia on exercise tests [2,3] and during ambulatory electrocardiographic monitoring [4] that interest in this subject increased [5].

My own interest in asymptomatic coronary artery disease began in the early 1970s and initially involved ECG responses during exercise testing. Our first study was reported at the American Heart Association meetings in 1975 [6] and was followed by a review in 1977 [7], which described the unexpectedly vast scope of the disorder. Introduction of the concept of a "defective anginal warning system" soon followed, with speculation as to its causes and effects on prognosis [8]. It became apparent to me that if this subject were to be investigated fully, a classification system for asymptomatic coronary artery disease was necessary. Accordingly, in 1981 [9], we proposed that silent myocardial ischemia be thought of as occurring in three types of patients with coronary artery disease (Table 1). The first group consisted of persons who were totally asymptomatic and the second group of persons who were asymptomatic after an infarction. In addition, silent myocardial ischemia can be seen in patients with angina who also have asymptomatic episodes. The key to this classification is in documentation of active ischemia; persons who have asymptomatic coronary artery disease but are not experiencing active ischemia are purposely not involved in this classification. Thus, someone with an infarction, a totally occluded vessel and no ongoing ischemia by objective criteria would be excluded.

The five major questions that were posed in the 1981 review [9] are still pertinent today and form the basis for this monograph, slightly modified. They are

1. What is the pathophysiological basis of silent myocardial ischemia and silent myocardial infarction?
2. What is the prevalence of the different types of silent myocardial ischemia, and of silent myocardial infarction?
3. What are the most reliable noninvasive methods of detecting the syndrome of silent myocardial ischemia, and what are the indications for cardiac catheterization in asymptomatic persons?
4. What is the prognosis of patients with silent myocardial ischemia and/or silent myocardial infarction?
5. How should silent myocardial ischemia be treated if at all? Others have also posed similar questions [10].

The first attempt of answering these questions in a systematic way was in a seminar that appeared in 1983 in the *Journal of the American College of Cardiology* [11]. This was followed by the first international symposium of Silent Myocardial Ischemia held in Geneva, Switzerland, in 1984 under the auspices

Table 1 Types of Cases in Which Silent Myocardial Ischemia
May Be Found

I. Persons who are totally asymptomatic.
II. Persons who are asymptomatic following a myocardial infarction, but still demonstrate active ischemia.
III. Persons with angina who are asymptomatic with some episodes of myocardial ischemia, but not others.

of the European Society of Cardiology [12]. Numerous other national and international symposia have been held since then. In 1986, the first edition of this book was published [13] and was soon joined by several other important state-of-the-art publications [14–16] and, in 1989, by the second edition of this work [17]. The 1990s saw the publication of the third edition of this book [18], as well as multiauthored text, [19] and a useful guide for the general public [20]. In addition to these publications (and the articles referred to in the current edition), there are three special reports that should be of particular interest to readers of this book. These are the recommendations of the combined American College of Cardiology/American Heart Association Task Force on Assessment of Diagnostic and Therapeutic Cardiovascular Procedures on exercise testing [21], coronary angiography and angioplasty [22,23], and Holter monitoring [24]. Each report contains a section on the indications for these procedures in (1) asymptomatic patients at high risk for latent coronary artery disease, and/or (2) those patients with symptoms but in whom silent ischemia is suspected or has been demonstrated.

REFERENCES

1. Roseman MD. Painless myocardial infarction: A review of the literature and analysis of 220 cases. Ann Intern Med 1954; 41:1.
2. Master AM, Geller AM. The extent of completely asymptomatic coronary artery disease. Am J Cardiol 1969; 23:173.
3. Froelicher VF, Yanowitz FG, Thompson AJ. The correlation of coronary angiography and the electrocardiographic response to maximal treadmill testing in 76 asymptomatic men. Circulation 1973; 48:597.
4. Stern S, Tzivoni D. Early detection of silent ischaemic heart disease by 24-hour electrocardiographic monitoring of active subjects. Br Heart J. 1974; 35:481.
5. Gettes LS. Painless myocardial ischemia. Chest 1974; 66:612.

6. Lindsey HE, Cohn PF. "Silent" ischemia during and after exercise testing in patients with coronary artery disease (abstr). Circulation 1975; 52(suppl 11): 46.

7. Cohn PF. Severe asymptomatic coronary artery disease: A diagnostic, prognostic and therapeutic puzzle. Am J Med 1977; 62:565.

8. Cohn PF. Silent myocardial ischemia in patitents with a defective anginal warning system. Am J Cardiol 1980; 45:697.

9. Cohn PF. Asymptomatic coronary artery disease: Pathophysiology, diagnosis, management. Mod Concepts Cardiovasc Dis 1981; 50:55.

10. Iskandrian AS, Segal BL, Anderson GS. Asymptomatic myocardial ischemia. Arch Intern Med. 1981; 141:95.

11. Cohn PF. Introduction to Seminar on Asymptomatic Coronary Artery Disease. J Am Coll Cardiol. 1983; 3:922.

12. Rutishauser W, Roskamm H, eds. Silent Myocardial Ischemia. Berlin: Springer-Verlag, 1984.

13. Cohn PF. Silent Myocardial Ischemia and Infarction. New York: Marcel Dekker, Philadelphia: 1986.

14. Pepine CJ, ed. Cardiology Clinics: Silent Myocardial Ischemia. Philadelphia: W. B. Saunders, 1986.

15. Cohn PF, Kannel W. Recognition, pathogenesis and management options in silent coronary artery disease. Circulation 1987; 75(suppl II):1–54.

16. von Armin T, Maseri A, eds. Silent Ischemia: Current Concepts and Management. Darmstadt: Steinkopff, 1987.

17. Cohn PF. Silent Myocardial Ischemia and Infarction, 2nd ed. New York: Marcel Dekker, 1989.

18. Cohn PF. Silent Myocardial Ischemia and Infraction. New York: Marcel Dekker, 1993.

19. Stern S, ed. Silent Myocardial Ischemia. London: Martin Dunitz, 1998.

20. Cohn PF, Cohn JK. Fighting the Silent Killer: How Men and Women Can Prevent and Cope with Heart Disease Today. Wellesley, MA: AK Peters, 1993.

21. Gibbons RJ, Balady GJ, Beasley JW, Bricker JT, Duvernoy WFC, Froelicher VF, Mark DB, Marwick TH, McCallister BD, Thompson PD, Winters WL Jr., Yanowitz FC. ACC/AHA Guidelines for exercise testing: A report of the American College of Cardiology/American Heart Association Task Force on Practice Guidelines (Committee on Exercise Testing). J Am Coll Cardiol 1997; 30:260–315.

22. Ryan TJ, Bauman WB, Kennedy JW, Kereiakes DJ, King SB III, McCallister BD, Smith SC Jr, Ullyot DJ. ACC/AHA Guidelines for percutaneous transluminal coronary angioplasty. A report of the American College of Cardiology/American Heart Association Task Force on Assessment of Diagnostic and Therapeutic Cardiovascular Procedures (Committee on Percutaneous Transluminal Coronary Angioplasty). J Am Coll Cardiol 1993; 22:2033–2054.

23. Scanlon PJ, Faxon DP, Audet AM, Carabello B, Dehmer GJ, Eagle KA, Legako RD, Leon DF, Murray JA, Nissen SE, Pepine CJ, Watson RM. ACC/AHA Guidelines for Coronary Angiography: A report of the American College of Cardiol-

ogy/American Heart Association Task Force on Practice Guidelines (Committee on Coronary Angiography). Circulation 1999; 99:2345–2357.

24. Crawford MH, Knoebel SB, Dunn MI, et al. A Report of the American College of Cardiology/American Heart Association Task Force on Assessment of Diagnostic and Therapeutic Cardiovascular Procedures: Guidelines for Clinical Use of Ambulatory Electrocardiography. J Am Coll Cardiol 1999; 100:886.

I

PATHOPHYSIOLOGY OF SILENT MYOCARDIAL ISCHEMIA

1
Cardiac Pain Mechanisms

We start with pain mechanisms because for many investigators that is really the key to understanding the pathophysiological basis for the enigma that is silent coronary artery disease. Because pain is subjective, it cannot be easily investigated with the kinds of experimental models that are usually employed in laboratory settings. In those experimental pain studies that can be performed, some pain modalities are easier to assess than others. Somatic pain is one of the "easier" types, whereas visceral pain is harder to categorize experimentally.

Therefore, cardiac pain, being visceral in nature, does not lend itself easily to reproducible studies in the animal laboratory.

I. NEUROANATOMY OF CARDIAC PAIN PATHWAYS

What has been established in the animal laboratory is the gross anatomy of the apparent cardiac nociceptive pathways. The afferent fibers that run in the cardiac sympathetic nerves are usually thought of as the essential pathway for the transmission of cardiac pain. The atria and ventricles are abundantly supplied with sympathetic sensory innervation; from the heart the sensory nerve endings connect to afferent fibers in cardiac nerve bundles which in turn connect to the upper five thoracic sympathetic ganglia and the upper five thoracic dorsal roots of the spinal cord (Fig. 1). However, examination of the extrinsic cardiac veins and ganglia by Janes and colleagues [1] suggests that the anatomic pattern of the innervation of the human heart is not as unique as traditionally defined (i.e., consisting of three major sympathetic cardiac nerves and ganglia). Instead, Janes and colleagues found the pattern to be very similar to that in other animals, especially the baboon. Within the spinal cord itself, impulses mediated by this sympathetic afferent route probably converge with impulses from somatic thoracic structures onto the same ascending spinal neurons. The contribution of cells of the spirothalamic tract have been studied extensively by Foreman and colleagues [2,3]. This would be the basis for cardiac-referred pain (i.e., pain referred to the chest, wall, arm, back, etc.). In addition to this "convergence-projection theory" (first proposed by Ruch [4] almost 40 years ago and more recently supported by Foreman's studies), the contribution of vagal afferent fibers must be acknowledged or else we have no explanation for cardiac pain referred to the jaw and neck. How these vagal fibers are activated remains unclear. Because experimental studies suggest a different spatial organization of afferent fibers (i.e., preferential location of sympathetic fibers in the anterior wall of the heart and vagal fibers in the inferior wall), it has been postulated that patients with anterior versus inferior infarcts will experience their pain in different somatic regions. This may hold true in the same patient but does not allow us to predict the site of myocardial ischemia from one patient to the next based on somatic localization of ischemic pain.

II. THEORIES OF CARDIAC PAIN

The links between disease of the coronary arteries and cardiac pain go back to the time of Heberden's original descriptions of the clinical picture of angina

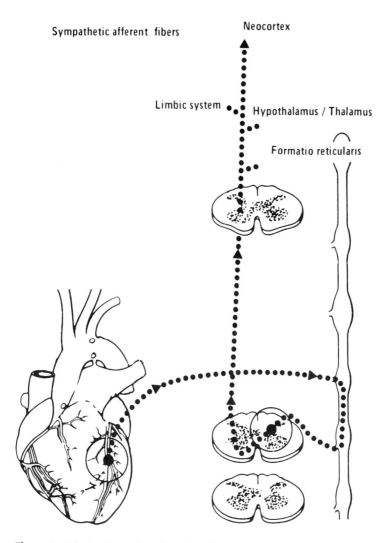

Figure 1   Mechanisms of cardiac pain. (From Droste C, Roskamm H. In: Rutishauser W and Roskamm H, eds., Silent Myocardial Ischemia. Berlin: Springer-Verlag, 1984.)

pectoris. Early writers believed that coronary spasm was common and that interruption in blood supply could produce pain. Lewis [5] has noted that Potain was the first to draw the analogy between pain arising from ischemic myocardium and an ischemic limb. But what was the actual "trigger" that stimulated the sensory nerve endings? Lewis proposed that a chemical pain stimulus was involved, the so-called "factor P" produced by exercise-induced ischemia. Others proposed that anoxia itself was the cause of the pain. The "trigger" is still unclear. In the last several years, there has been increasing attention to the role of peptides in cardiac innervation [6]. Distributed throughout cardiac and extracardiac nerves, they may be acting alone or in combination with classical adrenergic and cholinergic transmitters. Another chemical substance that has been linked to the production of angina-like chest pain is adenosine. Sylvan et al. [7] observed that an adenosine infusion resulted in chest pain in *patients* without coronary artery disease. Subsequently, they gave varying doses to healthy volunteers and caused dose-dependent chest pain in all the volunteers. Concomitant dipyridamole administration (which reduces cellular uptake of adenosine) increased the pain response while theophylline (a nonspecific adenosine antagonist) reduced the pain response [8]. When Crea et al. [9] gave via intracoronary infusion to 22 angina patients, it reproduced chest pain significantly in 20 of the 22 patients but without electrocardiographic evidence of ischemia (Fig. 2). When the drug was infused into the right atrium, it failed to reproduce the pain. From these studies and others [10–12] it appears that adenosine is a mediator of cardiac and muscular ischemic pain. The cardiac effects of adenosine are caused by the stimulation of surface membrane P_1 receptors. At one time, a mechanical stimulus (stretching of the coronary arteries) was also proposed as the cause of the pain even when ischemia itself was not induced. This was suggested after watching the behavior of laboratory animals whose coronary arteries were stretched. This theory has received increased support because it has been demonstrated that during coronary angioplasty in humans a greater balloon inflation pressure could cause more intense pain [13] (Fig. 3). Experiments by Malliani and others have also been helpful in elucidating the "afferent code for ischemic cardiac pain" [14,15] by recording electrical activity from cardiac afferent nerves.

Malliani [14,15] notes that the two main hypotheses for the peripheral (somatic) manifestation of pain are the "intensity" and "specificity" hypotheses (Fig. 4). The "intensity" hypothesis assumes that pain results from an excessive stimulation of receptive structures. The "specificity" hypothesis postulates that pain is conceived as a specific sensation by excitation of a well-defined nociceptive system that responds to noxious stimuli. Malliani poses the question: Do specific cardiac nociceptors exist? Are there really hundreds of

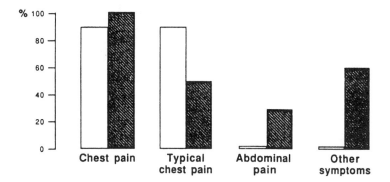

Figure 2 Symptoms caused by intracoronary (open bars) and intra-atrial (crossed bars) adenosine infusion. Chest pain was caused by adenosine in 13 of 15 patients during intracoronary infusion and in all 10 patients in whom this substance was infused into the right atrium. Chest pain was similar to the spontaneous anginal pain in all patients during intracoronary administration, but only in five during intra-atrial infusion. Furthermore, patients frequently complained of other symptoms such as abdominal pain, facial flushing, or anxiety during intra-atrial infusion, but never during intracoronary administration. (From Crea F, Pupita G, Galassi AR, El-Tamimi H, Kaski JC, Davies G, Maseri A. Circulation 1990; 81:164. Reproduced with permission of the American Heart Association.)

cardiac nerve fibers exclusively designed for signaling higher centers about certain kinds of coronary emergencies? Another theory of neuronal encoding of peripheral painful stimuli states that pain is felt as a result of an imbalance between different diameter fibers and central impulses. An element of inhibition is present in this schema (the "gate control" theory), most likely within the posterior horn of the spinal cord (Fig. 5) [16].

III. EXPERIMENTAL STUDIES

Electrophysiological studies of the afferent fibers that are most likely to convey cardiac nociception (the ventricular fibers) evaluated these fibers for absence of spontaneous impulse activity, unresponsiveness to normal physiological hemodynamic stimuli, and the ability to respond to stimuli of pathophysiological significance. In Malliani's experiments, multifiber recordings were obtained from afferent sympathetic fibers. As indicated in Figure 4, excitation could be demonstrated during interruption of coronary blood flow. In the early experi-

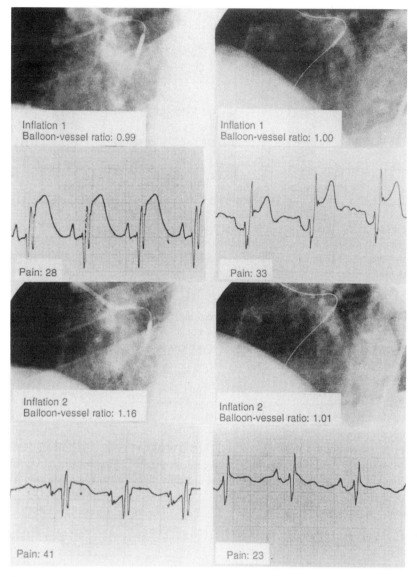

Figure 3 Representative example of the relation between ischemic changes on the intracoronary electrocardiogram and pain severity during balloon inflations in one patient from Group A [i.e., second inflation greater than first (left panel)] and one from Group B [i.e., two inflations at same pressure (right panel)]. Both patients had an isolated obstructive lesion of the left anterior descending coronary artery. The balloon/vessel ratio and cardiac pain severity are indicated for each inflation period in the two patients. In the patient in Group A, ST segment shift is less but vessel stretching and pain are greater during the second than during the first inflation. Conversely, in the patient in Group B, although ST segment shift is also less, vessel stretching is similar and pain severity is less during the second than during the first inflation. (From Tomai F, Crea F, Gaspardone A, Versaci F, Esposito C, Chiarello L, Gioffre PA. J Am Coll Cardiol 1993; 22:1892–1896.)

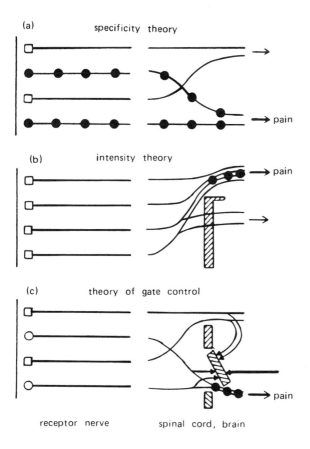

Figure 4   Theories of neural encoding of peripheral painful stimuli. (From Droste C, Roskamm H. In: von Arnim T, Maseri A, eds. Silent Ischemia: Current Concepts and Management. Darmstad: Steinkopff, 1987: 27.)

ments, recruitment of a few silent units (i.e., without obvious background discharge) could be demonstrated by computer-assisted techniques. This recruitment suggested to Malliani and coworkers that specific cardiac nociceptors were present. Reexamination of the data in later experiments casts doubts about this interpretation in light of the animal preparation used. In the preparation, the spinal cord was transsected and the baseline arterial pressure was low enough to "artificially" reduce the normal background discharge of the fibers. In other

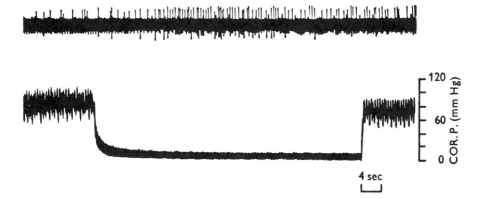

Figure 5 Effect of myocardial ischemia on an afferent unit in the inferior cardiac nerve. The sudden fall in coronary pressure (Cor. P. in mmHg) occurred when the inflow was stopped. There was some background activity that showed a marked increase during ischemia. (From Brown AM, Malliani A. J Physiol 1971; 212:685.)

experiments [17] using coronary occlusion or the intracoronary administration of bradykinin—a naturally occurring substance that is believed to play a role in the genesis of cardiac pain—no recruitment of silent afferent units could be demonstrated (Fig. 6). Thus, whether myelinated or not, the ventricular afferent fibers always possessed some degree of spontaneous impulse activity and a responsiveness to normal hemodynamic stimuli. Malliani concluded that the sensitivity to both mechanical and chemical stimuli, such as bradykinin, was not unique, as others [18] claimed.

Malliani has also commented on behavior of conscious animals exposed to intense excitation of cardiovascular sympathetic fibers. In one of his experiments, the thoracic aorta was stretched via an implanted and inflatable rubber cylinder [19]. A mechanical stimulus elicited a pressor reflex without any pain. In the other experiment, bradykinin was injected directly into a branch of the left coronary artery that had previously been cannulated. Despite pressor responses, there was no pain (Fig. 7). However, when the same experiment was performed 3 days after surgery, the animal was obviously in pain; the surgery had "facilitated" the cardiac pain. Under chronic conditions with an implanted occluder, Theroux et al. [20] reported pain responses are variable. Thus, as

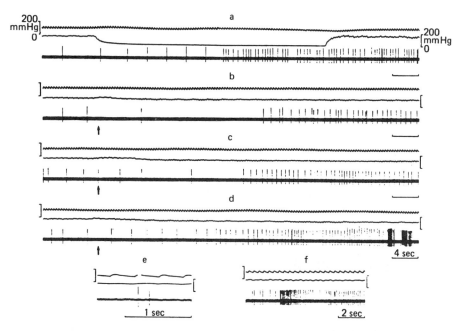

Figure 6 Activity of an afferent sympathetic unmyelinated nerve fiber with a left ventricular ending. Tracings represent from top to bottom: systemic arterial pressure, coronary perfusion pressure, nerve impulse activity (cathode-ray oscilloscope recordings). (a) Interruption of the left main coronary artery perfusion; (b) intracoronary administration, beginning at the arrow, of bradykinin 5 ng/kg; (c) intracoronary administration of bradykinin 10 ng/kg; (d) intracoronary administration of bradykinin 30 ng/kg; (e) electrical stimulation of the left inferior cardiac nerve activating the affering fiber to calculate the conduction velocity; (f) mechanical probing, marked by a bar, of an area of the external surface of the left ventricle. (From Lombardi F, Della Bella P, Casati R, Malliani A. Circ Res 1981; 48:69. Reproduced with the permission of the American Heart Association.)

noted earlier, Malliani has concluded that no specific cardiac nociceptive apparatus could be confirmed. Rather, the "intensity" hypothesis appears a more valid explanation, especially a modified version that is based on a unique spatiotemporal pattern of afferent discharges with central inhibitory modulation [21,22]. Based on their studies with adenosine infusion Crea and Gaspardone question this theory since the severity of adenosine-induced pain in their stud-

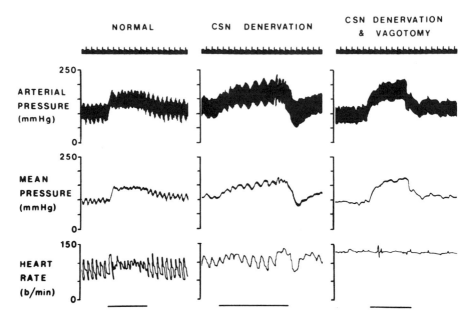

Figure 7   Reflex effects of aortic distension (indicated by the bottom bars) on systemic arterial pressure and heart rate in a conscious dog. The left panel depicts the control response, the middle panel the response after carotid sinoaortic denervation, and the right panel the response after further sectioning of both vagi. Note the progressive increase of the pressor response that follows the denervation procedures. "Pain" (i.e., agitation, etc.) was not observed in any of these experiments. (From Pagani M, Pizzinelli P, Bergamaschi M, Malliani A. Circ Res 1982; 50:125.)

ies was determined "primarily by the number of pain receptors stimulated rather than the intensity of their stimulation above a certain threshold" [23].

IV.   RELATION OF EXPERIMENTAL STUDIES TO THE CLINICAL SETTING

How does the "intensity" pain mechanism relate to the clinical setting and particularly to the occurrence of silent myocardial ischemia? Sufficient levels of afferent impulses must be reached and an appropriate activation of the central ascending pathway must be established before a breakthrough can occur and there is a conscious perception of pain. The level of impulses may be influenced by hypertension and tachycardia preceding the ischemia episodes—the more general the cardiac sympathetic afferent discharge, the more likely the intensity of discharges will reach the critical threshold necessary to convert a receptive process (nociception) into a conscious experience (angina pectoris). By not reaching this critical threshold, ischemia remains "silent." This is not the only mechanism possible. For example, after a transmural myocardial infarction, Barber et al. [24] and Dae et al. [25] showed areas of both sympathetic and vagal afferent "autodenervation" produced apical to the infarcted region. Ischemia can have the same effect [26–28].

V. CONCLUSIONS

The neurophysiology of the cardiac pain pathway is becoming better understood as is the link between pain perception and cardiac tissue damage [23,29].

REFERENCES

1. Janes RD, Brandys JC, Hopkins DA, Johnstone DE, Murphy DA, Armour JA. Anatomy of human extrinsic cardiac nerves and ganglia. Am J Cardiol 1986; 57:299.

2. Foreman RD, Ohata CA, Gerhard KD. Neural mechanisms underlying cardiac pain. In: Schwartz, PJ, Brown AM, Malliani A, Zanchetti A. eds., Neural Mechanisms in Cardiac Arrhythmias. New York: Raven Press, 1978:191.

3. Foreman RD. Spinal substrates of visceral pain. In: Yaksh TL, ed. Spinal Afferent Processing. New York: Plenum Press, 1986:217.

4. Ruch TC. Pathophysiology of pain. In: Fulton JF, ed. A Textbook of Physiology. Philadelphia: WB. Saunders Co., 1955:358.

5. Lewis T. Pain in muscular ischemia: Its relation to anginal pain. Arch Intern Med 1932; 49:713.

6. Weihe E. Peripheral innervation of the heart. In: von Arnim T, Maseri A, eds. Silent Ischemia: Current Concepts and Management. Darmstadt: Steinkopff, 1987:9.

7. Sylven C, Beermann B, Jonzon B, Brandt R. Angina pectoris-like pain provoked by intravenous adenosine in healthy volunteers. Br Med J 1986; 293:227–230.

8. Honeydew T, Ichihra K, Abiko Y, Onodera S. Release of adenosine and lactate from human hearts during atrial pacing in patients with ischemic heart disease. Clin Cardiol 1989; 12:76–82.

9.   Crea F, Pupita G, Galassi AR, El-Tamimi H, Kaski JC, Davies G, Maseri A. Role of adenosine in pathogenesis of anginal pain. Circulation 1990; 81:164.

10. Lagerqvist B, Sylven C, Beermann B, Helmius G, Walderstrom A. Intracoronary adenosine causes angina pectoris like pain: an inquiry into the nature of visceral pain. Cardiovasc Res 1990; 24:609–613.

11. Crea F, Gaspardone A, Kaski FC, Davies G, Maseri A. Relation between stimulation site of cardiac afferent nerves by adenosine and location of cardiac pain in patients with stable angina. J Am Coll Cardiol 1992; 20:1498–1504.

12. Sylven C, Jonzon B, Borg G, Fredholm BB, Kaijser L. Adenosine injection into the brachial artery produces ischemia-like pain or discomfort in the forearm. Cardiovasc Res 1988; 22:674–678.

13. Tomai F, Crea F, Gaspardone A, Versaci F, Esposito C, Chiariello L, Gioffre PA. Mechanisms of cardiac pain during coronary angioplasty. J Am Coll Cardiol 1993; 22:1892–1896.

14. Malliani A, Lombardi F. Consideration of the fundamental mechanisms eliciting cardiac pain. Am Heart J 1982; 103:575.

15. Malliani A. The elusive link between transient myocardial ischemia and pain. Circulation 1986; 73:201.

16. Droste C, Roskamm H. Experimental approach to painful and painless ischemia. In: von Arnim T, Maseri A. eds., Silent Ischemia: Current Concepts and Management. Darmstadt: Steinkopff, 1987:27.

17. Lombardi F, Dell Bella P, Casati R, Malliani A. Effects of intracoronary administration of bradykinin on the impulse activity of afferent sympathetic unmyelinated fibers with left ventricular endings in the cat. Circ Res 1981; 48:69.

18. Baker DG, Coleridge HM, Coleridge JCG, Terndrum T. Search for a cardiac nociceptor: Stimulation by bradykinin of sympathetic afferent nerve endings in the heart of the cat. J Physiol 1980; 306:519.

19. Pagani M, Pizzinelli P, Bergamaschi M, Malliani A. A positive feedback sympathetic pressor reflex during stretch of the thoracic aorta in conscious dogs. Circ Res 1982; 50:125.

20. Theroux P, Ross J, Franklin D, Kemper WS, Sassayama S. Regional myocardial function in the conscious dog during acute coronary occlusion and responses to morphine, propranolol, nitroglycerin, and lidocaine. Circulation 1976; 53:302.

21. Malliani A. Pathophysiology of ischemic cardiac pain. In: von Arnim T, Maseri A. eds., Silent Ischemia: Current Concepts and Management. Darmstadt: Steinkopff, 1987:21.

22. Malliani A, Pagani M, Lombardi F. Visceral versus somatic mechanisms. In: Wall PD, Melzack R, eds. Textbook of Pain. Edinburgh: Churchill Livingstone, 1989:128.

23. Crea F, Gaspardone A. New look to an old symptom: angina pectoris. Circulation 1997; 96:3766–3773.

24. Barber MJ, Mueller TM, Davies BG, Gill RM, Zipes DP. Interruption of sympathetic and vagal-mediated afferent responses by transmural myocardial infarction. Circulation 1985; 72:623.

25. Dae MW, Herre JM, O'Connell JW, Botvinick EH, Newman D, Munoz L. Scintigraphic assessment of sympathetic innervation after transmural versus nontransmural myocardial infarction. J Am Coll Cardiol 1991; 17:1416.
26. Inoue H, Skale BT, Zipes DP. Effects of ischemia on cardiac afferent sympathetic and vagal reflexes in dogs. Am J Physiol 1988; 255 (Heart Circ Physiol 24):H26.
27. Zipes DP. Influence of myocardial ischemia and infarction on autonomic innervation of heart. Circulation 1990; 82:1095.
28. Machac J, Vallabhajosula S, Gatley J, Schiyer D, Volkow N, Wolf A, Goldsmith SJ, Gomes JA, Gorlin R. Effect of ischemia at rest on myocardial sympathetic nerve integrity in humans (abstr). J Am Coll Cardiol 1992; 19:68A.
29. Masseri A, Crea F, Kaski JC, Davies G. Mechanisms and significance of cardiac ischemic pain. Prog Cardiovasc Dis 1992; 35:1.

2

Alterations in Sensitivity to Pain in Patients with Silent Myocardial Ischemia

The clearer elucidation of the cardiac pain mechanism is helpful in understanding why pain is not necessarily present during episodes of myocardial ischemia. In the clinical setting, one promising line of investigation is concerned with an alteration in the patient's sensitivity to pain, either centrally or peripherally.

I. STUDIES OF PAIN THRESHOLD AND PAIN PERCEPTION

The most thorough series of investigations of this subject to date has been that of Droste and Roskamm. In their first study [1], these investigators reported result in 42 men (mean age 51 years). All patients had angiographically confirmed coronary artery disease (i.e., ≥75% stenosis in at least one major coronary artery). In addition, they all had >1.0 mm ST segment depression on multiple exercise studies. Patients were divided into two groups depending on the occurrence of angina pectoris during the exercise tests. Factors such as digitalis medication, hypokalemia, valvular heart disease, etc., that could have been responsible for specious ST segment depression were excluded. All patients had normal neurological examinations. There were 20 patients in the asymptomatic group; 16 had ECG evidence of prior infarction, but only six had pain with the infarction. Furthermore, 16 of the patients had no angina during everyday activity; the other five had complained of pain in the past. By contrast, in the symptomatic group (22 patients), only 2 of 17 patients who had prior infarctions had no pain with the infarctions. Distribution of coronary risk factors was similar in both groups, as were angiographic features (Table 1).

   Droste and Roskamm studied three different modalities of pain perception. The first was an electrical pain threshold test in which the magnitude of pain current applied to the thigh was evaluated. The value of threshold was reported according to the degree of electrical current used (in mA). The second test was a standard cold pressor test in which patient's left arm was submerged in water cooled to 4°C. The third test was a modified form of the submaximal effort tourniquet technique in which the working muscle of the left arm is stressed. The endpoint in the first test was the actual amount of electrical current needed to produce pain. In the other two tests, the time that elapsed before the patient perceived pain, or was no longer able to tolerate pain, was measured. The results of these studies showed striking differences when the two groups were compared. For example, when pain threshold was determined, symptomatic patients demonstrated a mean electrical pain threshold of 0.57 mA (Fig. 1, top). This finding is in agreement with other studies performed in healthy men in which 0.55 mA was the average value. Asymptomatic patients had a much wider range of values with a mean value of 1.04 mA (Fig. 1, bottom). During the cold pressor tests, asymptomatic patients showed much greater values for pain tolerance than did symptomatic patients (Fig. 2, bottom). Pain thresholds showed a similar trend, but the differences were not statistically significant. During the arm muscle ischemic pain test, asymptomatic patients had a higher pain threshold and pain tolerance than symptomatic patients, though only the latter difference achieved statistical significance. In addition, asymp-

Table 1 Comparison of Selected Medical Variables Measured in Patients with Symptomatic and Asymptomatic Myocardial Ischemia

	Myocardial ischemia	
	Symptomatic (n = 22)	Asymptomatic (n = 20)
1-vessel disease	9	3
2-vessel disease	3 2.1 ± 0.9	3 2.5 ± 0.8
3-vessel disease	10	14
Friesinger score	8.6 ± 3.1	10.4 ± 2.6
Ejection fraction (%)	60 ± 16	58 ± 12
Heart volume (mL)	816 ± 142	856 ± 220
Heart volume related to body weight (mL/kg)	10.9 ± 1.2	11.1 ± 2.5
Previous myocardial infarction (no. of patients)	17	16
Risk factors		
age (yr)	51 ± 5.8	52 ± 9.6
smoking	17	10
hypertension (> 140 > 95 mmHg)	8	8
diabetes	1	2
cholesterol (mg/dL)	240 ± 40	237 ± 65
triglycerides (mg/dL)	195 ± 83	174 ± 79

All data are = standard deviation values.
Differences between the symptomatic and asymptomatic groups for each variable were not significant.
Source: Droste C, Roskamm H. J Am Coll Cardiol 1983; 1:940.

tomatic patients rated a strong stimulus as actually being less intense than did the symptomatic patients. (This was also true in the cold pressor test.) In later studies, measurements of transcutaneous partial oxygen tension in the occluded forearm were added [2]. This allowed information about oxygen supply and demand in the resting and working muscle to be obtained and the development of ischemia and anoxia quantitatively assessed. This is depicted in Figure 3, in which asymptomatic patients exhibited lower oxygen tensions at threshold and tolerance than symptomatic patients and needed more time to reach these levels.

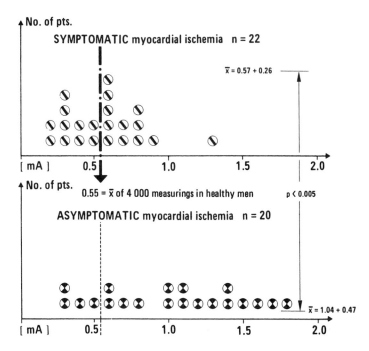

Figure 1 Electrical pain threshold in symptomatic and asymptomatic patients. (From Droste C, Roskamm H. J Am Coll Cardiol 1983; 1:940.)

The pain threshold studies of Droste and Roskamm were subsequently confirmed by Glazier et al. [3]. They studied 27 patients, 12 with predominantly painless ischemia and 15 with predominantly painful ischemia. Threshold and tolerance values were greater in the painless group, but overlap was considerable (Fig. 4). Using a different pain test, electrical dental pulp stimulation, Falcone et al. were able to show a significant difference in pain threshold between patients with and without painless ischemia [4]. Pain perception has also been evaluated in relation to advancing age. Miller et al. [5] used a "silent ischemia interval" (time of onset of angina, minus the time to onset of 1 mm ST depression) to demonstrate this point (Fig. 5). The clinical significance of somatic pain tolerance in patients with coronary artery disease was evaluated by Narins et al. [6]. In their study, 271 patients with a recent coronary event underwent pain tolerance tests using the arm tourniquet test described earlier. Narins et al. found that patients with lower tolerance to somatic pain

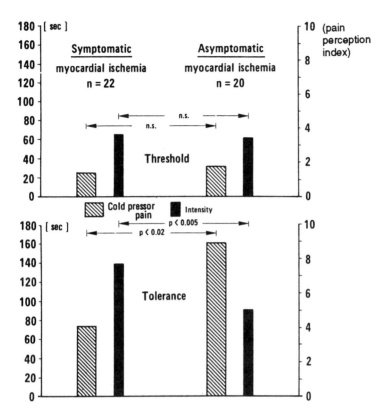

Figure 2 Cold pressor test: group differences for threshold and tolerance levels. (Hatched columns = stimulus intensity; solid columns = subjective experience of pain.) (From Droste C, Roskamm H. J Am Coll Cardiol 1983; 1:940.)

were "more likely to experience clinical symptoms and functional impairment" (on exercise electrocardiography) than the control patients, although prognosis appeared similar.

The issue of whether there is an abnormal handling by the central nervous system of afferent messages from the heart remains unresolved, but several new studies have shed additional light on the subject. Rosen et al. [7] studied regional cerebral blood flow changes with positron emission tomography (PET) scanning in two matched groups of patients—those with and without silent ischemia. As a result of their study, the authors concluded that "abnormal central processing of afferent pain messages from the heart may play a deter-

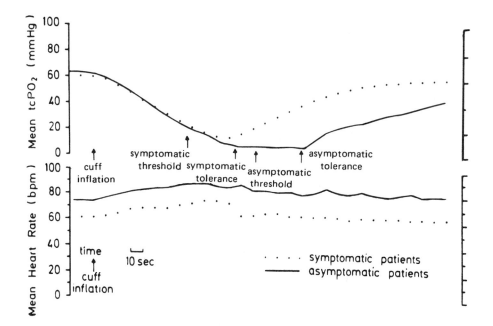

Figure 3 Time course of mean values of transcutaneous partial oxygen tension ($tcPO_2$) (upper traces) and heart rate (lower traces) for symptomatic (dotted lines; $n = 6$) and asymptomatic (solid lines; $n = 6$) patients. Time of cuff inflation denoted by arrows. Threshold and tolerance levels are depicted separately (arrows) for symptomatic and asymptomatic groups. (From Droste C, Greenlee MW, Roskamm H. Pain 1986; 26:199.)

mining role in silent myocardial ischemia" (Fig. 6). Central modulation of pain perception was also evaluated by Langer and O'Connor [8]. Using a different technique, they found that this complex interaction could not be adequately explained other than by a multiplicity of factors.

II. CLINICAL FEATURES THAT MAY EXPLAIN ABSENCE OF PAIN

Droste and Roskamm evaluated three arguments put forth as possible explanations for the lack of pain. The first has to do with destruction of nociceptive pathways by infarction, diffuse ischemia, or some type of neuropathy. In these patients, however, the frequency of myocardial infarctions, extensive multives-

(a) Threshold values

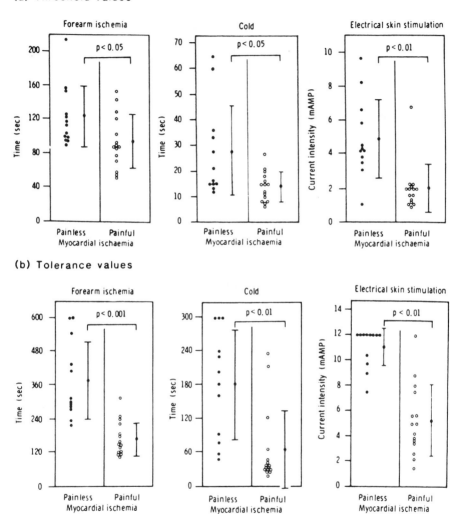

Figure 4 (a) Threshold and (b) tolerance values for a variety of painful stimuli in the two study patient groups. Although both threshold and tolerance values were, on average, greater in the patients with painless ischemia, overlap between the two groups was considerable. (From Glazier JJ, Chierchia S, Brown MJ, Maseri A. Am J Cardiol 1986; 58:667.)

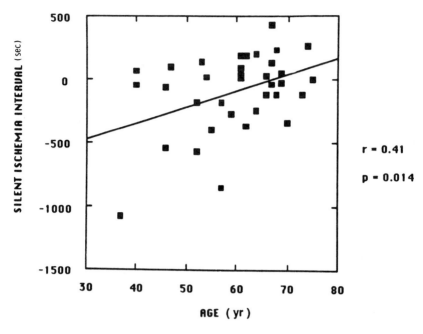

Figure 5 Relationship between pain perception index (time of onset of angina minus the time to onset of 1 mm ST segment depression) in seconds, and age in years. (From Miller PF, Sheps DS, Bragdon EE, Herbst MC, Dalton JL, Hinderliter AL, Koch GG, Maxiner W, Ekelund L-G. Am Heart J 1990; 120:22. Reproduced with permission.)

sel disease, diabetes, or alcoholism was similar in both the symptomatic and asymptomatic subgroups. The authors maintained that only radical surgical procedures—transplantation, autotransplantation, plexectomy—could sufficiently denervate a heart so that angina became absent. The authors also felt that their study amply demonstrated that the intensity of ischemia is not necessarily reduced in asymptomatic patients. They based this on the finding that the degree of ischemia—as determined by ST depression—was comparable in both groups. (We comment further on this factor—the amount of myocardium at jeopardy—in Chap. 4.) Thus, they concluded that the hyposensibility to pain in general that they reported best differentiated the asymptomatic from the symptomatic patients. This supported earlier, less quantitative data from studies of patients with silent myocardial infarction [9].*

---

*Pain mechanisms in silent myocardial infarctions are discussed further in Chapter 6.

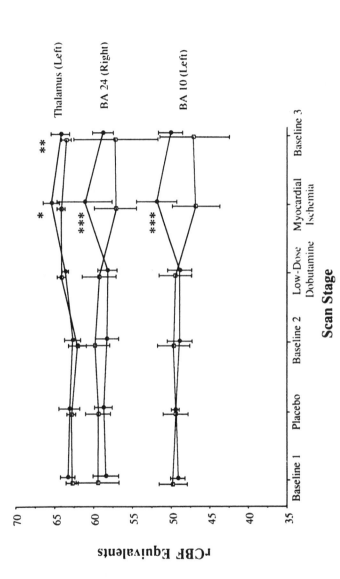

Figure 6 Time course of regional cerebral blood flow changes in selected regions of the brain. Changes in regional cerebral blood flow (rCBF) in the left thalamus, right Brodmann area 24 (BA24), and left Brodmann area 10 (BA10) over time. These areas show the difference in frontal activation between patients with silent ischemia and those with angina pectoris and the difference in the time course of activation between the frontal areas and the thalami. Thus, the regional cerebral blood flow changes in Brodmann area 24 and Brodmann area 10 during myocardial ischemia are significantly greater in patients with silent ischemia. Although the regional cerebral blood flow increases in Brodmann area 24 and Brodmann area 10 entirely resolved by the baseline 3 scan, thalamic regional cerebral blood flow remained increased in both patient groups during the scan done after ischemia. 0 = patients with angina; = patients with silent ischemia. *p = 0.001, baseline 1 and 2 (both groups); **p < 0.01, groups; ***p < 0.001, angina pectoris compared with silent ischemia. (Reproduced by permission from Rosen SD, Paulesu E, Nihoyannopoulos P, Tousoulis D, Frackowiak RSJ, Frith CD, Jones T, Camici PG. Ann Intern Med 1996; 124:939.

The authors then posed the question as to which mechanisms were involved in the decreased sensibility to pain: pain-discriminating ability versus individual response tendencies that categorize a stimulus as pain. The authors felt that some of their data, especially that dealing with the differences in electrically determined pain thresholds and thresholds for ischemic pain, supported the former mechanism. But the tendency for asymptomatic patients to rate painful stimuli as less intense—and thus tolerate the stimulus much longer—argues also for a difference in response tendencies. The two factors are not necessarily independent of each other. One should also consider the importance of psychological traits on under-reporting of anginal complaints [10].

III. POSSIBLE ROLE OF ENDORPHINS

Could endorphic mechanisms influence the difference in pain responses? Normally, varying concentrations of these opioid-like substances exist in plasma and cerebrospinal fluid and may be important in mediating pain sensitivity. VanRijn and Rabkin [11] reported that injection of the opioid-antagonist naloxone precipitated angina earlier during exercise-induced ischemia than a placebo. However, they only tested five patients. We were unable to reproduce these results in eight symptomatic patients, nor were we able to use this agent to precipitate angina during treadmill exercise tests in nine patients with documented silent myocardial ischemia [12]. In a similar study, Ellestad and Kuan [13] reported on their findings in 10 men with asymptomatic but positive stress tests. These men were given naloxone, 2 mg intravenously, and the tests repeated. No chest pain was reported by any patient and naloxone did not significantly alter exercise duration, heart rate, blood pressure, or ST segment changes compared to the control test.

Droste and Roskamm have reported results different from those cited above. They studied 60 patients [14] in a manner similar to their earlier studies in 42 patients [1]. The 60 patients were evenly divided between those with and those without asymptomatic ischemia. The asymptomatic patients had reproducible symptomatic manifestations of myocardial ischemia in several exercise tests. Mean ST depression was 3.8 mm (0.38 mV). Factors that could have indicated false-positive ST segment depression (such as other forms of heart disease or cardiac medications) were excluded. Most of these patients did not have angina during everyday activities and many had had prior myocardial infarctions. All patients had angiographically proven coronary artery disease. A control group of 30 patients with symptomatic coronary artery disease had less ST segment depression during exercise testing (mean 2.2 mm), but other selected mechanical variables showed no difference between the two groups. These variables included age, smoking history, and other clinical features, as well as angiographic measurements such as number of vessels diseased, ejection fraction, etc. The three different pain-receptive modalities employed in their previous studies were repeated in this study with similar results. In 10 asymptomatic patients, the tests were repeated following intravenous injection of 2 mg of naloxone and again after a placebo injection. There were no differences in parameters of exercise testing (maximum effort, heart rate, blood pressure, or ST segment depression) between the placebo tests and those employing naloxone. Two of the ten patients developed angina during the naloxone test, though one required 4 mg of the drug before this response was elicited. The most striking finding occurred during the ischemic pain test in which arm ischemia is produced by a tourniquet. Both the threshold to pain and tolerance to it were significantly altered after naloxone administration. The investigators concluded that the results lent support to their previous work showing a differential sensitivity to pain and suggested a possible role for endorphic mechanisms in silent myocardial ischemia. Several papers from different laboratories have dealt directly with this issue (i.e., via measurements of plasma endorphin levels). The study of Glazier et al. cited earlier found similar levels in symptomatic and asymptomatic ischemia. This was confirmed by two other studies (Fig. 7) [15,16]. The study of Sheps et al. [17], however, does suggest a causative role for endorphins, but even in this study, there was considerable overlap (Table 2). Higher levels were also reported by Falcone et al. [18] in patients with silent infarction, as well as those with silent ischemia. Additional data from Falcone et al. [19] from coronary angioplasty studies have suggested a link between endorphin levels and symptoms. Kurita et al. [20] have recently reported data confirming the relationship between endorphin levels and symptoms during exercise testing. By contrast, Oldroyd et al. [21] found endorphin release to be common during both spontaneous and provoked acute myocardial ischemia, but had no correlation with the intensity of chest pain. More recent studies of the role of endogenous opioids have again clouded the picture. For example, Garber et al. [22] used naloxone and essentially confirmed the studies of Droste et al. that opioids alone can regulate the absolute presence or absence of pain. By contrast, Hikita et al. [23,24] confirmed only that elevated beta-endorphin levels during exercise are associated with silent ischemia in nondiabetic patients (Table 3). Beta-endorphin levels have also been implemented during silent ischemia induced by psychological stress [25]. Whether beta-endorphin levels can account for the increased pain perception by African Americans during exercise testing in unclear [26]. For a detailed review of the control of pain by opioids, readers are referred to the review by Stein [27].

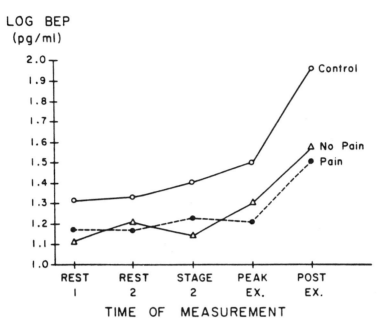

Figure 7 Effects of exercise on plasma beta-endorphin levels in control subjects and patients with silent myocardial ischemia (no pain) or symptomatic ischemia (pain). Beta-endorphin levels are the logarithmic transformation of the original data. Values are group means. Stage 2 = approximately 6 min of exercise; Peak Ex = peak exercise; Post Ex = 10 min after exercise. (From Heller GV, Garber CW, Connolly MJ, Allen-Rowlands CF, Siconolfi SF, Gann DS, Carleton RA. Am J Cardiol 1987; 159:735.)

In summary, the evidence linking endorphins to silent myocardial ischemia is suggestive, but not conclusive.

IV. CONCLUSIONS

There is evidence to suggest that some patients with silent myocardial ischemia have an altered sensibility to certain types of pain. It is still not clear, however, in how many patients endorphins influence this hyposensibility.

Table 2 Postexercise Endorphin Levels Versus Anginal Status

Age (yr) and sex	Cath CAD	History of MI	Time to angina (s)	Pos RNV	Rest EF (%)	Exercise-induced ST↓	Angina	Postexercise endorphin level
73M	0	+	140	+	72	+	+	8.3
64M	+	+	255	+	47	+	+	3.7
68M	+	+	...	+	58	+	0	19.5
56M	+	+	230	0	24	0	0	3.2
55M	0	0	...	+	75	+	+	7.3
63M	0	+	...	0	56	0	0	4.5
53F	+	0	375	0	56	+	+	3.5
43M	0	+	...	0	62	+	0	7.0
61M	0	+	270	+	62	+	+	5.9
36M	0	0	...	0	59	+	0	4.5
61M	+	+	192	+	51	+	+	13.0
64M	+	+	...	0	51	+	0	5.0
56F	0	0	200	0	61	+	+	7.1
58F	0	0	...	+	71	0	0	11.8
58M	0	0	267	+	49	0	+	3.2
67M	+	+	200	+	41	+	+	1.5
40F	+	+	180	+	62	+	+	11.5
64F	+	+	80	+	40	0	+	1.3
75F	0	0	...	+	72	+	0	8.5
67M	0	+	...	+	56	+	0	12.5
73M	+	0	130	0	59	+	+	0.0
60M	+	+	...	+	59	+	0	5.8
57M	0	0	585	0	57	+	+	2.6
61M	+	+	625	0	48	0	+	11.9
66F	+	+	120	+	47	+	+	2.6

CAD = coronary artery disease; Cath = catheterized; EF = ejection fraction; MI = myocardial infarction; RNV = radionuclide ventriculogram; ST↓ = ST segment depression; + = present; 0 = absent.

Source: Sheps DS, Adams KF, Hinderliter A, Price C, Bissette J, Orlando G, Margolis B, Koch G. Am J Cardiol 1987; 59:523.

Table 3   Plasma Beta-Endorphin Levels at Rest and Exercise

	Nondiabetic with overt myocardial ischemia	Nondiabetic with silent myocardial ischemia	Diabetic with overt myocardial ischemia	Diabetic with silent myocardial ischemia
Rest (pg/mL)	7.5 ± 3.2	7.6 ± 3.0	8.0 ± 3.6	6.8 ± 2.0
Exercise (pg/mL)	8.4 ± 4.2	13.2 ± 7.0[a,b]	8.5 ± 4.0	8.3 ± 2.0

[a] $p < 0.05$ vs. nondiabetic with overt myocardial ischemia and diabetic with silent myocardial ischemia.
[b] $p < 0.05$ vs. rest.
Source: Reproduced with permission from Hikita H, Kurita A, Takase B, Nakamura H. ANE 1997; 2(4):319.

REFERENCES

1. Droste C, Roskamm H. Experimental pain measurement in patients with asymptomatic myocardial ischemia. J Am Coll Cardiol 1983; 1:940.
2. Droste C, Greenlee MW, Roskamm H. A defective angina pectoris warning system: Experimental findings of ischemia and electrical pain test. Pain 1986; 26:199.
3. Glazier JJ, Chierchia S, Brown MJ, Maseri A. Importance of generalized defective perception of painful stimuli as a cause of silent myocardial ischemia in chronic stable angina pectoris. Am J Cardiol 1986; 58:667.
4. Falcone C, Sconocchia R, Guasti L, Codega S, Montemartini C, Specchia G. Dental pain threshold and angina pectoris in patients with coronary artery disease. J Am Coll Cardiol 1988; 12:348.
5. Miller PF, Sheps DS, Bragdon EE, Herbst MC, Dalton JL, Hinderliter AL, Koch GG, Maixner W, Ekelund L-G. Aging and pain perception in ischemic heart disease. Am Heart J 1990; 120:22.
6. Narins CR, Zareba W, Moss AJ, Brown MW, Case RB, Case N, Goldstein RE. The clinical significance of somatic pain tolerance in patients with coronary artery disease. ANE 1997; 2(4):338.
7. Rosen SD, Paulesu E, Nihoyannopoulos P, Tousoulis D, Frackowiak RSJ, Frith CD, Jones T, Camici PG. Silent ischemia as a central problem: Regional brain activation compared in silent and painful myocardial ischemia. Ann Intern Med 1996; 124:939.
8. Langer A, O'Oconnor P. Central modulation of pain perception in patients with silent myocardial ischemia. Am J Cardiol 1994; 74:182.
9. Procacei P, Zoppi M, Padeletii L, Maresca M. Myocardial infarction without pain. A study of the sensory function of the upper limbs. Pain 1976; 2:309.

10. Davies RF, Linden W, Klinke WP, Habibi H, Buttars JA, Dessain P, and CASIS Investigators. Under-reporting of somatic symptoms in patients with silent ischemia (abstr). J Am Coll Cardiol 1992; 19:284A.

11. VanRijn T, Rabkin SW. Effect of naloxone, a specific opioid antagonist, on exercise induced angina pectoris (Abstr). Circulation 1981; 65(suppl 4):149.

12. Cohn P F, Patcha R, Singh S, Vlay SC, Mallis G, Lawson W. Effect of naloxone on exercise tests in patients with symptomatic and silent myocardial ischemia (abstr). Clin Res 1985; 33:177A.

13. Ellestad MH, Kuan P. Naloxone and asymptomatic ischemia. Failure to induce angina during exercise testing. Am J Cardiol 1984; 54:928.

14. Droste C, Roskamm H. Pain measurement and pain modification by naloxone in patients with asymptomatic myocardial ischemia. In: Rutishauser W, Roskamm H, eds. Silent Myocardial Ischemia. Berlin: Springer-Verlag, 1984:14–23.

15. Weidinger F, Hammerle A, Sochor H, Smetna R, Frass M, Glogar D. Role of beta-endorphins in silent myocardial ischemia. Am J Cardiol 1986; 58:428.

16. Heller GV, Garber CE, Connolly MJ, Allen-Rowlands CF, Siconolfi SF, Gann DS, Carleton RA. Plasma beta-endorphin levels in silent myocardial ischemia. Am J Cardiol 1987; 59:735.

17. Sheps DS, Adams KF, Hinderliter A, Price C, Bissette J, Orlando G, Margolis B, Koch G. Endorphins are related to pain perception in coronary artery disease. Am J Cardiol 1987; 59:523.

18. Falcone C, Specchia G, Rondanelli R, Guasti L, Corsico G, Codega S, Montemartini C. Correlation between beta-endorphin plasma levels and anginal symptoms in patients with coronary artery disease. J Am Coll Cardiol 1988; 11:719.

19. Falcone C, Guasti L, Ochan M, Tortorici M, Specchia G. Anginal pain and beta-endorphin variations during PTCA (abstr). Circulation 1991; 84(suppl 2):293.

20. Kurita A, Takase B, Uehata A, Sugahara H, Nishioka T, Maruyama T, Satomura K, Mizuno K, Nakamura H. Differences in plasma beta-endorphin and bradykinin levels between patients with painless or with painful myocardial ischemia. Am Heart J 1992; 123:304.

21. Oldroyd KG, Harvey K, Gray CE, Beastall GH, Cobbe SM. Beta-endorphin release in patients after spontaneous and provoked acute myocardial ischemia. Br Heart J 1992; 67:230.

22. Garber CE, Barbour MM, Malkin RD, Ahlberg AW, Heller GV. Role of endogenous opioids in the determination of anginal pain. Am J Cardiol 1994; 74:815.

23. Hikita H, Kurita A, Takase B, Nagayoshi H, Uehata A, Nishioka T, Mitani H, Mizuno K, Nakamura H. Usefulness of plasma beta-endorphin level, pain threshold and autonomic function in assessing silent myocardial ischemia in patients with and without diabetes mellitus. Am J Cardiol 1993; 72:149.

24. Hikita H, Kurita A, Takase B, Nakamura H. Reexamination of the roles of beta-endorphin and cardiac autonomic function in exercise-induced silent myocardial ischemia. ANE 1997; 2(4):319.

25. Sheps DS, Ballenger MN, DeGent GE, Krittayaphong R, Dittman E, Maixner W,

McCartney W, Golden RN, Koch G, Light KC. Psychophysical responses to a speech stressor: correlation of plasma beta-endorphin levels at rest and after psychological stress with thermally measured pain threshold in patients with coronary artery disease. J Am Coll Cardiol 1995; 25:1499.

26. Sheffield D, Kriby S, Biles PL, Sheps DS. Comparison of perception of angina pectoris during exercise testing in African-Americans versus Caucasians. Am J Cardiol 1999; 83:106.

27. Stein C. The control of pain in peripheral tissue by opioids. N Engl J Med 1995; 332:1685.

3

The Sequence of Events During Episodes of Myocardial Ischemia

Where Does Pain Fit In?

How can we document the sequence of events during the "ischemic cascade"? Because of technical and ethical reasons, the direct manipulation of coronary blood flow to induce myocardial ischemia has been difficult to achieve in humans, compared to experimental animal models. Within the past 20 years, however, the advent of percutaneous transluminal coronary angioplasty (PTCA) has provided a unique tool for understanding the sequence of events leading up to the occurrence of pain during episodes of myocardial ischemia in humans. This understanding is an essential component for appreciating the pathophysiology of silent myocardial ischemia. Prior to PTCA, what was

39

known about the sequence of events had been learned from other types of studies. These will be reviewed first.

I. EXERCISE STUDIES

Upton and colleagues [1] used radionuclide ventriculography in 25 coronary artery disease patients and 10 normal controls to evaluate left ventricular dysfunction before angina occurred. These investigators provoked ischemia during two levels of an upright bicycle exercise test. The first radionuclide study during exercise was performed before the onset of ST segment depression and the second one after its appearance. As indicated in Figure 1, the mean ejection fraction increased in the normal subject during the first level of exercise but remained unchanged (an abnormal response) in the patients with coronary artery disease. At the second level of exercise, the control group continued to show an increase, while in the coronary artery disease group there was now a frank decrease for the group as a whole and all patients showed an abnormal response. Wall motion patterns showed a similar trend. A regional wall motion index was used to assess these changes. At the first level of exercise, 14 of the coronary patients (56%) developed a new wall motion abnormality or demon-

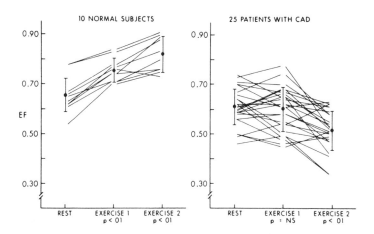

Figure 1   Changes in ejection fraction (EF) from rest to the first level of exercise (exercise 1) and the second level (exercise 2) in 10 normal subjects and 25 patients with coronary artery disease (CAD). (From Upton MT, Rerych SK, Newman GE, Port S, Cobb FR, Jones RH. Circulation 1980; 62:341.)

strated progression in a preexisting defect at rest. At the second level of exercise, wall motion was abnormal in all patients. Nine of the twenty-five patients with coronary artery disease did not experience angina during these studies. Thus, this study concluded that angina pectoris and ST segment shifts on the electrocardiogram are frequently late manifestations of myocardial ischemia. Another exercise study—this one involving recumbent exercise—showed that regional wall motion changes (determined by echocardiography) began at 30 ± 15 s after onset of exercise and preceded electrocardiographic changes by an average of 60 s [2]. Heller et al. [3] studied the effect of different levels of exercise on the presence of angina, ECG changes, and reversible thallium-201 perfusion defects. The same sequence of events in the ischemic cascade was observed during varying levels of exercise (Fig. 2). Increasingly higher levels of exercise were more likely to result in a higher proportion of patients demonstrating abnormalities at each point of the cascade, but the sequence remained the same.

II. CONTINUOUS HEMODYNAMIC MONITORING

Possibly the single most important of these studies emanated from Maseri's laboratory 20 years ago. This study by Chierchia et al. [4] is important because of the intensive invasive and noninvasive monitoring that the six patients in the study underwent. These six patients were admitted to the coronary care unit because of transient, recurrent episodes of angina at rest with atypical ST-T changes. To document the location and direction of ST segment changes, 12-lead ECG tracings were recorded in each patient during the course of several angina attacks. In addition to electrocardiographic monitoring, the left ventricular or aortic pressure was continuously monitored, as well as the coronary sinus oxygen saturation. The latter was assumed to reflect changes in myocardial blood flow, provided the arterial oxygen content and the myocardial oxygen consumption remained constant. Thirty-one episodes of ST segment or T-wave abnormalities (most involving ST segment elevation in these mainly Prinzmetal angina patients) were recorded. Only eight episodes were accompanied by typical angina pain.

Although the ischemic episodes were accompanied by different hemodynamic patterns in individual patients, some common features were striking. Pain when present occurred 50–120 s *after* the onset of ST-T wave changes. The authors concluded that pain did not appear to be a reliable and sensitive marker of transient, acute myocardial ischemia. In none of these patients with rest angina were the ST-T changes preceded by consistent increases in the

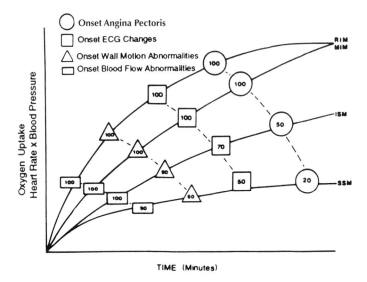

Figure 2   Theoretical relation between events of the ischemic cascade and intensity of exercise achieved. Three types of exercise are compared: maximal exercise, either with rapid or moderate incremental exercise (RIM, MIM); submaximal incremental exercise (ISM); and submaximal steady-state exercise (SSM). The relative onset of ischemic events (in the percentage observed in the patients being tested) is compared to time after onset of exercise and either rate-pressure product or oxygen uptake. Rapid incremental exercise and submaximal steady-state exercise are based on results of the present study, whereas moderate or submaximal incremental exercise was theoretically derived from prior studies. (From Heller GF, Ahmed I, Tikemeier PL, Barbour MB, Garber CE. Am J Cardiol 1991; 68:569. Reproduced with permission.)

hemodynamic determinants of myocardial oxygen consumption (such as increased heart rate or blood pressure). Hemodynamic changes reflecting acute left ventricular functional impairment did occur before ST changes but even earlier changes than these usually occurred in the coronary sinus oxygen saturation. This presumably reflected decreased myocardial blood flow. Figures 3 and 4 depict the sequence of events: primary reduction in coronary blood flow, fall in left ventricular systolic pressure and left ventricular dP/dt, and a rise in left ventricular end-diastolic pressure, and then ST-T changes. Pain was the final event, when it occurred. The truly ischemic nature of these episodes was confirmed by thallium-201 scintigrams during painless episodes in four patients that showed perfusion defects relative to control tracings. Levy et al.

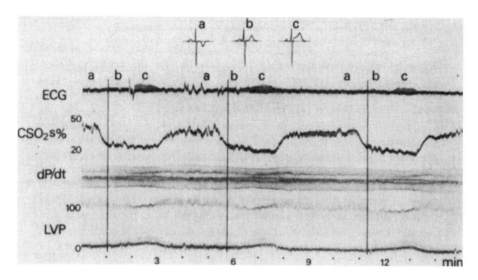

Figure 3   Low-speed playback (paper speed 0.3 mm/s) of ECG, coronary sinus O_2 saturation (CSO_2S), left ventricular pressure (LVP), and dP/dt during three successive asymptomatic episodes recorded over a period of about 15 min. At the top are electrocardiographic patterns (lead V_2) in resting conditions (a), at the onset (b), and at the peak (c) of the ischemic episode. Vertical lines correspond to the onset of the ST-T changes. A sharp drop of CSO_2s (denoting reduction in coronary blood flow) consistently precedes the onset of ECG and hemodynamic changes. (From Chierchia S, Simonetti I, Lazzari M, Maseri A. Circulation 1980; 61:759. Reproduced with permission of the American Heart Association.)

[5] used ambulatory pulmonary artery monitoring during spontaneous, pacing-induced and exercise-induced ischemia to document a similar sequence. Pain was the final event, occurring after the rise in pulmonary artery diastolic pressure and ST segment depression (Fig. 5). Continuous monitoring of left ventricular function is now also possible using ambulatory radionuclide monitoring (the VEST) [6]. This technique is discussed further in Chapter 4. Data from VEST studies confirms the occurrence of left ventricular dysfunction before the onset of ECG changes. More recent studies have been concerned with the relationship between blood pressure changes and the development of spontaneous myocardial ischemia (i.e., do hemodynamic changes precede or follow the ischemic marker of ST depression?) Rehman et al. [7] used an ambulatory monitoring device that triggered blood pressure recordings for the level of the ST segment. They were thus able to document systolic and diastolic blood pres-

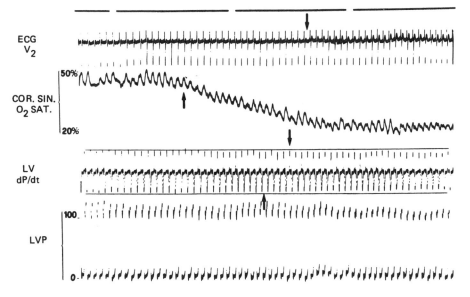

Figure 4   High-speed playback (paper speed 10 mm/s) of the transient phase of an ischemic episode characterized by peaking of T waves. Arrows indicate the onset of change for each recorded parameter. A drop in CSO_2s (denoting reduction in coronary blood flow) precedes the onset of ECG and hemodynamic changes. (From Chierchia S, Brunelli C, Simonetti I, Lazzari M, Maseri A. Circulation 1980; 61:759. Reproduced with permission of the American Heart Association.)

sure and heart rate changes. They found that significant increases in myocardial oxygen demand, including systolic blood pressure, occurred during episodes of spontaneous myocardial ischemia. (Fig. 6). These changes followed a circadian variation (Fig. 7). The influence of systolic blood pressure at the time of ECG evidence of ischemia, especially the dynamic increase in systolic blood pressure—is an important factor in the sensory perception of ischemia (i.e., acute activation of baroreceptors may result in anti-nociception). This is the conclusion of studies by Go et al. [8].

III.   TRANSIENT CORONARY ARTERY OBSTRUCTION DURING BALLOON ANGIOPLASTY

Sigwart and colleagues [9] were among the first to use this procedure to shed additional light on the sequence of ischemic events. In a classic study they care-

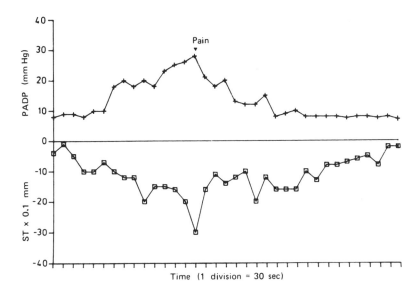

Figure 5   Changes in pulmonary artery diastolic pressure (PADP) and the ST segment during an episode of angina recorded during ambulatory monitoring. (From Levy RD, Shapiro LM, Wright C, Mockus L, Fox KM. Br Heart J 1986; 56:12.)

fully monitored several variables during balloon obstruction of the coronary arteries in humans. This technique—the key part of the transluminal coronary angioplasty procedure—allows the onset of ischemia to be precisely defined in a controlled setting. In 12 patients, one catheter was placed in the pulmonary artery, and a high-fidelity micromanometer was placed in the left ventricle via the transseptal approach. The time of coronary occlusion was identified by a sudden pressure drop at the distal end of the balloon catheter. Duration of the balloon occlusion was adjusted according to the alteration in the contractility and relaxation variables that were measured. Left ventricular dimensional changes were obtained in five patients with M-mode echocardiography and in five patients with biplane angiography. The time course of various hemodynamic changes is shown in Figure 8. Heart rate and blood pressure changes were small during the first 15 s of the balloon occlusion (which usually involved the left anterior descending coronary artery), but dP/dt_{max} and dP/dt_{min} (the latter an index of relaxation) fell. Left ventricular end-diastolic pressure changed little. Ejection fraction measured 10 s after occlusion in five patients was reduced by over one-third of the control value. Angina, when it occurred,

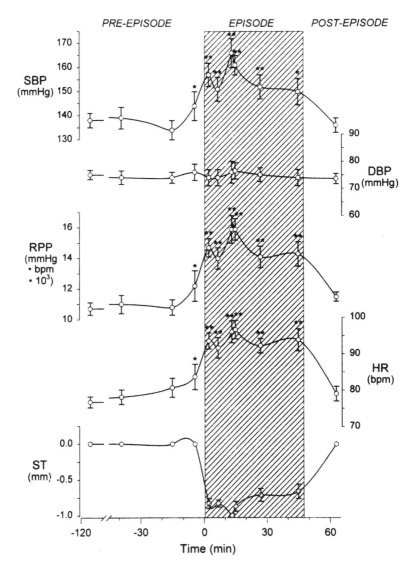

Figure 6 Mean hemodynamic changes observed during 64 episodes of spontaneous myocardial ischemia. Systolic blood pressure (SBP), diastolic blood pressure (DBP), rate-pressure product (RPP), heart rate (HR), and ST segment level (ST) are shown before, during (shaded), and after termination of the ischemic episodes. Mean values ± SEM of the data obtained before (1 to 4 h, 20 to 59 min, 10 to 19 min, and <10 min), during (<5 min, 5 to 10 min, 11 to 20 min, 21 to 40 min, and >40 min), and after the end of the episode are tabulated. Significant changes in systolic blood pressure, heart rate, and rate pressure product occurred during the episodes ($p < 0.001$ by analysis of variance). *$p < 0.05$; **$p < 0.001$ compared with a period >10 min before the onset of ST segment depression. Bpm = beats/min. (Reproduced with permission from Rehman A, Zalos G, Andrews NP, Mulcahy D, Quyyumi AA. J Am Coll Cardiol 1997; 30: 1249–1255.)

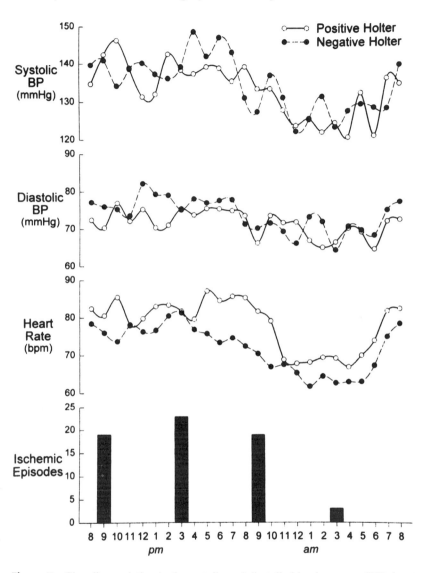

Figure 7 Circadian variation in the systolic and diastolic blood pressure (BP), heart rate, and transient ischemic episodes (6 AM to 12 PM, 12 PM to 6 PM, 6 PM to 12 AM, 12 AM to 6 AM) in patients with positive exercise test results and no episodes (solid circle) and those with episodes of transient ischemia (open circles). Bpm = beats/min. (Reproduced with permission from Rehman A, Zalos G, Andrews NP, Mulcahy D, Quyyumi AA. J Am Coll Cardiol 1997; 30:1249–1255.)

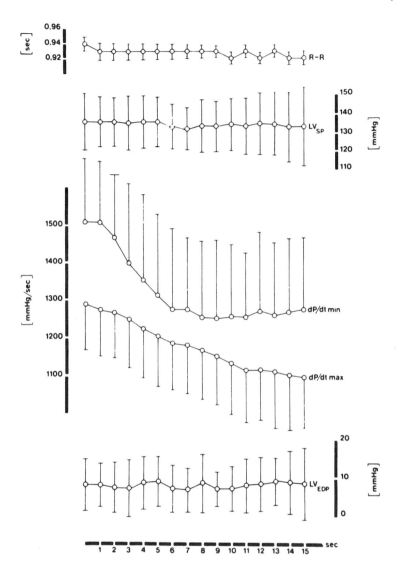

Figure 8 Heart rate (R-R), left ventricular systolic pressure (LV$_{sp}$), dP/dt$_{min}$, dP/dt$_{max}$, and left ventricular end-diastolic pressure (LV$_{EDP}$) during the first 15-s coronary balloon obstruction in 12 patients (mean ± 1 SD). (From Sigwart U, Grbic M, Payot M, Goy JJ, Essinger A, Fischer A. In: Rutishauser W, Roskamm H, eds. Silent Myocardial Ischemia. Berlin: Springer-Verlag, 1984.)

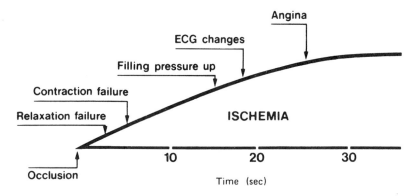

Figure 9   Appearance of events during transient coronary occlusion. (From Sigwart U, Grbic M, Payot M, Goy J-J, Essinger A, Fischer A. In: Rutishauser W, Roskamm H, eds. Silent Myocardial Ischemia. Berlin: Springer-Verlag, 1984.)

was later than 25 s after balloon occlusion and was usually preceded by ECG changes.

Figure 9 shows the actual sequence of events over the course of the first 30 s after occlusion. This sequence is similar to that depicted in Figure 2. It was of interest that the relaxation parameters were the most sensitive of all the variables. This confirmed earlier reports in experimental animals, as well as other studies of transluminal angioplasty in humans. The authors concluded that "ischemia in conscious man is always characterized by a transition period during which it remains silent." As we shall see from other clinical studies in subsequent chapters, the transition to a symptomatic stage does not necessarily occur in many instances of transient myocardial ischemia. Serruys et al. [10] reported similar findings in their studies using cine left ventriculography, but it has been the echocardiogram that has emerged as the prime investigational tool for documenting left ventricular wall motion changes. For example, Hauser et al. [11] studied 18 patients with echocardiography during PTCA. Left ventricular wall motion was originally normal in 14. During 22 episodes of angioplasty, hypokinesis, usually rapidly progressing to dyskinesis, occurred 19 ± 8 s after coronary occlusion. ST segment shifts occurred after 30 ± 5 s and pain occurred after 39 ± 6 s (in nine episodes) (Table 1). Similar findings were reported by Visser et al. [12] Alam et al. [13] and Wohlgelernter et al. [14] while Labovitz et al. [15] documented changes in both diastolic and systolic left ventricular function with echocardiographic techniques. In the last several years there has been an outpouring of additional articles on the relationship between

Table 1 Clinical, Electrocardiographic, and Echocardiographic Findings in Patients Undergoing Coronary Angioplasty

Case	Age (yr) and sex	Symptoms	PCA vessel (obstruction)	Mean time to dyssynergy (s)	Mean time to normal- ization (s)	Mean time to ST shift (↑↓) (s)	Mean time to pain (s)	Wall motion pre-PCA	Wall motion during PCA
1	45M	Stable angina	LAD (95%)	20.5	39	30 ↑	40	Normal	Apical dys
2	71M	Unstable angina	LAD (80%)	11.5	9	—	52	Mild apical dys	Marked dys
3	59M	Postinfarction	LAD (75%)	10	22	30 ↑	30	Mild apical hypo	Apical dys
4	60M	Unstable angina	LAD (90%)	22.5	9	—	—	Normal	Apical dys
5	68F	Unstable angina	RCA (95%)	22.5	20	—	—	Normal	Inferior dys
6	46M	Unstable angina	LAD (95%)	27.5	15	—	55	Normal	Apical hypo
			RCA (80%)	22.5	7.5	—	—		Inferior hypo
7	58M	Stable angina	LAD (90%)	No change	—	—	—	Normal	Normal[a,b]
8	46M	Stable angina	LAD (80%)	32.5	16	40 ↓	45	Normal	Apical dys[c]
			LAD (70%)	30	—	—	—	Normal	Apical dys
9	63M	Stable angina	LCx (60%)	No change	—	—	—	Normal	Normal[a]
			RCA (90%)	30	—	—	—		Inferior hypo

#	Age/Sex	Diagnosis	Vessel						
10	55M	Stable angina	LAD (90%)	20	80	30 ↑	30	Normal	Apical dys
11	70F	Unstable angina	LAD (95%)	13.5	15	25 ↓	30	Normal	Apical dys
12	53M	Unstable angina	LAD (95%)	20	20	—	—	Normal	Apical dys
13	42M	Stable angina	LAD (90%)	22.5	24.5	—	35	Normal	Apical dys
14	53F	Unstable angina	LAD (85%)	12	28.5	30 ↓	—	Normal	Apical dys
			RCA (70%)	25	10	30 ↑	—		Inferior dys
15	40M	Unstable angina	LAD (75%)	15	12	—	—	Normal	Apical dys
16	54M	Stable angina	LAD (95%)	No change	—	—	—	Anterior apical akin	No change
17	60M	Stable angina	RCA (90%)	18	12.5	—	35	Inferior hypo[d]	Inferior akin
18	41M	Stable angina	LAD (75%)	13.5	27.5	25 ↓	—	Normal	Apical dys

[a] Balloon inflations limited to 30 s duration.
[b] Percutaneous coronary angioplasty vessel highly collateralized.
[c] Mitral valve prolapse normalizes during percutaneous coronary angioplasty (see text).
[d] Normal wall motion after conclusion of percutaneous coronary angioplasty.

Akin = akinesia; dys = dyskinesia; F= female; hypo = hypokinesia; LAD = left anterior descending coronary artery; LCx = left circumflex coronary artery; M = male; PCA = percutaneous coronary angioplasty; RCA = right coronary artery; ↑↓ = ST segment elevation or depression, respectively.

Source: Hauser AM, Gangadharan V, Ramos RG, Gordon S, Timmis GC. J Am Coll Cardiol 1985; 5:193.

PTCA and silent ischemia. Some of these are related to the genesis of cardiac pain during the procedure, with Tomai et al. [16] attributing the pain to stretching of the coronary artery wall. If the stretching is maintained at a constant level during repeated coronary occlusions, the cardiac pain is predicted by the severity of the ischemia as determined by ST segment changes. Falcone et al. [17] measured beta-endorphin levels during PTCA and found that they were higher and more stable in patients with silent ischemia, thereby suggesting to these investigators that variations in opiate levels can be linked to differing patient-to-patient perception of pain during PTCA. In a later study, the same group of investigators conducted tooth pulp stimulation tests of dental pain to verify whether reactivity to the pulp test could help identify patients prone to having angina during PTCA, and they did indeed find such a relationship [18]. Two groups of investigators from Japan have studied cardiac pain experienced with PTCA and, in particular, the effect of aminophylline and theophylline. They are both antagonists of the adenosine receptor described earlier in Chapter 1. In the study of Hashimura et al. [19] cardiac ischemia pain was reduced by intravenous aminophylline administered during a sequence of balloon inflations. ST segment abnormalities were similar; by contrast Hashimura et al. found that theophylline did reduce ST segment abnormalities [20]. Complicating the hypothesis concerning vessel expansion, however, is the recent observation by Jeremias et al. [21] that not only is stent implantation more likely to result in chest pain than PTCA but the pain is *not* ischemic in nature. The echocardiogram has also been used in other than PTCA studies to define the timing of ischemic events. The experience of Distante and colleagues has been particularly impressive in documenting the "pre-ECG phase" in which left ventricular dysfunction is the only abnormality (Table 2) [22] similar to the VEST study findings discussed earlier. This "pre-ECG phase" of silent ischemia has also been termed "truly silent" or "clandestine" ischemia [23].

IV. CONCLUSIONS

Based on exercise studies, hemodynamic monitoring and, most importantly, transient coronary artery obstruction during PTCA, it is clear that pain is the *final* event in the sequence of events that characterizes the ischemic episode. In primary ischemia, there is first a reduction in coronary blood flow followed by hemodynamic evidence of left ventricular dysfunction and then ECG changes. In secondary ischemia, increases in the work of the heart lead to the hemodynamic abnormalities that are followed by ECG changes. Angina—when it occurs—follows the ECG changes.

Table 2   Time Sequence of Echocardiographic Signs During Acute Ischemia with ST-Segment Elevation in Humans (Prinzmetal's Patients)

	Pre-ECG phase	ECG phase	Post-ECG phase
Electrocardiogram	ST =	ST ↑	ST =
Echocardiogram (M-Mode)			
Wall signs			
Motion	↓	↓↓	↑
End-diastolic thickness	↓	↓	=
End-systolic thickness	↓	↓↓	↑
% systolic thickening	↓	↓↓	↑
Cavity signs			
End-diastolic diameter	=/↑	↑	=/↓
End-systolic diameter	↑	↑↑	↓
% fractional shortening	↓	↓↓	↑
Anginal pain	No	Yes/No	No

ST = no change; ST ↑ = ST-segment elevation; ↓ = reduction; ↓↓ = marked reduction; ↑ = increase; ↑↑ = marked increased; = no change; No = absent; Yes = present.
Source: Distante A. In: von Arnim T, Maseri A, eds. Silent Ischemia: Current Concepts and Management. Darmstadt: Steinkopff, 1987: 98.

REFERENCES

1. Upton MT, Rerych SK, Newman GE, Port S, Cobb FR, Jones RH. Detecting abnormalities in left ventricular function during exercise before angina and ST-segment depression. Circulation 1980; 62:341.
2. Sugishita Y, Koseki S, Matsuda M, Tamura T, Yamaguchi I, Ito I. Dissociation between regional myocardial dysfunction and ECG changes during myocardial ischemia induced by exercise in patients with angina pectoris. Am Heart J 1983; 106:1.
3. Heller GV, Ahmed I, Tikemeier PL, Barbour MM, Garber CW. Comparison of chest pain, electrocardiographic changes and thallium-201 scintigraphy during varying exercise intensities in men with stable angina pectoris. Am J Cardiol 1991; 68:569.
4. Chierchia S, Brunelli C, Simonetti I, Lazzari M, Maseri A. Sequence of events in angina at rest: Primary reduction in coronary flow. Circulation 1980; 61:759.
5. Levy RD, Shapiro LM, Wright C, Mockus L, Fox KM. Haemodynamic response to myocardial ischaemia during unrestricted activity, exercise testing, and atrial pacing assessed by ambulatory pulmonary artery pressure monitoring. Br Heart J 1986; 56:12.

6. Tamaki N, Yasuda T, Moore RH, Gill JB, Boucher CA, Hutter Jr AM, Gold HK, Strauss HW. Continuous monitoring of left ventricular function by an ambulatory radionuclide detector in patients with coronary artery disease. J Am Coll Cardiol 1988; 12:669.

7. Rehman A, Zalos G, Andrews NP, Mulcahy D, Quyyumi AA. Blood pressure changes during transient myocardial ischemia: insights into mechanisms. J Am Coll Cardiol 1997; 30:1249–55.

8. Go BM, Sheffield D, Krittayaphong R, Maixner W, Sheps DS. Association of systolic blood pressure at time of myocardial ischemia with angina pectoris during exercise testing. Am J Cardiol 1997; 79:954–956.

9. Sigwart U, Grbic M, Payot M, Goy J-J, Essinger A, Fischer A. Ischemic events during coronary artery balloon occlusion. In: Rutishauser W, Roskamm H, eds. Silent Myocardial Ischemia. Berlin: Springer-Verlag, 1984: 29–36.

10. Serruys PW, Wijns W, van Brand M. Left ventricular performance, regional blood flow, wall motion and lactate metabolism during transluminal angioplasty. Circulation 1984; 70:25.

11. Hauser AM, Gangadharan V, Ramos RG, Gordon S, Timmis GC. Sequence of mechanical, electrocardiographic and clinical effects of repeated coronary artery occlusion in human beings: Echocardiographic observations during coronary angioplasty. J Am Coll Cardiol 1985; 5:193.

12. Visser CA, David GK, Kan G. Two-dimensional echocardiography during percutaneous transluminal coronary angioplasty. Am Heart J, 1986; 111:1035.

13. Alam M, Khaja F, Brymer J, Marzelli M, Goldstein S. Echocardiographic evaluation of left ventricular function during coronary artery angioplasty. Am J Cardiol 1986; 57:20.

14. Wohlgelernter D, Jaffe CC, Cabin HS, Yeatman LA, Jr., Cleman M. Silent ischemia during coronary occlusion produced by balloon inflation: Relation to regional myocardial dysfunction. J Am Coll Cardiol 1987; 10:491.

15. Labovitz AJ, Lewen MK, Kern M, Vandormael M, Deligonal U, Kennedy HL. Evaluation of left ventricular systolic and diastolic dysfunction during transient myocardial ischemia produced by angioplasty. J Am Coll Cardiol 1987; 10:743.

16. Tomai F, Crea F, Gaspardone A, Versaci F, Esposito C, Chiariello L, Gioffre PA. Mechanisms of cardiac pain during coronary angioplasty. J Am Coll Cardiol 1993; 22:1892–1896.

17. Falcone C, Guasti L, Ochan M, Codega S, Tortorici M, Angoli L, Bergamaschi R, Montemartini C. Beta-endorphins during coronary angioplasty in patients with silent or symptomatic myocardial ischemia. J Am Coll Cardiol 1993; 22: 1624–1620.

18. Falcone C, Auguadro C, Sconocchia R, Catalano O, Ochan M, Angoli L, Montemartini C. Susceptibility to pain during coronary angioplasty: usefulness of pulpal test. J Am Coll Cardiol 1996; 28:903–909.

19. Hashino T, Ikeda H, Ueno T, Imaizumi T. Aminophylline reduces cardiac ischemic pain during percutaneous transluminal coronary angioplasty. J Am Coll Cardiol 1996; 28:1725–1731.

20. Hashimura K, Kijima Y, Matsu-ura Y, Ueda T, Kato Y, Mori I, Minamino T, Kitakaze M, Masatsugu H. Effect of theophylline on adaptation of the heart to myocardial ischemia during percutaneous transluminal coronary angioplasty in patients with stable angina pectoris. Am J Cardiol 1997; 79:475–477.
21. Jeremias A, Kutscher S, Haude M, Heinen D, Holtmann G, Wolfgang S, Erbel R. Nonischemic chest pain induced by coronary interventions: A prospective study comparing coronary angioplasty and stent implantation. Circulation 1998; 98:2656–2658.
22. Distante A. Noninvasive detection of silent myocardial ischemia with echocardiography. In: von Arnim, T, Maseri, A, eds. Silent Ischemia: Current Concepts and Management. Darmstadt: Steinkopff, 1987: 98.
23. Candell-Riera J, Santana-Boado S, Bermejo B, Castell-Conesa J, Aguade-Bruix S, Canela T, Soler-Soler J. Prognosis of "clandestine" myocardial ischemia, silent myocardial ischemia, and angina pectoris in medically treated patients. Am J Cardiol 1998; 82:1333–1338.

4

Left Ventricular Dysfunction and Myocardial Blood Flow Disturbances During Episodes of Silent Myocardial Ischemia

Is Less Myocardium at Jeopardy Than During Symptomatic Ischemia?

This chapter will consider an alternative hypothesis for the etiology of silent ischemic episodes in humans. Altered pain perception by itself is probably not sufficient to explain all episodes of silent myocardial ischemia, as discussed in Chapter 2. For that reason, it has been postulated that in some instances ischemia is "silent" because less myocardium is ischemic compared to that involved in symptomatic episodes. This chapter will review studies that have

57

compared left ventricular function and myocardial blood flow in symptomatic and asymptomatic myocardial ischemia.

The left ventricular studies can be categorized into three major types: (1) hemodynamic changes recorded with catheters in the right and/or left heart chambers; (2) ventriculography performed either invasively, with contrast agent, or noninvasively, with radionuclide ventriculography; and (3) echocardiography.

I. HEMODYNAMIC CHANGES DURING SILENT MYOCARDIAL ISCHEMIA

One of the earliest and still most comprehensive of these studies was the 1983 report by Chierchia and colleagues [1]. These investigators studied 14 patients admitted to the coronary care unit because of rest angina. Left ventricular (or pulmonary artery) pressures and systemic arterial hemodynamics were measured for a mean of 13.6 h during continuing electrocardiographic monitoring. Eighty-four percent (or 247) of the 293 episodes of transient ST segment and T-wave changes were completely asymptomatic. Figure 1 shows a computer plot of hemodynamic variables recorded in these episodes. Most (63%) of these asymptomatic episodes were associated with an elevation in the left ventricular end-diastolic or pulmonary artery diastolic pressure of 5 mmHg or more; a smaller number (15%) had elevations of 2 to 4 mmHg. In 22%, there were no changes or less than a 2-mmHg rise in pressure. Peak contraction and relaxation indices using dP/dt (the first derivative of left ventricular pressure) were reduced considerably (to 100 mmHg/s or more) in over 88% of the asymptomatic episodes. That these hemodynamic changes represented ischemia in these patients was confirmed by primary reductions in coronary sinus blood flow calculated from changes in coronary sinus oxygen saturation. (Although the patients in this series represented examples of coronary vasospasm, not all instances of silent myocardial ischemia are due to this mechanism.)

The hemodynamic changes during the 247 asymptomatic episodes were compared to those occurring during the 46 symptomatic episodes (Fig. 2). Comparisons were also made by type of ST segment changes (depression or elevation). It was of interest that the mean duration of the asymptomatic episodes was significantly shorter than the symptomatic episodes (253 $\pm$ 19 s vs. 674 $\pm$ 396 s; $p < 0.001$). Furthermore, the left ventricular end-diastolic pressure did not rise as high in the asymptomatic episodes (5.9 $\pm$ 5.0 mmHg vs. 16.5 $\pm$ 6.9 mmHg; $p < 0.001$). Using peak contraction dP/dt as an index of contractility, the authors also reported less of an impairment in systolic func-

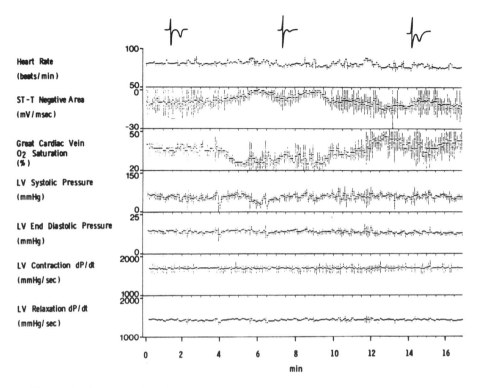

Figure 1 Computer plot of an asymptomatic episode of pseudonormalization of an inverted T wave (decrease in ST-T negative area) in a patient with anterior ischemia. In this patient, there was no increase of left ventricular (LV) end-diastolic pressure and the peak contraction and relaxation dP/dt were not altered, although there was a reduction of great cardiac vein oxygen saturation preceding and accompanying the electrocardiographic change. (From Chierchia S, Lazzari M, Freedman B, Brunelli C, Maseri A. J Am Coll Cardiol 1983; 1:924.)

tion during the asymptomatic episodes (252 ± 156 mmHg/s vs. 395 ± 199 mmHg/s; $p < 0.001$). Diastolic function was characterized by peak relaxation dP/dt; again, the reduction in this measurement was less in the asymptomatic episodes (259 ± 191 mmHg/s vs. 413 ± 209 mmHg/s; $p < 0.001$). These trends were observed regardless of the type of ST segment abnormality. The authors concluded that in their study population "asymptomatic episodes were usually characterized by a shorter duration and a lesser degree of ischemic left ventricular dysfunction than the symptomatic episodes, although there is a consider-

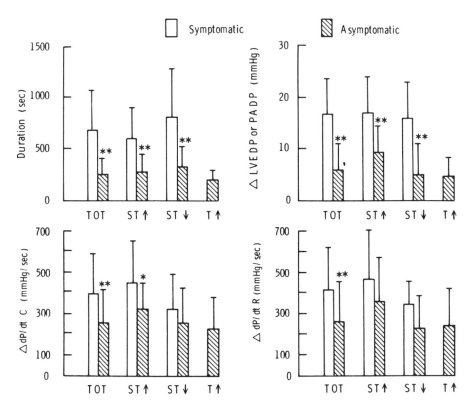

Figure 2 Comparison of symptomatic and asymptomatic episodes of ST segment and T-wave changes. The mean values and standard deviation are plotted for the duration of episodes, the increases in left ventricular end-diastolic (LVEDP) [or pulmonary artery diastolic (PADP)] pressure and reductions of left ventricular peak contraction (C) and relaxation (R) dP/dt. P values for comparison of symptomatic and asymptomatic episodes: * = < 0.01; ** = < 0.001. Overall, asymptomatic episodes were shorter and were accompanied by lesser degrees of left ventricular impairment. ST↑ or ST↓ = transient ST segment elevation or depression; T = transient pseudonormalization or peaking of inverted or flat T waves; TOT = total. (From Chierchia S, Lazzari M, Freedman B, Brunelli C, Maseri A. J Am Coll Cardiol 1983; 1:924.)

able degree of overlap both in the group data and the results from individual patients." The authors speculated that asymptomatic episodes may represent lesser degrees of myocardial ischemia, though they acknowledged that the wide overlap in duration of episodes and degree of left ventricular impairment observed in the group data (as well as multiple episodes in individual patients) indicated that the severity of ischemia was not the only factor involved in the genesis of anginal pain.

II. RADIONUCLIDE AND CONTRAST VENTRICULOGRAPHY

Other investigators have utilized radionuclide ventriculography to evaluate left ventricular function in asymptomatic subjects. In one of the earliest studies, our laboratory [2] employed a computerized program to calculate regional ejection fractions at rest and during exercise. Figure 3 depicts the computer-generated left ventricular regions of interest that were evaluated in 40 patients, 16 with and 24 without silent myocardial ischemia. The clinical and arteriographic features of these two groups of patients were similar (Table 1) and so was their ejection fraction response to exercise (Table 2). None of the asymptomatic patients had pain with their test nor were they receiving any antianginal medications that could have modified the pain response. During exercise, global ejection fraction decreased by 0.06 in both groups. Even when differences in resting (baseline) values were considered, the relative decreases were not significant (9% vs. 12%). Analysis of each of the three ventricular regions of interest showed no significant differences in the degree of reduction during exercise. In addition, the percent of normal regions at rest (i.e., with ejection fraction >0.50), that demonstrated a decrease during exercise was 60% in both groups (19/33 vs. 22/46). We concluded that in these 40 patients—in whom the prevalence of myocardial infarction and multivessel disease was similar—no discernible differences in wall motion abnormalities or ejection fraction were present.

Iskandrian and Hakki [3] approached this problem in a slightly different manner. They compared left ventricular function during exercise radionuclide ventriculography in anginal patients who either did or did not have their usual angina during the exercise procedure. Thirty-one patients had angina during the test and 43 did not. Multivessel disease was present in equal percentages in both groups of patients, as were a variety of clinical factors. Although the global ejection fraction was similar at rest in both groups, it fell to a greater

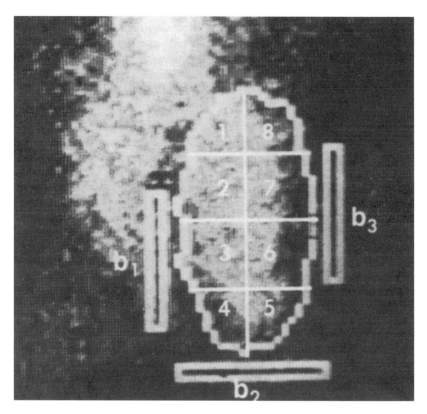

Figure 3 End-diastolic image of heart in left anterior oblique position with hand-drawn left ventricular outline. Eight regions of interest (subdivisions within the left ventricle) are indicated by the numbers 1 to 8. Regions 2 and 3 represent the anteroseptal, 4 and 5 the apical, and 6 and 7 the inferoposterior regions. Regions 1 and 8 are not used in analysis of regional ejection fraction because of the overlying cardiac valves and other structures. Three background regions (rectangles b_1, b_2, and b_3 located outside the left ventricular perimeter) are considered using an automated background correction algorithm. (From Cohn PE, Brown EJ, Wynne J, Holman BL, Atkins HL. J Am Coll Cardiol 1983; 1:931.)

extent in the symptomatic group (-0.045 ± 0.076 vs. -0.01 ± 0.094; $p < 0.01$). Other measurements (wall motion score, end-systolic volume, etc.) showed similar trends (Figs. 4 and 5).

The authors concluded that even though asymptomatic myocardial ischemia may occur in patients with extensive coronary artery disease and be

Table 1 Clinical and Arteriographic Features in Patients with (Group 1) and Without (Group 2) Silent Myocardial Ischemia

	Group 1 (16 patients)	p	Group 2 (24 patients)
Age (yr)	55 ± 3[a]	NS	54 ± 2
Male	13	NS	19
Prior MI	10	NS	15
CAD			
3 vessel	7	NS	11
2 vessel	6	NS	7
1 vessel	3	NS	6

[a]Mean value ± standard error of the mean.
CAD = coronary artery disease; MI = myocardial infarctions; NS = not significant; p = probability value.
Source: Cohn PF, Brown EJ, Wynne J, Holman BL, Atkins HL. J Am Coll Cardiol 1983; 1:931.

Table 2 Radionuclide Ejection Fraction in Patients with (Group 1) and Without (Group 2) Silent Myocardial Ischemia

	Group 1 (16 patients)	p	Group 2 (24 patients)
Global			
Rest	0.60 ± 0.04	NS	0.53 ± 0.04
Exercise	0.54 ± 0.04	NS	0.47 ± 0.04
Anteroseptal region			
Rest	0.60 ± 0.04	NS	0.51 ± 0.04
Exercise	0.56 ± 0.04	NS	0.45 ± 0.04
Apical region			
Rest	0.65 ± 0.06	NS	0.57 ± 0.05
Exercise	0.62 ± 0.06	NS	0.52 ± 0.05
Inferoposterior region			
Rest	0.70 ± 0.07	NS	0.66 ± 0.05
Exercise	0.64 ± 0.04	NS	0.59 ± 0.05

NS = not significant; p = probability value.
Source: Cohn PF, Brown EJ, Wynne J, Holman BL, Atkins HL. J Am Coll Cardiol 1983; 1: 931.

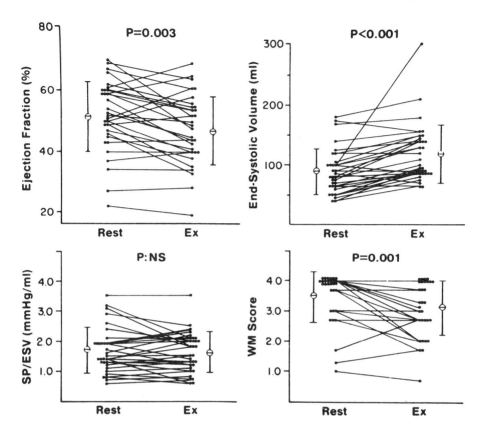

Figure 4 Left ventricular ejection fraction, end-systolic volume, systolic blood pressure–end systolic volume ratio (SP/ESV), and wall motion (WM) score at rest and during exercise (Ex) in patients with angina during the test. The means and standard deviations are also shown. NS = not significant. (From Iskandrian AS, Hakki A-H. Am J Cardiol 1984; 53:1239.)

associated with abnormal exercise left ventricular function, in general patients with symptomatic episodes have worse exercise left ventricular function than those with asymptomatic episodes.

Ratib and colleagues [4] performed isotope ventriculography in 25 patients who did not develop chest pain during exercise and found no differences in left ventricular function when compared to 14 patients who did develop angina with exercise (Fig. 6). These results are similar to those from

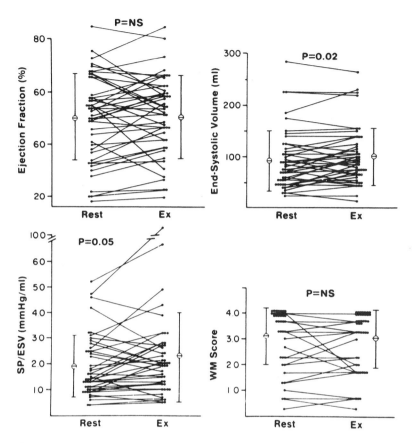

Figure 5 Left ventricular ejection fraction, end-systolic volume, systolic blood pressure–end-systolic volume ratio (SP/ESV), and wall motion (WM) score at rest and during exercise in patients without angina. NS = not significant. (From Iskandrian AS, Hakki A-H. Am J Cardiol 1984; 53:1239.)

our laboratory, as opposed to those of Iskandrian and Hakki. The phase analysis techniques used in this study are different from those of regional ejection fraction analysis, but the results are equally valid.

Gleichmann and colleagues [5] studied wall motion disorders during contrast ventriculography with bicycle exercise in 141 patients with coronary artery disease. Four combinations were used: angina with wall motion disorders (25% of total group); angina without wall motion disorders (16%); no

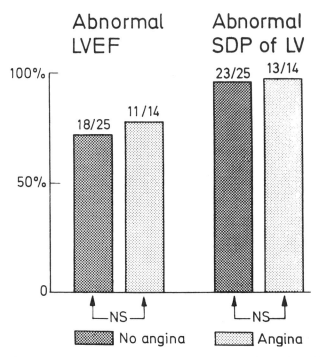

Figure 6 The numbers of patients with an abnormal response of left ventricular (LV) function during exercise. A failure to increase left ventricular ejection fraction (LVEF) by 5% or more was considered abnormal. Using this criterion, 72% of the patients without angina and 78% of the patients with angina had an abnormal LVEF during exercise. The authors established the upper limit of normal for standard deviation of peak (SDP) of LV as 14°, which is the mean plus 2 standard deviations measured in 10 normals at maximum exercise. There was no statistical difference between the two groups. SDP is an index of the degree of synchronicity of LV wall motion. (From Ratib O, Righetti A, Rutishauser W. In: Rutishauser W, Roskamm H, eds. Silent Myocardial Ischemia. Berlin: Springer-Verlag, 1984:84–89.)

angina with wall motion disorders (22%); and neither angina nor wall motion disorders (37%). Thus, the presence of angina could not clearly differentiate normal and abnormal left ventricular function with exercise. For example, more than 50% of the patients with one-vessel disease and no prior infarction had no angina but had hypokinesis or akinesis. This combination was less frequent in patients with two-vessel disease (3%) or three-vessel disease (25%). The four possible combinations are depicted in Figure 7. The severe nature of these silent episodes was further confirmed by the rise in left ventricular end-

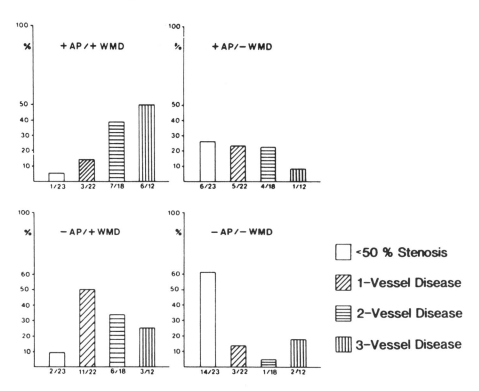

Figure 7 Left ventricular exercise angiography: frequency of angina pectoris (AP) and wall motion disorders (WMD) in 75 patients with coronary artery disease (CAD) without scar. (From Gleichmann U, Faßbender D, Mannebach H, Vogt J, Trieb G. In: Rutishauser W, Roskamm H, eds. Silent Myocardial Ischemia. Berlin: Springer-Verlag, 1984:71–77.)

diastolic pressure during exercise in many of the patients with wall motion disorders. However, the higher prevalence of one-vessel disease does suggest less myocardium at jeopardy.

Hirzel and colleagues [6] also reported on both wall motion disorders and hemodynamic changes in their series of 36 patients with exercise-induced silent ischemia and 36 matched patients with exercise-induced angina. All patients had a history of angina, but only the latter patients continued to have angina at time of admission, despite the disparity in symptoms. Under similar exercise conditions, comparable hemodynamic and wall motion abnormalities indicative of ischemia were observed in both groups of patients (Fig. 8). The

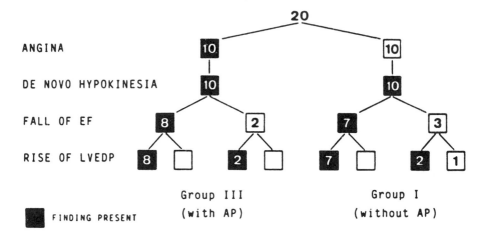

Figure 8 Clinical, hemodynamic, and angiographic characteristics during exercise in 20 patients with proven coronary artery disease but without prior myocardial infarction. Ten patients were limited by angina, 10 tolerated the exercise test without anginal symptoms. Both patient groups were carefully matched for extent and severity of coronary artery lesions. No differences in prevalence of either regional de novo hypokinesia, decrease of left ventricular ejection fraction (EF), or increase in end-diastolic pressure (LVEDP) were noted between the two groups during exercise at comparable external work loads and rate-pressure products. (From Hirzel HO, Leutwyler R, Krayenbuehl HP. J Am Coll Cardiol 1985; 6:275.)

authors concluded that "angina pectoris cannot be considered a prerequisite for hemodynamically significant ischemia during exertion." Vassiliadis et al. [7] came to similar conclusions when they studied 77 patients with radionuclide ventriculography during exercise. Wall motion abnormalities can also be induced by mental stress. Rozanski and colleagues [8] demonstrated this in 23 of 59 patients with coronary artery disease using radionuclide ventriculography to document the abnormalities, most of which occurred in the absence of symptoms. Even in the 1990s radionuclide testing continued to be a popular technique for assessing areas of ischemia. Klein et al. [9] argued that patient selection biases may influence the clinical significance of exercise-induced chest pain. In their analysis of SPECT studies in 117 patients, they reported that patients with angina during exercise had more severe indices of ischemia compared to patients with silent ischemia (Figs. 9 and 10). Two 1997 studies also concluded that patients with painless ischemia had less severe and less extensive reversible defects on stress thallium scintigraphy, as well other indices of

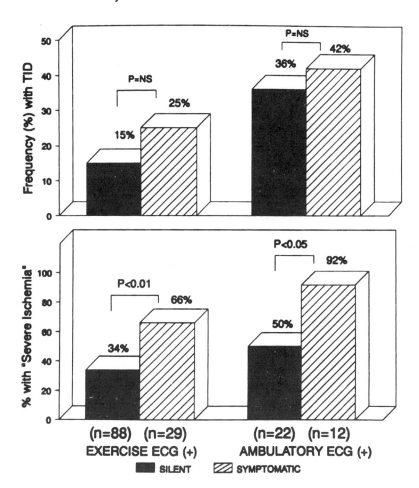

Figure 9 Top graph: Frequency of transient ischemic dilation (TID) of the left ventricle after stress (on the vertical axis) in the exercise and ambulatory ECG subgroups. Note the high frequency of TID in the patients with a positive ambulatory ECG study regardless of the presence or absence of chest pain during ischemic episodes. Bottom graph: Percent of patients manifesting severe ischemia (five or more reversible thallium defects) on the vertical axis. Patients with chest pain and exercise-induced ST-segment depression had nearly twice the frequency of severe ischemia on thallium scintigraphy compared with patients with silent ST segment depression. (Reproduced by permission from Klein J, Chao SY, Berman DS, Rozanski A. Circulation 1994; 89:1958–1966.)

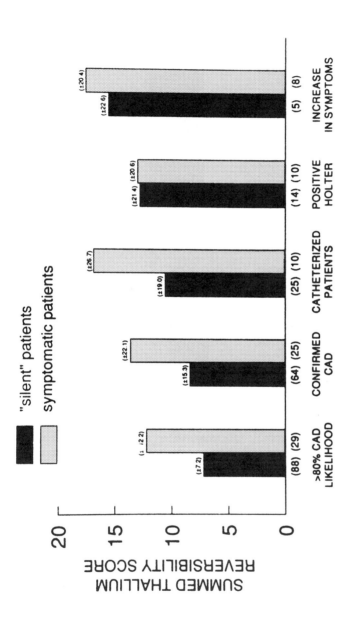

Figure 10   Bar graph: Summed thallium reversibility score (vertical axis) is shown for silent and symptomatic patients in five groups as increasing selection criteria were applied to define the population of interest. There was a substantial difference in the summed thallium reversibility score between symptomatic and silent cohorts of patients having a high likelihood of coronary artery disease (CAD) ($p = 0.002$); confirmed CAD ($p = 0.004$); or recent catheterization ($p = 0.06$) (first three groups on the left). By contrast, in the patients defined on the basis of having a positive Holter or increasing anginal symptoms, no significant differences were noted. Note that the absolute values for the summed thallium reversibility scores increased progressively as the population became increasingly selected. (Reproduced by permission from Klein J, Chao SY, Berman DS, Rozanski A. Circulation 1994; 89: 1958–1966.)

ischemia, than did patients with angina. In one study all 936 patients had experienced an acute coronary event 1 to 6 months earlier [10] (Table 3) and, in the other, 300 patients had a well-established history of ischemic heart disease [11] (Table 4).

As described in Chapter 3, a technique using an ambulatory left ventricular function monitoring device (VEST) has been used to record left ventricular ejection fraction during daily activities. Tamaki et al. [12] reported 36 episodes of transient fall in ejection fraction in 16 angina patients; only 12 were accompanied by typical anginal symptoms. Transient left ventricular dysfunction after myocardial infarction—often silent—has been reported after thrombolytic therapy for myocardial infarction [13]. Most recently, Mohiuddin et al. [14] reported VEST studies in 26 subjects evaluated at rest and during exercise both before and after anti-ischemic therapy. Left ventricular function abnormalities were often severe, even in the absence of angina. Davies et al. [15] used a precordial scintillation probe to record ventricular volumes in painful and painless ischemia. No significant differences were found.

III. ECHOCARDIOGRAPHY

As noted in Chapter 3, wall motion abnormalities recorded by echocardiography during coronary angioplasty have shown no difference between painful and painless episodes. This was most clearly reported by Wohlgelernter et al. [16] in their comparison of regional and global indices of left ventricular dysfunction (Figs. 11 and 12), but was also alluded to by others [17]. Exercise echocardiography has also demonstrated that the occurrence of exertional angina is unrelated to extent or severity of ischemia [18]. However, a 1995 report by Nihoyannopoulos et al. [19] casts doubt on earlier reports. New wall motion abnormalities on exercise echocardiography were seen in 93% of patients with painful vs. 55% with painless ischemia ($p < 0001$). Hecht [20] found the opposite in their group of 130 patients. They also had a population of patients with "truly silent ischemia" cited earlier (i.e., echocardiographic abnormalities without chest pain or ECG abnormalities). These patients *did* have less ischemia than patients with ECG indicators of ischemia, with or without chest pain.

IV. MYOCARDIAL BLOOD FLOW STUDIES

Myocardial blood flow (perfusion) studies are generally of two types: quantitative (invasive) vs. qualitative (noninvasive). A prime example of the former

Table 3 Diagnostic Test Results

	Ischemia on noninvasive testing			p Value	
	None (n = 433)	Silent (n = 378)	Symptomatic (n = 125)	3-tailed	Silent vs. symptomatic
ETT					
Exercise duration (s)	616 ± 198	640 ± 173	529 ± 190	<0.001	<0.001
Time to 1-mm ST segment depression (s)	NA	530 ± 215	420 ± 205	NA	<0.001
STS					
Ischemia				<0.001	0.04
None (%)	100	30	21		
Mild (%)	0	19	16		
Moderate (%)	0	21	21		
Severe (%)	0	30	42		
Scar (%)	41	55	57	<0.001	NS[a]
Ischemia on ambulatory ECG (%)	4	9	19	<0.001	<0.005
Mean 75% coronary angiographic jeopardy score	3.1	3.8	4.2	<0.001	<0.05

[a] $p > 0.05$. Data presented are mean value ±SD, unless otherwise indicated.

ECG = electrocardiogram; NA = not applicable; other abbreviations as in Table 1.

Source: Reproduced by permission from Narins CR, Zareba W, Moss AJ, Goldstein RE, Jackson Hall W. J Am Cardiol 1997; 29:756–763.

Table 4 Clinical Findings in Patients with Painful or Silent Reversible Sestamibi Perfusion Defects During Exercise

	Painful ischemia $n = 97(32\%)$	Silent ischemia $n = 203 (68\%)$	p Value
Age (yr)	58 ± 8	56 ± 10	NS
Male/female	77/20	182/21	NS
History			
Hypertension	23 (24%)	56 (27%)	NS
Diabetes	5 (5%)	11 (5%)	NS
Hypercholesterolemia	24 (25%)	52 (26%)	NS
Body mass index (kg/m^2)	27 ± 3	25 ± 3	<0.001
Previous MI	36 (37%)	116 (57%)	<0.05
Effort angina	71 (73%)	53 (26%)	<0.001
Rest and effort angina	13 (13%)	16 (8%)	NS
Medications			
Nitrates	49 (51%)	69 (34%)	<0.01
Beta-blockers	46 (47%)	73 (36%)	<0.01
Calcium antagonists	41 (42%)	59 (29%)	<0.01
Angiography	46	95	
Single-vessel disease	14 (32%)	32 (34%)	
Multivessel disease	30 (68%)	62 (66%)	NS
Occluded vessels	25 (54%)	36 (38%)	0.09
Proximal LAD occlusion	5 (11%)	10 (11%)	NS
Left ventricular ejection fraction[a]	55 ± 11	52 ± 12	NS

[a]On biplane two-dimensional echocardiography or contrast ventriculography. Data are reported as mean values $\pm$SD or number (%) of patients.
LAD = left anterior descending coronary artery; MI = myocardial infarction.
Source: Reproduced by permission from Marcassa C, Galli M, Baroffio C, Campini R, Gianuzzi P. J Am Cardiol 1997; 29:948–954.

type is the xenon-133 clearance technique for measuring regional myocardial blood flow. Because of physiological restraints, this technique has been shown in several centers around the world to be most reliable when the same patient is used as his or her own control. One of the pioneers in this work is Lichtlen. He and his colleagues reported their results in 11 patients with coronary artery disease not experiencing angina during ischemia by rapid atrial pacing [21]. Fifteen patients had angina during these studies and served as a control group. Figure 13 depicts the results: blood flow increased in poststenotic areas much

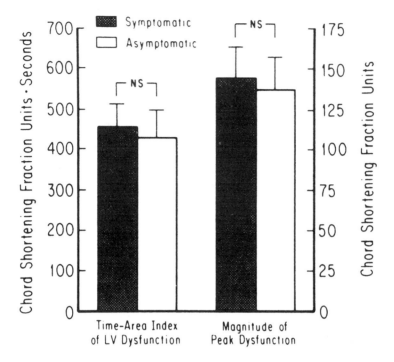

Figure 11   Comparison of regional dysfunction variables in the symptomatic and asymptomatic groups. Brackets represent ± 1 SD. There were no differences between the groups in the time-area index of left ventricular (LV) dysfunction or the magnitude of peak dysfunction. (From Wohlgelernter D, Jaffe CC, Cabin HS, Yeatman LA, Jr., Cleman M. J Am Coll Cardiol 1987; 10:491.)

less than in normal regions during rapid atrial pacing, but no differences were found between the angina and nonangina groups. However, individual responses did show a tendency for flow to be actually reduced in some patients with angina (Fig. 14). The reason for this is not clear, but a vasospastic mechanism may be implicated.

The prime example of a qualitative, noninvasive method for evaluating myocardial perfusion is the thallium-201 scintigram. Righetti and colleagues [22] found that coronary patients showing perfusion defects without angina had a smaller number of ischemic segments despite a higher double product. Kurata et al. [23], Travin et al. [24] and Patterson et al. [25] also found less ischemia in those patients who experienced silent exercise-induced thallium defects. By contrast, Reisman et al. [26] reported similar degrees of thallium perfusion

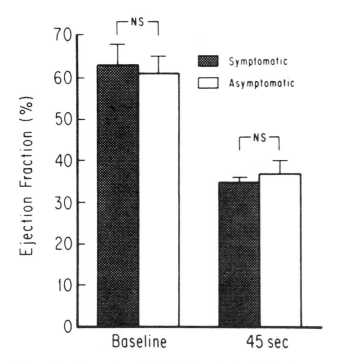

Figure 12 Comparison of global left ventricular ejection fraction responses to balloon inflation in the symptomatic and asymptomatic groups. T represents ± 1 SD. There were no differences between the groups in ejection fraction values at baseline or at 45 s into inflation. (From Wohlgelernter D, Jaffe CC, Cabin HS, Yeatman LA, Jr., Cleman M. J Am Coll Cardiol 1987; 10:491.)

defects in their patient groups, as did Gasperetti et al. [27] (Fig. 15) and Mahmarian et al. [28], the latter using the single-photon emission computed tomography (SPECT) technique.

Hinrichs and colleagues [29,30] correlated results of lactate extraction and thallium scintigraphy in nine asymptomatic patients with angiographically proven coronary artery disease. In three patients, no myocardial lactate production at rest or after atrial pacing was observed and thallium scintigraphy was normal. Six other patients had both significant defects and lactate production. Coronary sinus blood flow increased to the same degree in both groups of patients. The authors concluded that the absence of metabolic and perfusion abnormalities probably indicated less myocardium at jeopardy, despite the same degree of ST segment depression during atrial pacing or exercise ECG.

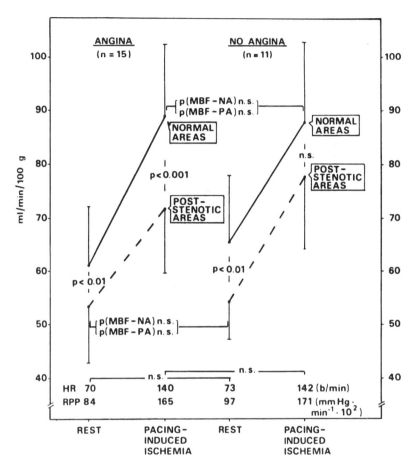

Figure 13   Regional myocardial blood flow (MBF) at rest and during rapid atrial pacing in 15 patients with and 11 patients without angina pectoris during ischemia. NA = normal areas; PA = poststenotic area; HR = heart rate; RPP = rate-pressure product. (From Daniel WG, Engel H-J, Hundeshage H, Lichtlen PR. In: Rutishauser W, Roskamm H, eds. Silent Myocardial Ischemia. Berlin: Springer-Verlag, 1984:45–49.)

Another type of myocardial perfusion technique utilizes an intravenous infusion of rubidium-82. Positron tomograms of rubidium uptake were made for five regions of interest by Deanfield et al. [31] during 24-h ambulatory monitoring, exercise tests, and cold pressor tests in 34 patients with histories of angina. An example of the ECG and perfusion abnormalities with and without angina is depicted in Figure 16. There was no significant difference in the

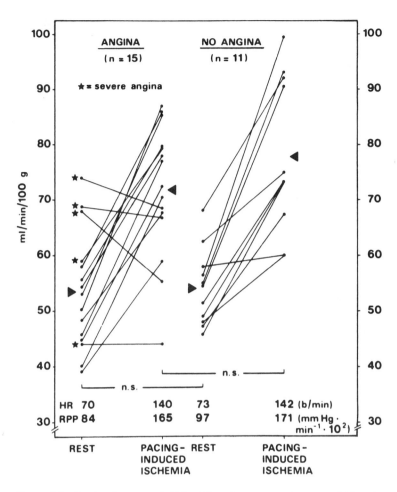

Figure 14   Regional myocardial blood flow in poststenotic areas of 15 patients with and 11 patients without angina pectoris during rapid atrial pacing-induced ischemia. * = severe angina. (From Daniel WG, Engel H-J, Hundeshage H, Lichtlen PR. In: Rutishauser W, Roskamm H, eds. Silent Myocardial Ischemia. Berlin: Springer-Verlag: 45–49.)

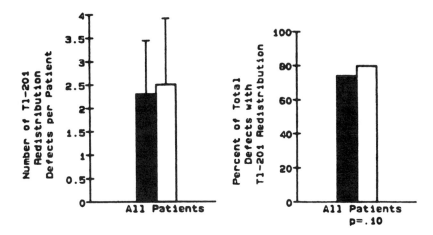

Figure 15 Comparison of silent ischemia (solid bars) and angina (open bars) groups with respect to extent of thallium-201 (^{201}Tl) redistribution. (From Gasperetti CM, Burwell LR, Beller GA. J Am Coll Cardiol 1990; 16:115. Reproduced with permission.)

change in uptake of rubidium-82 in the abnormal segment of myocardium between exercise tests accompanied by angina and those without pain (uptake changed from 47 ± 9.8 to 38 ± 10.6 for episodes of ST segment depression with angina vs. 52 ± 13 to 44 ± 12 for episodes of painless ST depression). Similarly, regional uptake changes in the abnormal segment of myocardium during unprovoked episodes of ST depression with angina were not significantly different from those found during painless episodes (from 48 ± 8.5 to 36 ± 6.6 for episodes of ST segment depression with angina vs. 48 ± 7 to 37.5 ± 8.3 for episodes of painless ST depression). The same investigative group has also documented impressive perfusion abnormalities when silent myocardial ischemia occurred during mental arithmetic [32] (Fig. 17) and smoking [33]. These studies tend to refute the hypothesis that lesser amounts of myocardium are injured during painless ischemia. The same conclusions can be inferred from the coronary angioplasty studies cited earlier, even though myocardial blood flow was not measured in these studies. At similar durations of occlusion and at similar occlusion pressures (with presumably similar degrees of reduction in myocardial blood flow), there were no differences in degree of left ventricular dysfunction or other indices of myocardial performances.

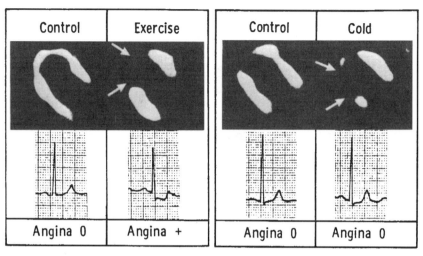

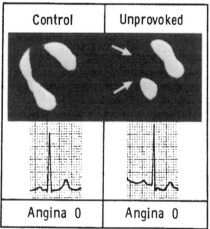

Figure 16 The tomographic slices for a single patient through the midleft ventricle showing the regional myocardial uptake of rubidium-82 in the posterior wall (PW), free wall (FW), anterior wall (a), and interventricular septum (S_1 and S_2) of the left ventricle. This demonstrates the distribution of regional perfusion during control, cold pressor, unprovoked ST depression, and exercise. Evidence of regional ischemia occurred during all three tests and supported the ST segment changes as evidence of ischemia whether or not chest pain occurred. (From Deanfield JE, Ribiero P, Oakley K, Krikler S, Selwyn AP. Am J Cardiol 1984; 54:1195.)

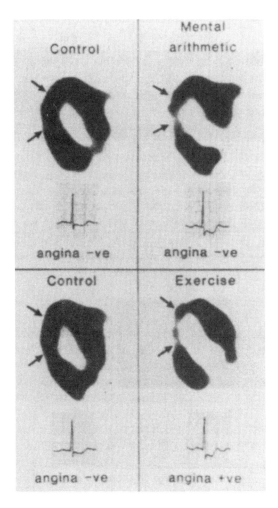

Figure 17   Changes in regional myocardial uptake of rubidium-82 and in ECG in relation to chest pain before and after mental arithmetic or exercise. Control scans show homogeneous regional cation uptake. Patient No. 9 shows anterior and free-wall ischemia and ST segment depression with mental arithmetic and exercise, but angina only after exercise (−ve = negative; +ve = positive). (From Deanfield JE, Kensett M, Wilson RA, Shea M, Horlock P, deLandsheere CM, Selwyn AP. Lancet 1984; 2:1001.)

V. SILENT MYOCARDIAL ISCHEMIA AND "STUNNED"
OR "HIBERNATING" MYOCARDIUM

The terms "stunned" [34] or "hibernating" myocardium [35] have been used to describe, respectively, (1) a state of prolonged postischemic myocardial dysfunction following severe transient ischemia and (2) reduced myocardial inotropy due to a persistent state of reduced coronary blood flow (i.e., chronic ischemia). It is thought that the reduced inotropy in the latter state may be a protective mechanism whereby the reduced oxygen demand secondary to the reduced inotropy minimizes the extent of ischemia, necrosis, or both [36]. That the myocardium in both postulated states is not irreversibly damaged is suggested by a series of studies documenting contractile reserve (after appropriate stimuli) in coronary patients with depressed left ventricular function [37–40]. The clinical relevance of these syndromes, especially "stunning," is further demonstrated by exercise studies in which hemodynamic and metabolic evidence of ischemia presents long after the symptoms and ECG findings have disappeared [40]. How can silent ischemia contribute to this picture and what are the clinical implications? If patients are unaware of the ischemic episodes that lead to stunned or hibernating myocardium, they may not take the necessary anti-ischemic agents that can reverse the hemodynamic and metabolic abnormalities. Thus, multiple episodes of silent ischemia may lead to a chronic ischemic state marked by persistent left ventricular dysfunction and perhaps even electrical instability. Whether an actual ischemic cardiomyopathy—with pathological changes as well—can result is still unclear, but reported cases of ischemic cardiomyopathy presenting de novo without prior angina or infarction suggests this is possible. Complicating this picture is the concept of "ischemic preconditioning" (i.e., brief periods of myocardial ischemia enhance myocardial tolerance to subsequent and more prolonged ischemic episodes). In humans, this adaptation to ischemia has been demonstrated by Deutsch et al. [40] during coronary angioplasty. The importance of preconditioning in the pathophysiology of silent ischemia is unclear. All the studies in the literature appear to be related to symptomatic chest pain rather than silent ischemia [41–44]. These studies indicate that preconditioning exists in humans with several possible mechanisms cited (e.g., involvement of adenosine, nitric oxide, prostacyclin, and free radicals).

VI. CONCLUSIONS

The majority of studies evaluating hemodynamic, ventriculographic, and myocardial blood flow changes during silent myocardial ischemia do not show any clearcut evidence that less myocardium is at jeopardy during painless episodes compared to symptomatic episodes. Whether these painless ischemic changes can account for some of the left ventricular dysfunction observed in "stunned" or "hibernating" myocardium is an intriguing concept. If so, "chronic" ischemia may be a real entity after all.

REFERENCES

1. Chierchia S, Lazzari M, Freedman B, Brunelli C, Maseri A. Impairment of myocardial perfusion and function during painless myocardial ischemia. J Am Coll Cardiol 1983; 1:924.
2. Cohn PF, Brown EJ, Wynne J, Holman BL, Atkins HL. Global and regional left ventricular ejection fraction abnormalities during exercise in patients with silent myocardial ischemia. J Am Coll Cardiol 1983; 1:931.
3. Iskandrian AS, Hakki A-H. Left ventricular function in patients with coronary heart disease in the presence or absence of angina pectoris during exercise radionuclide ventriculography. Am J Cardiol 1984; 53:1239.
4. Ratib O, Righetti A, Rutishauser W. Isotope ventriculography during asymptomatic ischemia. In: Rutishauser W, Roskamm H, eds. Silent Myocardial Ischemia. Berlin: Springer-Verlag, 1984. 84–89.
5. Faβbender D, Vogt J, Mannebach H, Gleichmann U. Regional wall motion disorders during exercise with and without angina. In: von Arnim T, Maseri A. eds. Silent Ischemia: Current Concepts and Management. Darmstadt: Steinkopff, 1987:88.
6. Hirzel HO, Leutwyler R, Krayenbuehl HP. Silent myocardial ischemia: Hemodynamic changes during dynamic exercise in patients with proven coronary artery disease despite absence of angina pectoris. J Am Coll Cardiol 1985; 6:275.
7. Vassiliadis IV, Machac J, O'Hara M, Sezhiyan T, Horowitz SF. Exercise-induced myocardial dysfunction in patients with coronary artery disease with and without angina. Am Heart J 1991; 121:1403.
8. Rozanski A, Biarey CN, Krantz DS, Friedman J, Resser KJ, Morell M, Hilton-Chalfen S, Hestrin L, Bietendorf J, Berman DS, Mental stress and the induction of silent myocardial ischemia in patients with coronary artery disease. N Engl J Med 1988; 318:1005.
9. Klein J, Chao SY, Berman DS, Rozanski A. Is "silent" myocardial ischemia really as severe as symptomatic ischemia? The analytical effect of patient selection biases. Circulation 1994; 89:1958–1966.
10. Narins CR, Zareba W, Moss AJ, Goldstein RE, Jackson Hall W. Clinical implications of silent versus symptomatic exercise-induced myocardial ischemia in patients with stable coronary disease. J Am Cardiol 1997; 29:756–763.
11. Marcassa C, Galli M, Baroffio C, Campini R, Giannuzzi P. Ischemic burden in silent and painful myocardial ischemia: a quantitative exercise sestamibi tomographic study. J Am Cardiol 1997; 29:948–954.

12. Tamaki N, Yasuda T, Moore RH, Gill JB, Boucher CA, Hutter AH, Jr., Gold HG, Strauss HW. Continuous monitoring of left ventricular function by an ambulatory radionuclide detector in patients with coronary artery disease. J Am Coll Cardiol 1988; 12:669.

13. Kayden DS, Wackers FJ Th, Zaret BL. Silent left ventricular dysfunction during routine activity after thrombolytic therapy for acute myocardial infarction. J Am Coll Cardiol 1990; 15:1500.

14. Mohiuddin IH, Kambara H, Ohkusa T, Nohara R, Fudo T, Ono S, Tamaki N, Ohtani H, Yonekura Y, Kawai C, Konishi J. Clinical evaluation of cardiac function by ambulatory ventricular scintigraphic monitoring (VEST): Validation and study of the effects of nitroglycerin and nifedipine in patients with and without coronary artery disease. Am Heart J 1992; 123:386.

15. Davies GJ, Bencivelli W, Fragasso G, Chierchia S, Crea F, Crow J, Crean PA, Pratt T, Morgan M, Maseri A. Sequence and magnitude of ventricular volume changes in painful and painless myocardial ischemia. Circulation 1988; 78:310.

16. Wohlgelernter D, Jaffee CC, Cabin HS, Yeatman LA, Jr., Cleman M. Silent ischemia during coronary occlusion produced by balloon inflation: Relation to regional myocardial dysfunction. J Am Coll Cardiol 1987; 10:491.

17. Hauser AM, Gangadhran V, Ramos RG, Gordon S, Timmis GC. Sequence of mechanical, electrocardiographic and clinical effects of repeated coronary artery occlusion in human beings: Echocardiographic observations during coronary angioplasty. J Am Coll Cardiol 1985; 5:193.

18. Marwick TH, Nemec JJ, Torelli J, Salcedo EE, Stewart WJ. Extent and severity of abnormal left ventricular wall motion detected by exercise echocardiography during painful and silent ischemia. Am J Cardiol 1992; 69:1483.

19. Nihoyannopoulos P, Marsonis A, Joshi J, Athanassopoulos G, Oakley C. Magnitude of myocardial dysfunction is greater in painful than in painless myocardial ischemia: an exercise in echocardiographic study. J Am Cardiol 1995; 25:1507–12.

20. Hecht HS, DeBord L, Sotomayor N, Shaw R, Ryan C. Truly silent ischemia and the relationship of chest pain and ST segment changes to the amount of ischemic myocardium: evaluation by supine bicycle stress echocardiography. J Am Coll Cardiol 1994; 23:369–376.

21. Faniel WG, Engel H-J, Hundeshage H, Lichtlen PR. Regional myocardial blood flow under rapid atrial pacing in patients with ST-segment depression without angina pain. In: Rutishauser W, Roskamm H, eds. Silent Myocardial Ischemia. Berlin: Springer-Verlag, 1984:45–49.

22. Righetti A, Ratib O, El-Harake B, Rutishauser W. Thallium-201 myocadial scintigraphy and electrographic findings in asymptomatic coronary patients during exercise testing. In: Rutishauser W, Roskamm H, eds. Silent Myocardial Ischemia. Berlin: Springer-Verlag, 1984;79–83.

23. Kurata C, Sakata K, Taguchi T, Kobayashi A, Yamazaki N. Exercise-induced silent myocardial ischemia: Evaluation by thallium-201 emission computed tomography. Am Heart J 1990; 119:557.

24. Travin MI, Flores AR, Boucher CA, Newell JB, Raia PJ. Silent versus symptomatic ischemia during a thallium-201 exercise test. Am J Cardiol 1991; 68:1600.
25. Patterson RE, Eisner RL, Shonkoff D, Clininger KG, Cedarholm J, Martin SE, Churchwell AL, Battey LL, Liberman HA, Morris DC. Exercise-induced ischemia may remain "silent" because it involves a smaller mass of the left ventricle: Tomographic thallium studies in dogs and humans (abstr). J Am Coll Cardiol 1991; 17:91A.
26. Reisman S, Berman DS, Maddahi J, Swan HJC. Silent myocardial ischemia during treadmill exercise. Thallium scintigraphic and angiographic correlates (abstr). J Am Coll Cardiol 1985; 5:406.
27. Gasperetti CM, Burwell LR, Beller GA. Prevalence and variables associated with silent myocardial ischemia on exercise thallium-201 stress testing. J Am Coll Cardiol 1990; 16:115.
28. Mahmarian JJ, Pratt CM, Cocanougher MK, Verani MS. Altered myocardial perfusion in patients with angina pectoris or silent ischemia during exercise as assessed by quantitative thallium-201 single-photon emission computed tomography. Circulation 1990; 82:1305.
29. Hinrichs A, Kupper W, Hamm CLV, Bleifeld W. Detection of silent myocardial ischemia in correlation to hemodynamic and metabolic data. In: Rutishauser W, Roskamm H, eds. Silent Myocardial Ischemia. Berlin: Springer-Verlag, 1984: 50–57.
30. Hamm CW, Kupper W, Hinrichs A, Bleifeld W. Identification of patients with silent myocardial ischemia by metabolic, scintigraphic and angiographic findings. In: von Arnim T, Maseri A, eds. Silent Ischemia: Current Concepts and Management. Darmstadt: Steinkopff, 1987:72.
31. Deanfield JE, Shea M, Ribiero P, deLandsheere CM, Wilson RA, Horlock P, Selwyn AP. Transient ST segment depression as a marker of myocardial ischemia during daily life: A physiological validation in patients with angina and coronary disease. Am J Cardiol 1984; 54:1195.
32. Deanfield JE, Kensett M, Wilson RA, Shea M, Horlock P, deLandsheere CM, Selwyn AP. Silent myocardial ischemia due to mental stress. Lancet 1984; 2:1001.
33. Deanfield JE, Shea MT, Wilson R, deLandsheere CM, Jonathan A, Selwyn AP. Direct effect of smoking on the heart: Silent ischemic disturbances of coronary flow. Am J Cardiol 1986; 57:1005.
34. Braunwald E, Kloner RA. The stunned myocardium: prolonged, post-ischemic ventricular dysfunction. Circulation 1982; 66:1146.
35. Braunwald E, Rutherford JD. Reversible ischemic left ventricular dysfunction: Evidence for the hibernating myocardium. J Am Coll Cardiol 1986; 8:1467.
36. Iskandrian AS, Heo J, Helfant RH, Segal BL. Chronic myocardial ischemia and left ventricular function. Ann Intern Med 1987; 107:925.
37. Patel B, Kloner RA, Przyklenk K, Braunwald E. Postischemic myocardial "stunning": A clinically relevant phenomenon. Ann Intern Med 1988; 108:626.
38. Lewis SJ, Sawada SG, Ryan T, Segar DS, Armstrong WF, Feigenbaum H. Segmental wall motion abnormalities in the absence of clinically documented

myocardial infarction: Clinical significance and evidence of hibernating myocardium. Am Heart J 1991; 121:1088.

39. Kloner RA, Allen J, Cox TA, Zheng Y, Ruiz CE. Stunned left ventricular myocardium after exercise treadmill testing in coronary artery disease. Am J Cardiol 1991; 68:329.

40. Deutsch E, Berger M, Kussmaul WG, Hirshfeld JW, Jr., Herrmann HC, Laskey WK. Adaptation to ischemia during percutaneous transluminal coronary angioplasty: Clinical, hemodynamic and metabolic features. Circulation 1990; 82:2044.

41. Marzullo P, Parodi O, Sambeceti G, Marcassa C, Gimelli A, Bartili M, Neglia D, L'Abbate A. Does the myocardium become "stunned" after episodes of angina at rest, angina on effort, and coronary angioplasty. Am J Cardiol 1993; 71: 1045–1051.

42. Kloner RA, Yellon D. Does ischemic preconditioning occur in patients? J Am Coll Cardiol 1994; 24:1133–1142.

43. Nakagawa Y, Ito H, Kitakaza M, Kusuoka H, Hori M, Kuzuya T, Higashino Y, Fugii K, Minamino T. Effect of angina pectoris on myocardial protection in patients with reperfused anterior wall myocardial infarction: retrospective clinical evidence of "preconditioning." J Am Coll Cardiol 1995; 25:1076–1083.

44. Ottani F, Galvani M, Ferrini D, Sorbello, F, Limonetti P, Pantoli D, Rusticali F. Prodromal angina limits infarct size: a role for ischemic preconditioning. Circulation 1995; 91:291–297.

II

PREVALENCE OF ASYMPTOMATIC CORONARY ARTERY DISEASE

5
Prevalence of Silent Myocardial Ischemia

The actual number of persons with silent myocardial ischemia may never be known, but intelligent estimates are possible based on data available in the medical literature. These data suggest that the presence of pain in persons with coronary artery disease is just the "tip of the iceberg" (i.e., many individuals are free of pain during most ischemic episodes). Some never have pain.

I. SILENT MYOCARDIAL ISCHEMIA IN PERSONS WITH TOTALLY ASYMPTOMATIC CORONARY ARTERY DISEASE

This is the most difficult area to obtain "hard data" in. How are persons who are free of symptoms to be convinced of the need to undergo coronary arteriography in order to confirm the diagnosis of asymptomatic coronary artery disease? It is true that fortuitous—and anecdotal—"case finding" in this syndrome occurs commonly enough to draw attention to the problem, but systematic surveys are rare. This is because of concerns raised about subjecting asymptomatic individuals to an invasive procedure with a small, but definite, morbidity and mortality.

Another approach to estimating the prevalence of asymptomatic disease is through pathological surveys of atherosclerotic heart disease in adult populations who were apparently free of clinical coronary artery disease at time of death, and died of trauma or noncardiac causes. Diamond and Forrester conducted a comprehensive review in 1979 [1]. They summarized their data in Table 1, which breaks down the autopsy studies by age and sex. In the nearly 24,000 persons studied, the mean prevalence of coronary artery disease was 4.5%. The

Table 1 Prevalence of Coronary Artery Stenosis at Autopsy

	Men		Women	
Age (yr)	Proportion affected	Pooled mean ± SEP[a] (%)	Proportion affected	Pooled mean ± SEP[a] (%)
30–39	57/2954	1.9 ± 0.3	5/1545	0.3 ± 0.1
40–49	234/4407	5.5 ± 0.3	18/1778	1.0 ± 0.2
50–59	488/5011	9.7 ± 0.4	62/1934	3.2 ± 0.4
60–69	569/4641	12.3 ± 0.5	130/1726	7.5 ± 0.6
Totals	1348/17013		215/6983	
Population-weighted mean[b]		6.4 ± 0.2		2.6 ± 0.2

[a]Standard error of the percent.
[b]Population weighting was performed by use of the 1970 U.S. Census figures.
Source: Diamond GA, Forrester JS. N Engl J Med 1979; 300:1350.

population-weighted mean (obtained by use of the 1970 U.S. Census figures) was $6.4 \pm 0.2\%$ for men aged 30 to 69 and $2.6 \pm 0.2\%$ for women aged 30 to 69. This percentage increased with increasing age. Since these figures are obtained from autopsy data, they may overestimate the true incidence of this syndrome for two reasons. First, unless the autopsy procedure employs techniques for injecting the coronary arteries, the "collapsed" lumen examined by the pathologist may exaggerate the luminal narrowing caused by a given lesion during life. Second, even when the degree of narrowing is as it was during life, there is no certainty that lesions in the 50 to 60% category were hemodynamically significant when the person was alive. In other words, not all asymptomatic coronary artery disease present at autopsy is necessarily ischemia-producing coronary artery disease. Just as those lesions were not hemodynamically significant, others may represent "end-stage" or "burned-out" stages of the disease process: arteries became occluded, infarctions occurred, scar tissue formed, but there is no longer evidence of active ischemia.

Another approach to estimating the prevalence of coronary artery disease in asymptomatic persons is by reviewing coronary angiographic data. In their report, Diamond and Forrester [1] also performed that type of analysis. Their data suggested that the prevalence of coronary artery disease in asymptomatic adults was about 4%. These patients had undergone cardiac catheterization for reasons other than chest pain (evaluation of valvular heart disease, abnormal ECGs, etc.). Since these catheterization laboratory figures reflect a skewed population in that they were selected to undergo the procedure, one might argue that the 4% figure is too low. Perhaps an "average" of the autopsy and angiographic figures (about 5%) would be more useful. However, in neither the autopsy review nor the angiographic review are data supplied about the prevalence of active ischemia in these asymptomatic subjects.

Screening large numbers of asymptomatic persons with exercise tests and *then* subjecting positive responders to coronary angiography is a useful technique for estimating the number of individuals with *both* asymptomatic disease and active ischemia. Several such studies have been reported. In one small study, investigators at Yale University [2] exercised 129 workers in a nearby industrial plant. Sixteen subjects had an abnormal exercise test and 13 of these also had coronary artery calcification on fluoroscopy. The 13 men underwent coronary arteriography; 12 had at least 50% stenosis in one coronary artery. Thus, 12 of the anginal 129 subjects, or about 9%, had both symptomatic coronary artery disease and silent myocardial ischemia. U.S. Air Force studies in 1390 men revealed 111 with positive exercise tests in a single lead, of which 34 (or about 2.5%) had lesions of at least 50% stenosis [3]. The mean age of these patients was 43 years; all were males. In Norway, Erikssen and

Thaulow [4] studied 2014 male office workers who were aged 40 to 59 years (mean age 50). Sixty-nine had at least 50% stenosis in one coronary artery and 50 of these (or 2.8% of the total) were completely asymptomatic. This percentage is very similar to that in the U.S. Air Force study.

These figures must be considered as conservative estimates, since it is possible that some asymptomatic individuals did not manifest silent ischemia on the one screening exercise test and, therefore, were not selected for coronary angiographic studies. Furthermore, exercise tests in general have a certain percentage of false-negative tests, whereas coronary angiography tends to underestimate the severity of lesions. Thus, the figure of 5% cited earlier for the prevalence of asymptomatic anatomical disease probably exaggerates only slightly the true prevalence of hemodynamically significant asymptomatic disease (i.e., disease capable of producing ischemia during physiological stress). If one assumes that 4% of asymptomatic middle-aged males in the United States have silent myocardial ischemia, then we are considering a total of nearly 2 million men, not an insignificant sum. One of the most ambitious of the recent epidemiological studies was organized in Italy by Fazzini and associates, The Epidemiology and Clinics of Silent Heart Disease (ECCIS) project [5]. They studied 4842 presumably healthy men, most of whom were engaged in clerical work in Florence and Rome. Nearly 8000 men were screened in the initial phase with cardiovascular history, physical examination, lipid profile, noninvasive tests, and Holter monitoring. The 4842 men noted above were then selected for the second stage based on abnormalities in the first stage that suggested silent ischemic heart disease. The purpose of the second phase was to elicit even more strongly suggestive responses on electrocardiographic and nuclear stress tests. The third phase featured coronary angiography. The final "positive criteria" not only included evidence of stress-induced ischemia in conjunction with >50% luminal obstruction but also markers that might indicate prior unrecognized myocardial infarction. After adjustments for participant rates (i.e., dropouts, etc.) in the various stages a final estimate of less than 1% was reached (Table 2). This figure is smaller than that reported by the USAF School of Aerospace Medicine and Oslo Ischemia studies. The authors attributed this to the need for at least two perfusional and mechanical markers plus a positive coronary angiogram, as well as selection biases in the other two populations. Further studies from this group reported similar coronary angiographic anatomy when compared to that of a cohort of "matched" men with angina [6]. Another large-scale study that reported a lower prevalence than previously reported involved 5000 clinically asymptomatic English men aged 30 to 65 [4]. One hundred and seventy-two men (3.2%) had abnormal ST segment responses during or immediately after exercise tests. Seventy-seven (1.3%) had subsequent angiographically demonstrable disease, of whom 33 underwent

Table 2 Summary of Participation Rates at Subsequent Stages of the Study

	Number of Patients	%
A. Enrolled at entry	7781	
B. Participants to the study	5163	66.3% of A
C. Excluded for heart disease (known or unknown), handicaps, serious illnesses, chest pain	321	6.2% of B
D. Examined at first stage and eligible for diagnosis of silent ischemic heart disease	4842	93.8% of B
E. First-degree suspect of silent ischemic heart disease	439	9.1% of D; 8.5% of B
F. Healthy at first stage	4403	90.9% of D
G. Examined at second stage	387	88.1% of E
H. Second-degree suspect of silent ischemic heart disease	104	26.9% of G; 2.1% of D
I. No more suspect of silent ischemic heart disease	283	73.1% of G
J. Examined at third stage	62	59.6% of H
K. Final diagnosis of silent ischemic heart disease	25	40.3% of J; 0.52% of D
L. No more suspect of silent ischemic heart disease at third stage	37	59.7% of J

Source: Reproduced from Fazzini P F, Prati P L, Rovelli F, Antoniucci D, Menghini F, Seccareccia F, Menotti A. Am J Cardiol 1993; 72: 1383–1388.

coronary revascularization procedures. Figure 1 depicts the decision tree with the results of the initial screening, exercise ECGs, and further investigation leading to management choices. These investigators pointed out—as others have also done—that prevalence is higher when multiple coronary risk factors are present. This was also emphasized in the most recent U.S. study, performed in Cleveland between 1990 and 1993 and reported in 1995 [8]. Initial screening was with exercise tests in 4334 asymptomatic adults of whom 741 were men. Based on abnormal test results, a second test (thallium testing or coronary angiogram) was performed. Significant coronary artery disease was found in 71 patients or 1.6% of the original cohort with 50 requiring revascularization. The authors noted that when pretest probability is low (based on absence of risk factors), the cost is high and the diagnostic yield minimal. By contrast, when used in asymptomatic siblings of patients with premature coronary artery disease, thallium testing produces significantly higher numbers of abnormal

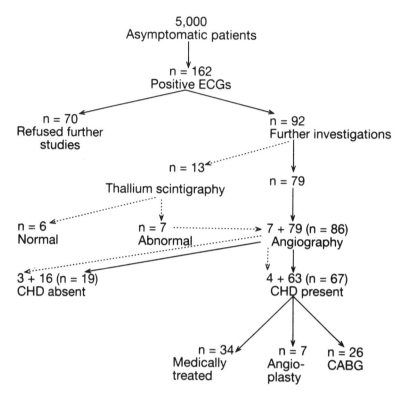

Figure 1 Noninvasive test results, coronary angiography, and thallium scintigraphy findings for subjects with positive exercise tests (*n* = 162). CHD = coronary heart disease; CABG = coronary artery bypass grafting. (From Davies B, Ashton WD, Rowlands DJ, El-Sayed M, Wallace PC, Duckett K, Coley J, Daggett AM. Clin Cardiol 1996; 19:303–308.)

responders with 29% of men and 9% of women having highly suggestive results. Coronary angiography was not used in this study.

In addition to the studies in which coronary artery disease is documented at autopsy or by coronary angiography, there are other studies in which the presence of asymptomatic disease is suggested by abnormal responses to exercise testing, etc. Although these are discussed in more detail in Part III of this book (Detection of Asymptomatic Coronary Artery Disease), it is important to cite several Johns Hopkins studies in particular because they combine exercise-induced ECG abnormalities with exercise-induced thallium defects [9–11].

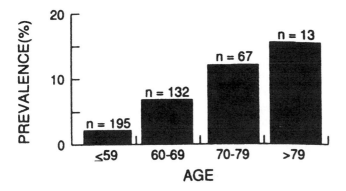

Figure 2 Prevalence of concordant positive exercise ECG and thallium-201 results by age decade. (From Fleg JL, Gerstenblith G, Zonderman AB, Becker LC, Weisfeldt ML, Costa PT, Jr., Lakatta EG. Circulation 1990; 81:428. Reproduced with permission of American Heart Association.)

Fleg et al. [9] reported a progressive increase in the prevalence of silent ischemia in apparently healthy individuals from one age decade to the next (Fig. 2). In a later report from the same institution, Blumenthal et al. [10] reported an increased prevalence of silent ischemia in an especially high-risk asymptomatic population (siblings of coronary artery disease patients). Katzel et al. [11] found that well-established risk factors for coronary artery disease also increased the chances of finding exercise-induced silent ischemia. In addition to exercise testing, other investigational procedures have been used to detect asymptomatic coronary artery disease. Ultrasound measured increased carotid artery intimal-medial thickness is one such parameter. The Johns Hopkins group has correlated this finding with abnormal exercise ECG and thallium scans [12]. Ultrafast (also called electron-beam) computed tomography is another new technique. The total calcium "score" can be correlated with the degree of coronary artery narrowing at autopsy or angiography. How well this promising technique can be used to predict severe stenoses in asymptomatic but high-risk populations remains to be seen [13,14].

II. SILENT MYOCARDIAL ISCHEMIA IN INDIVIDUALS ASYMPTOMATIC AFTER A MYOCARDIAL INFARCTION

It has been estimated that at least 500,000 hospitalized patients survive myocardial infarctions annually in the United States. Of these, 30 to 40% have their courses complicated by persistent angina, heart failure, or serious arrhythmias. The rest are asymptomatic at time of discharge. Of these 300,000 or so individuals, about one-third (100,000) have evidence of ischemia on various postinfarction tests. For example, the proportion that are pain-free on exercise tests differs from study to study, ranging from one-third to two-thirds [15–18]. Thus, based on exercise test data, about 50,000 asymptomatic postinfarction patients per year have silent myocardial ischemia in the initial 30-day postinfarction period. In patients who are unable to exercise, Holter monitoring has been used with increasing popularity to document the occurrence of silent ischemia. Again, the reported frequency of silent ischemia varies from 30% [19] to 42% [20], with one group finding the incidence increased the later the patients were monitored after the infarction [21]. Stress echocardiography (with dipyridamole as the pharmacological "stress") was used by Bolognese et al. [22] to induce wall-motion abnormalities in postinfarction patients. They were able to induce such abnormalities in 189 of 217 patients; in 94 of the 189 (43%), the abnormalities were unaccompanied by angina. Destruction of sympathetic nerves after infarction may play a role in all of these reports [23].

III. SILENT MYOCARDIAL ISCHEMIA IN PATIENTS WITH ANGINA

The number of patients with angina who also have symptomatic episodes of myocardial ischemia is large, but the exact percentage is unknown. About 5 to 6 million patients per year in the United States are seen by physicians because of anginal complaints. When I initially reviewed the literature on positive exercise tests, lactate determinations, abnormal ventriculograms, etc., in those studies that reported symptoms, I found that about one-third of asymptomatic patients (Table 3) had at least one documented episode of silent myocardial ischemia [24]. The widespread use of Holter monitoring in the angina population has provided additional data [25–33], though not all patients have coronary artery disease documented by coronary arteriography or prior myocardial infarction. In general, about half of the patients with angina (stable or unstable) have silent ischemia on Holter monitoring, with some series reporting much higher frequencies in their study population. In apparently adequately treated patients, the figure drops to about one-third. A good example is the study by Yeung et al. [30]. Off medication, 62 of 105 patients (59%) had ST segment depression on Holter monitoring, compared with 22 of 54 patients (38%) on medications. If 12-lead ST monitoring is used in patients hospitalized for unstable angina, more episodes of silent ischemia are detected than when standard 3-lead systems are explored. Thus, Klootwijk et al. [34] reported 77% of their 130 patients had such episodes compared to 62% detected by three leads.

Table 3 Myocardial Ischemia Without Anginal Symptoms

| | Patients with CAD manifesting abnormality | | |
| | | Group with angina[a] | |
Abnormality suggestive of myocardial ischemia	Total group (n)	no.	%
Abnormal left ventricular wall motion	87	33	39%
Pacing contrast ventriculogram[1]	8	3	38%
Pacing contrast ventriculogram[2]	8	6	75%
Exercise radionuclide ventriculogram[5]	63	18	29%
Exercise radionuclide ventriculogram[6]	8	6	75%
Abnormal lactate metabolism	36	9	25%
Pacing study[7]	14	1	7%
Pacing study[8]	22	8	36%
Abnormal myocardial perfusion scintigrams	64	26	40%
Thallium-201 study[9]	35	20	57%
Rubidium-81 study[10]	29	6	19%
Electrocardiographic stress test	568	186	32%
Treadmill test[11]	135	23	17%
Treadmill test[12]	122	32	26%
Bicycle and two-step test[13]	59	15	26%
Treadmill test[14]	146	68	45%
Treadmill test[15]	102	48	47%
Total	755	254	34%

[a] Although not symptomatic during this test, almost all patients in these studies had a history of angina or prior myocardial infarction (see text).

CAD = coronary artery disease.

Source: Cohn P F. Am J Cardiol 1980; 45:697. (Numbers in superscript refer to studies cited in this article.)

Finally, the silent episodes outnumber the painful ones at least three or four to one in both stable and unstable angina. This is discussed in Chapter 8.

IV. SUDDEN DEATH AND MYOCARDIAL INFARCTION IN PATIENTS WITHOUT PRIOR HISTORIES OF ANGINA

Although this in an "indirect" way of estimating the population with asymptomatic coronary artery disease, it provides important data. Presumably, individuals who die suddenly or experience a myocardial infarction as their initial

manifestation of coronary artery disease and who have extensive coronary atherosclerosis at autopsy or coronary angiography did not develop those lesions
overnight. Much of the disease must have been present, silent and undetected,
for weeks, months, or even years prior to the actual event. This is the natural
history—amply documented—of coronary atherosclerosis. That the precipitat-
ing event, such as rupture of a plaque into a vessel lumen, could have been sudden is not in dispute, but the atherosclerotic substrate took months and years to
develop. With that in mind, it is important to note that in most series one-quarter to one-half of the individuals who die suddenly each year with coronary
artery disease found at autopsy had no prior cardiac history [35–37], though
some series report a smaller percentage [38]. It is estimated that between
250,000 and 350,000 deaths per year are sudden; therefore, the number of persons without overt coronary artery disease is large by any standard. As Kuller
[36] has written, "The large pool of individuals currently over the age of 30 or
40 with silent, but significant, coronary atherosclerosis and stenosis will contribute to a high incidence of sudden death, at least for the next 20 or 30 years."
Savage et al. [39] provide a graphic example of death in one such individual
recorded on an ambulatory monitor that was performed fortuitously as part of
a Framingham study protocol (Fig. 3). Rarely, sudden death occurs from free
wall rupture [40].

Nearly half the patients presenting with their first myocardial infarctions
have not had angina beforehand [41–42]. Midwall and colleagues [42] noted
that, in general, these patients were more likely to be younger female, and have
a greater prevalence of one-vessel disease (Table 4). Pierard et al. [43] reported
a 39% prevalence in a series of 732 consecutive patients. Patients without preceding angina were younger, more likely to be men, and had a higher frequency
of inferior infarction and a lower frequency of postinfarction angina (Table 5).
Matsuda et al. [44] reported a lower ejection fraction in patients without
antecedent angina, even when coronary anatomy was similar. The same investigators also showed an almost equal likelihood of the infarction occurring at
rest as with exertion [45]. Behar et al. [46] found a higher prevalence of chronic
angina in women, hypertensives, and diabetics. Barbash et al. [47] also found
a higher incidence in hypertensives and diabetics. In a report from our hospital
[48], we studied 43 consecutive patients presenting with their initial myocardial infarction; 23 had no history of angina prior to the infarction, whereas 20
did. The two groups did not differ in age, smoking history, diabetes, hypertension, or cholesterol levels. The prevalence of Q and non-Q-wave infarcts was
similar, but there was a trend toward more inferior infarctions in the asymptomatic group (65% vs. 47%) and more single-vessel disease (40% vs. 11%).
Multivessel coronary artery disease is frequent enough, however, in patients

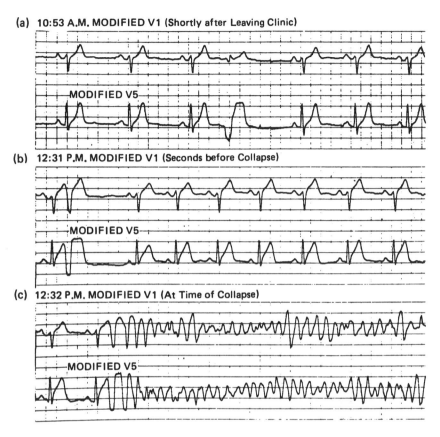

(a) 10:53 A.M. MODIFIED V1 (Shortly after Leaving Clinic)

MODIFIED V5

(b) 12:31 P.M. MODIFIED V1 (Seconds before Collapse)

MODIFIED V5

(c) 12:32 P.M. MODIFIED V1 (At Time of Collapse)

MODIFIED V5

Figure 3 (a) The subject's first ventricular premature depolarization, which was detected approximately a half hour after he left the clinic. No significant changes in the ST segment were noted at the time of this late-cycle premature depolarization. (b) The second form of ventricular premature depolarization, which was uniformly early-cycle and associated with increased ST segment elevation and convex ST segment morphology. (c) The electrocardiogram at the instant of the subject's collapse. The same early-cycle ventricular premature form detected earlier initiated a four-beat run of ventricular tachycardia, which rapidly degenerated to ventricular flutter-fibrillation. (From Savage DD, Castelli WP, Anderson SJ, Kannel WB. Am J Med 1983; 74:148.)

Table 4   Catheterization Data in Myocardial Infarction Patients

Parameter	Group 1: No prior AP	Group 2: AP prior to MI	Sig
Mean EDP (mmHg)	15.8 ± 6.9	14.5 ± 6.5	NS
Mean LVEF (%)	58.7 ± 14.7	58.5 ± 14.8	NS
Collaterals	46%	71%	$p < 0.05$
One-vessel disease	38/63 (60%)	3/34 (9%)	$p < 0.005$
Two-vessel disease	18/63 (29%)	18/34 (53%)	$p < 0.05$
Three-vessel disease	7/63 (11%)	13/34 (38%)	$p < 0.005$

Abbreviations: AP, angina pectoris; Sig, significance; MI, myocardial infarction; EDP, end-diastolic pressure; LVEF, left ventricular ejection fraction; NS, not significant.
Source: Midwall J, Ambrose J, Pichard A, Abedin Z, Herman MV. Chest 1982; 81:6.

without prior angina to suggest that an infarction without prior angina does not necessarily indicate less advanced coronary artery disease and, therefore, should not be considered a unique subset of coronary artery disease.

Whether it is the coronary arteries with the most advanced lesion that subsequently results in complete occlusion is unclear; increasing data suggest less severe and "softer" lesions progress more rapidly via hemorrhagic rupture, etc. [49,50].

V.   PREVALENCE OF SILENT MYOCARDIAL ISCHEMIA IN DIABETICS

These data are presented in the following chapter on silent myocardial infarctions.

VI.   CONCLUSIONS

Silent myocardial ischemia is a ubiquitous phenomenon, present in 1.5 to 15% of the asymptomatic population depending on risk-factor profiles, about one-third of uncomplicated asymptomatic postinfarction patients, and in many patients with angina. The scope of the problem is further indicated—albeit indirectly—by the large number of individuals dying suddenly or experiencing an infarction without a prior anginal history.

Table 5 Comparison Between Patients with and Without Angina Pectoris Before Infarction

	Patients with angina before infarction	Patients without angina before infarction	p value
Patients (n)	447	285	
Time interval between onset of pain and admission (h)	13 ± 24	10 ± 16	<0.05
Mean age (yr)	59 ± 9	57 ± 11	<0.05
Sex (%) women)	22	12	<0.001
Prior history of diabetes mellitus (%)	11	8	NS
Tobacco abuse (%)	80	86	<0.05
Medications before infarction			
Beta-blockers (%)	15	3	<0.001
Diuretics (%)	12	7	<0.05
Digitalis (%)	5	4	NS
Antiarrhythmics (%)	3	1	<0.05
Site of infarction			
Non-Q-wave (%)	11	11	NS
Anterior (%)	43	33	<0.01
Inferior (%)	44	55	<0.01
Unknown (%)	2	1	NS
Peak creatinine kinase (IU/L)	1454 ± 1142	1569 ± 1099	NS
Worst LV function score during hospital stay	1.0 ± 1.2	1.0 ± 1.1	NS
Early postinfarction angina (%)	21	10	<0.001
In-hospital recurrent infarction (%)	2	1	NS
Pericardial friction rub (%)	26	25	NS
Bradycardia (%)	17	17	NS
Atrial fibrillation (%)	16	11	NS
Frequent PVCs (%)	42	44	NS
Ventricular tachycardia (%)	6	5	NS
Ventricular fibrillation (%)	9	9	NS
Atrioventricular block (%)	11	15	NS
Bundle branch block (%)	9	10	NS
In-hospital mortality (%)	10	8	NS
3-year post-hospital mortality (%)	16	7	<0.001

LV = left ventricular; NS = difference not significant; PVCs = premature ventricular complexes.
Source: Pierard LA, Dubois C, Smeets J-P, Boland J, Carlier J, Kulbertus HE. Am J Cardiol 1988; 61:984.

REFERENCES

1. Diamond GA, Forrester JS. Analysis of probability as an aid in the clinical diagnosis of coronary artery disease. N Engl J Med 1979; 300:1350.
2. Langou RA, Huang EK, Kelley MJ, Cohen LS. Predictive accuracy of coronary artery calcification and abnormal exercise test for coronary artery disease in asymptomatic men. Circulation 1980; 62:1196.
3. Froelicher VF, Thompson AJ, Longo MR, Jr., Triebwasser JH, Lancaster MC. Value of exercise testing for screening symptomatic men for latent coronary artery disease. Prog Cardiovasc Dis 1976; 16:265.
4. Erikssen J, Thaulow E. Follow-up of patients with asymptomatic myocardial ischemia. In: Rutishauser W, Roskamm H, eds. Silent Myocardial Ischemia. Berlin: Springer-Verlag, 1984:156–164.
5. Fazzini PF, Prati PL, Rovelli F, Antoniucci D, Menghini F, Seccareccia F, Menotti A. Epidemiology of silent myocardial ischemia in symptomatic middle-aged men (the ECCIS Project). Am J Cardiol 1993; 72:1383–1388.
6. Antoniucci D, Seccareccia F, Fazzini PF, Prati PL, Rovelli F, Menotti A. Coronary angiographic findings in asymptomatic men with suspected silent myocardial ischemia (the ECCIS Project). Am J Cardiol 1994; 73:960–962.
7. Davies B, Ashton WD, Rowlands DJ, El-Sayed M, Wallace PC, Duckett K, Coley J, Daggett AM. Association of conventional and exertional coronary heart disease risk factors in 5000 apparently healthy men. Clin Cardiol 1996; 19:303–308.
8. Pilote L, Pashkow F, Thomas JD, Snader CE, Harvey SA, Marwick TH, Lauer MS. Clinical yield and cost of exercise treadmill testing to screen for coronary artery disease in asymptomatic adults. Am J Cardiol 1998; 81:219–224.
9. Fleg JL, Gerstenblith G, Zonderman AB, Becker LC, Weisfeldt ML, Costa PT, Jr., Lakatta EG. Prevalence and prognostic significance of exercise-induced silent myocardial ischemia detected by thallium scintigraphy and electrocardiography in asymptomatic volunteers. Circulation 1990; 81:428.
10. Blumenthal RS, Becker DM, Moy TF, Coresh J, Wilder LB, Becker LC. Exercise thallium tomography predicts future clinically manifest coronary heart disease in a high-risk asymptomatic population. Circulation 1996; 93:915–923.
11. Katzel LI, Sorkin JD, Colman E, Goldbert AP, Busby-Whitehead MJ, Lakatta LE, Becker LC, Lakatta EG, Fleg JL. Risk factors for exercise-induced silent myocardial ischemia in healthy volunteers. Am J Cardiol 1994; 74:869–874.
12. Nagai Y, Metter J, Earley CJ, Kemper MK, Becker LC, Lakatta EG, Fleg JL. Increased carotid artery intimal-medial thickness in asymptomatic older subjects with exercise-induced myocardial ischemia. Circulation 1998; 98:1504–1509.
13. Rumberger JA, Behrenbeck T, Breen JF, Sheedy PF II. Coronary calcification by electron beam computed tomography and obstructive coronary artery disease: A model for costs and effectiveness of diagnosis as compared with conventional cardiac testing methods. J Am Coll Cardiol 1999; 33:453–462.

14. Gidding SS, Bookstein LC, Chomka EV. Usefulness of electron beam tomography in adolescents and young adults with heterozygous familial hypercholesterolemia. Circulation 1998; 98:2580–2583.

15. Theroux P, Waters DD, Halphen C, Debaisieux J-C, Mizgala HF. Prognostic value of exercise testing soon after myocardial infarction. N Engl J Med 1979; 301:341.

16. Miller DH, Borer JD. Exercise testing early after myocardial infarction: Risks and benefits. Am J Med 1982; 72:427.

17. Weiner DA, Ryan RJ, McCabe CH, Luk S, Chaitman BR, Sheffield LT, Tristani F, Fisher LD. Significance of silent myocardial ischemia during exercise testing in patients with coronary artery disease. Am J Cardiol 1987; 59:725.

18. Falcone C, DeServi S, Poma E, Campana C, Scire A, Montemartini C, Specchia G. Clinical significance of exercise-induced silent myocardial ischemia in patients with coronary artery disease. J Am Coll Cardiol 1987; 9:295.

19. Gottlieb SO, Gottlieb SH, Achuff SC, Baumgardner R, Mellits ED, Weisfeldt ML, Gerstenblith G. Silent ischemia on Holter monitoring predicts mortality in high-risk postinfection patients. JAMA 1988; 259:1030.

20. Petretta M, Bonaduce D, Bianchi V, Vitagliano G, Conforti G, Rotandi F, Themistocklakis S, Morgano G. Characterization and prognostic significance of silent myocardial ischemia on predischarge electrocardiographic monitoring in unselected patients with myocardial infarction. Am J Cardiol 1992; 69:579.

21. Currie P, Saltissi S. Transient myocardial ischaemia after acute myocardial infarction. Br Heart J 1990; 64:299.

22. Bolognese L, Rossi L, Sarasso G, Prando MD, Sante Bongo A, Dellavesa P, Rossi P. Silent versus symptomatic dipyridamole-induced ischemia after myocardial infarction: Clinical and prognostic significance. J Am Coll Cardiol 1992; 19:953.

23. Hartikainen J, Kuikka J, Mantysaari Matti, Lansimies E, Pyorala K. Sympathetic reinnervation after acute myocardial infarction. Am J Cardiol 1996; 77:5–9.

24. Cohn PF. Silent myocardial ischemia in patients with a defective anginal warning system. Am J Cardiol 1980; 45:697.

25. Cecchi AC, Dovellini EV, Marchi F, Pucci P, Santoro GM, Fazzini PF. Silent myocardial ischemia during ambulatory electrocardiographic monitoring in patients with effort angina. J Am Coll Cardiol 1983; 1:934.

26. Mulcahy D, Keegan J, Crean P, et al. Silent myocardial ischemia in chronic stable angina: A study of its frequency and characteristics in 150 patients. Br Heart J 1988; 60:41.

27. Gottlieb SO, Weisfeldt ML, Ouyang P, Mellits ED, Gerstenblith G. Silent ischemia predicts infarction and death during 2 year follow-up of unstable angina. J Am Coll Cardiol 1987; 19:756.

28. Nademanee K, Intarachot V, Josephson MA, Rieders D, Mody FV, Singh BN. Prognostic significance of silent myocardial ischemia in patients with unstable angina. J Am Coll Cardiol 1987; 10:1.

29. Deedwania PC. Carbajal EV. Prevalence and patterns of silent myocardial

ischemia during daily life in stable angina patients receiving conventional antianginal drug therapy. Am J Cardiol 1990; 65:1090.

30. Yeung AC, Barry J, Orav J, Bonassin E, Raby KE, Selwyn AP. Effects of asymptomatic ischemia on long-term prognosis in chronic stable coronary disease. Circulation 1991; 83:1598.

31. Mulahy D, Parameshwar J, Holdright D, Wright C, Sparrow J, Sutton G, Fox KM. Value of ambulatory ST segment monitoring in patients with chronic stable angina: Does measurement of the "total ischaemic burden" assist with management? Br Heart J 1992; 67:47.

32. Panaza JA, Quyyumi AA, Diodati JG, Callahan TS, Bonow RO, Epstein SE. Long-term variation in myocardial ischemia during daily life in patients with stable coronary artery disease: Its relation to changes in the ischemic threshold. J Am Coll Cardiol 1992; 19:500.

33. Romeo F, Rosano GMC, Martuscelli E, Valente A, Reale A. Unstable angina: Role of silent ischemia and total ischemic time (silent plus painful ischemia); a 6-year follow-up. J Am Coll Cardiol 1992; 19:1173.

34. Klootwijk P, Meij S, Est Gav, Muller J, Umanss VAWM, Lenderick T, Simoons ML. Comparison of usefulness of computer assisted continuous 48-h 3-lead with 12-lead ECG ischaemia monitoring for detection and quantitation of ischaemia in patients with unstable angina. Eur Heart J 1997; 18:931–940.

35. Lown B. Sudden cardiac death: The major challenge confronting contemporary cardiology. Am J Cardiol 1979; 43:313.

36. Kuller LH. Sudden death: Definition and epidemiologic considerations. Prog Cardiovasc Dis 1980; 23:1.

37. Kannel WB, Cupples LA, D'Agostino RB. Sudden death risk in overt coronary heart disease: The Framingham Study. Am Heart J 1987; 113:799.

38. Goldstein S, Medendorp SV, Landis JR, Wolfe RA, Leighton R, Ritter G, Vasu CM, Acheson A. Analysis of cardiac symptoms preceding cardiac arrest. Am J Cardiol 1986; 58:1195.

39. Savage DD, Castelli WP, Anderson SJ, Kannel WB. Sudden unexpected death during ambulatory electrocardiographic monitoring: The Framingham study. Am J Med 1983; 74:148.

40. Shirani J, Berezowski K, Roberts WC. Out-of-hospital sudden death from left ventricular free wall rupture during acute myocardial infarction as the first and only manifestation of atherosclerotic coronary artery disease. Am J Cardiol 1994; 73:88–92.

41. Harper RW, Kennedy G, DeSanctis RW, Hutter AM. The incidence and pattern of angina prior to acute myocardial infarction: A study of 577 cases. Am Heart J 1979; 97:178.

42. Midwall J, Ambrose J, Pichard A, Abedin Z, Herman MV. Angina pectoris before and after infarction: Angiographic correlations. Chest 1982; 81:6.

43. Pierard LA, Dubois C, Smeets J-P, Boland J, Carlier J, Kulbertus HE. Prognostic significance of angina pectoris before first acute myocardial infarction. Am J Cardiol 1988; 61:984.

44. Matsuda Y, Ogawa H, Moritani K, Matsuda M, Naito H, Matsuzaki M, Ikee Y, Kusukawa R. Effects of the presence or absence of preceding angina pectoris on left ventricular function after acute myocardial infarction. Am Heart J 1984; 108:955.

45. Matsuda M, Matsuda Y, Ogawa H, Moritani K, Kusukawa R. Angina pectoris before and during acute myocardial infarction: Relation to degree of physical activity. Am J Cardiol 1985; 55:1255.

46. Behar S, Reicher-Reiss H, Abinader E, Agmon J, Friedman Y, Barzilai J, Kaplinsky E, Kauli N, Kishon Y, Palant A, Peled B, Rabinovich B, Reisin L, Zahavi I, Zion M, Goldbourt U. The prognostic significance of angina pectoris preceding the occurrence of a first acute myocardial infarction in 4166 consecutive hospitalized patients. Am Heart J 1992; 123:1481.

47. Barbash GI, White HD, Bodan M, Van de Werf F. Antecedent angina pectoris predicts worse outcome after myocardial infarction in patients receiving thrombolytic therapy: Experience gleaned from the International Tissue Plasminogen Activator/Streptokinase Mortality Trial. J Am Coll Cardiol 1992; 20:36.

48. Samuel SA, Cohn PF. Myocardial infarction without a prior history of angina pectoris: A unique subset of coronary artery disease? (abstr). Clin Res 1985; 33:224A.

49. Little WC, Downes TR, Applegate RJ. The underlying coronary lesion in myocardial infarction: Implications for coronary angiography. Clin Cardiol 1991; 14:868.

50. Kullo IJ, Edwards WD, Schwartz RS. Vulnerable plaque: Pathobiology and clinical implications. Ann Intern Med 1998; 129:1050–1060.

6

Prevalence and Distinguishing Features of Silent Myocardial Infarctions

If one accepts the premise that myocardial ischemia can occur without symptoms, then it should not be surprising to learn that myocardial infarction can do the same. In fact, the literature on the latter predates the former, extending back almost 90 years! Herrick was aware of it in his landmark paper published in 1912 [1] and anecdotal reports throughout the 1930s and 1940s maintained interest in this seeming paradox [2–5]. In 1954, Roseman reviewed the literature and analyzed 220 cases of this syndrome [6]. He concluded that its prevalence ranged from 20 to 60% of all infarctions depending on the particular population surveyed either with electrocardiograms or by autopsy.

I. ELECTROCARDIOGRAPHIC STUDIES

One of the problems in assessing the frequency of silent infarctions is in their definition. Unlike transient episodes of silent myocardial ischemia that can be documented during exercise tests, radionuclide procedures, Holter monitoring, etc., unrecognized infarctions are not witnessed at the time they occur—except for the few that are detected via use of 24-h ambulatory electrocardiographic monitoring. Reliance on patients' memory of possible cardiac symptoms does not provide the best type of data, nor are physicians' office notes sufficient. In the final analysis, we are usually left with electrocardiographic evidence of a myocardial infarction that occurred at some point between two standard ECG examinations. Nevertheless, several groups have attempted to assess the frequency of this phenomenon using ECG tracings. Probably the best example of these surveys is the Framingham study, a long-term prospective study of cardiovascular disease which began in 1948 in Framingham, Massachusetts, under the auspices of the National Institutes of Health. In this study, a standard cardiovascular examination was performed twice a year on 5209 subjects who ranged from 30 to 62 years at time of entry into the study. Cardiovascular endpoints were noted on these examinations, as well as by reviewing admission lists at the town's hospital.

The initial report on unrecognized infarctions was published in 1970 [7] and supplemented in 1984 [8] and 1986 [9]. The last report represents a 26-year follow-up. At this time, over 28% of infarctions in men and 35% in women were unrecognized (Fig. 1). Of these, half were truly silent, while in the other half some atypical symptoms were present but were not sufficient for either the patient or physician to consider that an infarction was occurring or had occurred. What this report also shows is that these unrecognized infarctions were uncommon in patients with prior angina. In a preliminary report concerning unrecognized infarction in the age group 65–94 in the Framingham Study, Vokonas et al. [10] found that 33% of infarctions in men and 36% in women were unrecognized.

Other groups have also studied this problem. Muller et al. [11] found a 42% incidence of unrecognized infarction in their patients (aged 64 or older), again with a higher percentage in women. The incidence in the Honolulu Heart Program (aged 45–68) was 33% [12]. The Multiple Risk Factor Intervention Trial (MRFIT) found 25% of infarctions to be unrecognized [13]. Another large

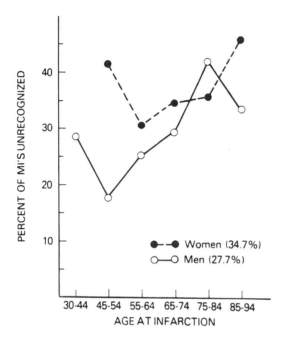

Figure 1 Proportion of myocardial infarctions unrecognized by age and sex in a 30-year follow-up in the Framingham study. (From Kannel WB. Cardiol Clin 1986; 4:583.)

study, that of the Western Collaborative Group, found a 30% rate of unrecognized infarction [14]. Studies are not confined to the United States. Medalie and Goldbourt [15] performed a prospective analysis in 9509 healthy government employees in Israel. Almost 40% of the subsequent 427 infarctions in this group were unrecognized. One difference between this study and that of the Framingham group was that these ECGs were read independently of prior tracings. This might tend to overestimate the number of unrecognized infarctions. Like the Framingham study, half of the unrecognized infarctions were totally silent. Also, like the Framingham study [16], increasing age and blood pressure were significantly associated with the development of unrecognized infarctions (Fig. 2). In analyzing the age issue more closely, Aronow initially reported 68% of infarcts in an elderly population (64–100 years) were unrecognized [17]. He subsequently revised this figure to 21% in a prospective study (Table 1) when physicians were instructed to look more carefully for nonpain presentations (dyspnea, neurological symptoms, etc.) [18]. This is important, since symp-

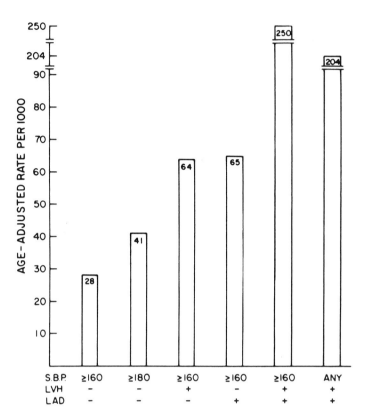

Figure 2   Five-year incidence of unrecognized (silent) myocardial infarction related to systolic blood pressure (SBP), left ventricular hypertrophy (LVH), and left axis deviation (LAD). (From Medalie JH, Goldbourt U. Ann Intern Med 1976; 284:256.)

toms due to the complications of silent infarctions—such as pulmonary edema or dyspnea [19,20]—can be the first clue to the underlying problem. The most recent reports are from Iceland: the Reykjavik study. Sigurdsson et al. [21] performed a prospective population-based cohort study of 9141 men born between 1907 and 1934. The follow-up period was 4 to 20 years. As with earlier studies, they found that at least one-third of all infarcts were unrecognized, with higher numbers in older patients. Again, prognosis was similar for patients with recognized compared to unrecognized infarcts. However, the latter had a lower incidence of angina prior to the infarctions. In a later communication, this group looked specifically at women [22]. They reported that age dependency

Table 1 Prevalence of Presenting Symptoms of Recognized Acute Myocardial Infarction and of Unrecognized Healed Myocardial Infarction in 110 Documented Myocardial Infarctions in Elderly Patients

	n	(%)
Chest pain	24	(22)
Dyspnea	38	(35)
Neurological symptoms	20	(18)
Gastrointestinal symptoms	5	(4)
Unrecognized Q-wave myocardial infarction	23	(21)

Source: Aronow WS. Am J Cardiol 1987; 60:1182.

was again an important factor (Fig. 3) and that this form of coronary artery disease was as common in women as in men.

II. AUTOPSY STUDIES

In addition to the reports cited earlier [2–5], more pertinent pathological studies have since been made available comparing the extent of coronary narrowing and size of the healed infarct in these patients. Cabin and Roberts [21] studied 61 patients with a healed transmural myocardial infarction. Medical records were reviewed in detail and the patients were divided into two groups according to the presence (33 patients) or absence (28 patients) of a clinical history of acute myocardial infarction. Patients with equivocal or inadequate histories were excluded. The group with unrecognized infarcts had a significantly higher prevalence of death from noncardiac causes, posterior wall infarcts, and small infarctions, as well as diabetes (Tables 2 and 3). However, the extent of narrowing of the coronary arteries was similar, as was the involvement of the various vessels (Table 4). The authors also addressed the question of whether patients with unrecognized infarcts had angina less frequently than did patients with symptomatic infarctions. Their results suggested this was the case, but the differences were not statistically significant.

III. MECHANISMS TO EXPLAIN THE ABSENCE OF PAIN: IS DIABETES MELLITUS A FACTOR?

Chapter 1 discussed cardiac pain pathways and Chapter 2 discussed possible alterations in pain sensibility during silent myocardial ischemia. In addition,

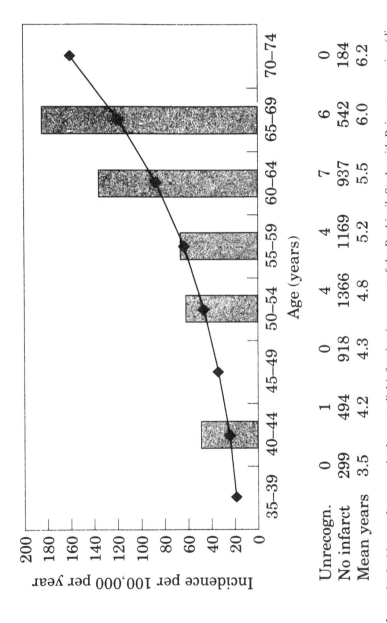

Figure 3 Incidence of unrecognized myocardial infarction in women of the Reykjavik Study with Poisson regression (diamonds) superimposed. (Reproduced with permission from Jonsdottir LS, Sigfusson N, Sigvaldason H, Thorgeirson G. Eur Heart J 1998; 19:1011–1018.)

Table 2 Clinical Findings in 33 Patients with Clinically Recognized and in 28 with Clinically Unrecognized Acute Myocardial Infarction (MI) and Healed Transmural Infarction at Necropsy

	Clinically recognized acute MI (33 patients)		Clinically unrecognized acute MI (28 patients)		
	n	%	n	%	p value
Age (yr)					
Mean	61	—	60	—	NS
Range	27–81	—	25–82	—	
Male–female ratio	25:8	—	21:7	—	NS
Angina pectoris	14	42	6	21	NS
Chronic congestive heart failure	14	42	9	32	NS
Systemic hypertension	11	33	12	43	NS
Diabetes mellitus (adult onset)	5	15	12	43	0.05
Mode of death					
Sudden	13	39	6	21	NS
Acute MI	8	24	7	25	NS
Chronic congestive heart failure	5	15	1	4	NS
Cardiac operation	2[a]	6	2[b]	7	NS
Cardiac catheterization	2	6	1	4	NS
Noncardiac	3	9	11	39	0.01

[a] Coronary artery bypass grafting in one and left ventricular aneurysmectomy in one.
[b] Coronary artery bypass grafting in both.
Source: Cabin HS, Roberts WC. Am J Cardiol 1982; 50:677.

some investigators have studied pain mechanisms in patients with prior silent infarctions. Procacci et al. [24] studied 18 such subjects. They tested their cutaneous pain thresholds in the arm and found them to be significantly higher than in normals, but not higher than in patients with painful infarctions. They also studied upper limb ischemia via cuff inflation and again found different onsets of pain and altered pain patterns compared to normals. They chose the arm because of the similar peripheral innervation found in "referred" cardiac pain.

Table 3 Myocardial Infarct (MI) Size and Location in 33 Patients with and in 28 Without a Clinical History of Acute MI and a Healed Transmural MI at Necropsy

Clinical history of acute MI	Patients (n)	MI size (%)		Number of patients with major (minor)[a] involvement of each left ventricular wall by MI			
		Range	Mean	Anterior	Posterior	Septal	Lateral
+	33	1–55	17	16 (1)	15 (3)	1 (12)	1 (14)
0	28	1–23	7	5 (1)	22 (1)	1 (8)	0 (9)
p value	—	0.001		0.01	0.025	NS	NS

[a] For each patient, major involvement refers to the left ventricular wall with the most scarring and minor involvement refers to 1 or more additional walls with scarring. In all but 3 patients, the anterior or posterior wall of left ventricle was the site of major involvement.
Source: Cabin HS, Roberts WC. Am J Cardiol 1982; 50:677.

These authors did not evaluate the effect of diabetes mellitus but others have. For example, Bradley and Schonfeld [25] reported that 42 of 100 nondiabetic patients had painless infarctions compared with 6 of 100 nondiabetic patients. This relationship was confirmed in the previously cited autopsy study of Cabin and Roberts [23]. As seen in Table 2, there was a significantly increased prevalence of diabetes mellitus among the patients in the unrecognized infarct group (43%) compared with those in the recognized infarct group. However, in two epidemiological studies cited earlier [9,14], the association of diabetes with unrecognized myocardial infarction did not reach a statistically significant level.

Pathological involvement of the autonomic nervous system by diabetes was demonstrated by Faerman et al. [26]. Abnormal morphology was found in cardiac sympathetic and parasympathetic nerves (Fig. 4–6). None of the changes were found in specimens taken from a control group. These findings of a visceral neuropathy may help to explain the absence of pain during transient ischemia, as well as during infarction. Raper et al. [20] postulated that diabetes was responsible for painless infarction in one of four cases that they reported as presenting to the hospital with acute life-threatening cardiac illness. These patients came to the hospital because of complications of cardiac ischemia (such as pulmonary edema) but were pain-free.

Table 4 Number of Major Epicardial Coronary Arteries (CA) Narrowed 76 to 100% in Cross-Sectional Area (XSA) by Atherosclerotic Plaque in 33 Patients with and 28 Without a History of Acute Myocardial Infarction (MI) and a Healed Transmural MI at Necropsy

Clinical history acute MI	Patients (n)	Total CA (n)	Patients with CA narrowed 76–100% in XSA											Mean CA per patient narrowed 76–100%
			LM		LAC		LC		R		Totals			
+	33	132	6	18	32	97	23	70	32	97	93	70		2.8
0	28	112	8	29	24	86	21	75	28	100	81	72		2.9
p value	—	—	NS		NS		NS		NS		NS			NS

LAD = left anterior descending; LC = left circumflex; LM = left main; R = right.
Source: Cabin HS, Roberts WC. Am J Cardiol 1982; 50:677.

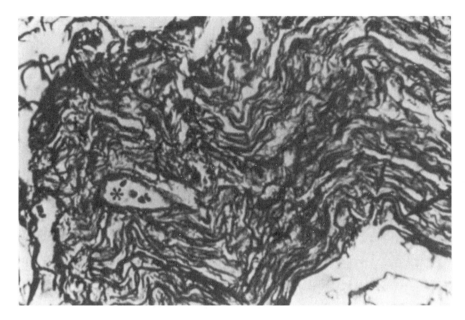

Figure 4 Abnormal appearance of a nerve fiber of a diabetic patient with painless myocardial infarction. Many fibers with hyperargentophilia, alterations of thickness, and fragmentation (arrows). Abnormally small numbers of fibers. A vasa nervorum with normal wass (asterisk). Strain: trichrome and argentic impregnation ×300. (From Faerman I, Fraccio E, Milei J, Nunez R, Jadzinsky M, Fox D, Rapaport M. Diabetes 1977; 26:1147.)

Diabetic neuropathy may also explain the occurrence of silent ischemia in certain patients. Several studies have been reported detailing the prevalence of silent ischemia (as documented by exercise testing and/or Holter monitoring) in diabetics and vice versa. Even in patients with angina and diabetes, the anginal perceptual threshold is often prolonged [27]. Nesto et al. have been particularly interested in diabetics with ischemic heart disease and have documented the high frequency of unexpected silent ischemia in diabetic populations without apparent heart disease [28], especially when peripheral vascular disease is present[29]. Dipyridamole thallium-201 scintigraphy is particularly useful diagnostically in this latter group of patients who cannot perform stan-

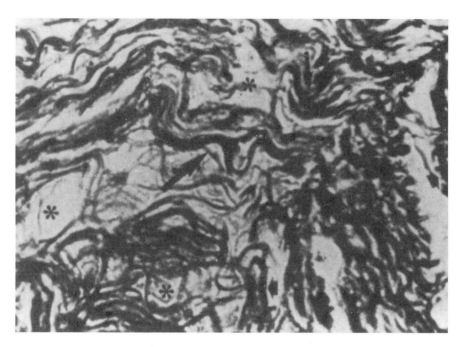

Figure 5 Abnormal nerve fiber in a diabetic patient with painless myocardial infarction. Note the spindle shape of many of the fibers (arrows), the interruption of fibers, and the enlarged interfibrillar spaces (asterisks). Trichrome and argentic impregnation ×1000. (From Faerman I, Faccio E, Milei J, Nunez R, Jadzinsky M, Fox D, Rapaport M. Diabetes 1977; 26:1147.)

dard exercise tests (Fig. 7). However, disease of the small, intramyocardial arteries may contribute to the "false–positive" scans seen in diabetics [30]. This latter factor may also account for the relatively low predictive value of thallium stress tests in estimating cardiovascular risk when diabetics undergo renal transplantation for end-stage renal disease [31]. Holter monitoring studies are also used to estimate the prevalence of silent ischemia in diabetics, and asymptomatic ST segment depression can be as high as 87% in elderly patients [32].

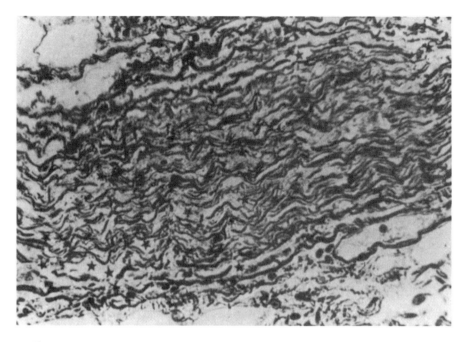

Figure 6 Diffuse abnormalities in a nerve fiber of the heart in a diabetic patient with painless myocardial infarction. Note the many fragmentations of the fibers (stars), hyperargentophilia, and smaller number of fibers. Trichrome and argentic impregnation ×300. (From Faerman I, Faccio E, Milei J, Nunez R, Jadzinsky M, Fox D, Rapaport M. Diabetes 1977; 26:1147.)

IV. CONCLUSIONS

The data have remained consistent throughout the past decade. One-quarter to one-third of myocardial infarctions are clinically unrecognized. Increasing age and hypertension are associated features. At autopsy the extent of coronary artery disease is similar to that seen with symptomatic infarctions. The etiology of painless infarctions is unclear, but the presence of diabetes appears to be a factor in some studies.

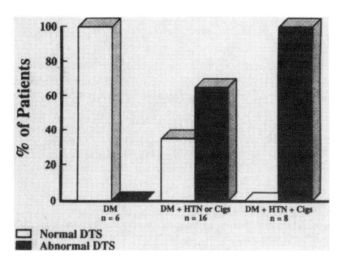

Figure 7 Comparison of the percent of patients with normal (light columns) and abnormal (dark columns) dipyridamole-thallium scans according to associated coronary artery disease risk factors ($p = 0.001$). Cigs, history of cigarette smoking; DM, diabetes mellitus; DTS, dipyridamole-thallium scintigraphy; HTN, hypertension. (From Nesto RW, Watson FS, Kowalchuk GJ, Zarich SW, Hill T, Lewis SM, Lane SE. Am Heart J 1990; 120:1073. Reproduced with permission.)

REFERENCES

1. Herrick JB. Clinical features of sudden obstruction of the coronary arteries. JAMA 1912; 59:2015.
2. Kennedy JA. The incidence of myocardial infarction without pain in autopsied cases. Am Heart J 1937; 14:703.
3. Boyde LD, Weblow SC. Coronary thrombosis without pain. Am J Med Sci 1937; 194:814.
4. Gorham LE, Martin SJ. Coronary artery occlusion with and without pain. Arch Intern Med 1938; 112:812.
5. Stroud WD, Wagner JA. Silent or atypical coronary occlusion. Ann Intern Med 1941; 15:25.
6. Roseman MD. Painless myocardial infarction: A review of the literature and analysis of 220 cases. Ann Intern Med 1954; 41:1.

7. Kannel WB, McNamara PM, Feinleib M, et al. The unrecognized myocardial infarction: 14-year follow-up experience in the Framingham study. Geriatrics 1970; 25:75.

8. Kannel WB, Abbott RD. Incidence and prognosis of unrecognized myocardial infraction. Based on 26 years follow-up on the Framingham study. In: Rutishauser W, Roskamm H, eds. Silent Myocardial Ischemia Berlin: Springer-Verlag, 1984: 131–137.

9. Kannel WB. Silent myocardial ischemia and infarction: Insights from the Framingham study. Cardiol Clin 1986; 4:583.

10. Vokonas PS, Kannel WB, Cupples LA. Incidence and prognosis of unrecognized myocardial infarction in the elderly, The Framingham Study (abstr). J Am Coll Cardiol 1988; 11:51A.

11. Muller RT, Gould LA, Betzu R, Vacek T, Pradeep V. Painless myocardial infarction in the elderly. Am Heart J 1990; 119:202.

12. Yano K, MacLean CJ. The incidence and prognosis of unrecognized myocardial infarction in the Honolulu, Hawaii, Heart Program. Arch Intern Med 1989; 149:1528.

13. Grimm RH, Jr., Tillinghast S, Daniels K, Neaton JD, Mascoli S, Crow R, Pritzker M, Prineas RJ. Unrecognized myocardial infarction: Experience in the Multiple Risk Factor Intervention Trial (MRFIT). Circulation, 1987; 75(suppl II):6.

14. Rosenman RH, Friedman M, Jenkins CD, et al. Clinically unrecognized infarction in the Western Collaborative Study. Am J Cardiol 1967; 19:776.

15. Medalie JH, Goldbourt U. Unrecognized myocardial infarction: Five-year incidence, mortality, and risk factors. Ann Intern Med 1976; 84:526.

16. Kannel WB, Dannenberg AL, Abbott RD. Unrecognized myocardial infarction and hypertension. the Framingham study. Am Heart J 1985; 109:581.

17. Aronow WS, Starling L, Etienne F, D'Alba P, Edwards M, Lee NH, Parungao RF. Unrecognized Q-wave myocardial infarction in patients older than 64 years in a long-term health-care facility. Am J Cardiol 1985; 56:483.

18. Aronow WS. Prevalence of presenting symptoms of recognized acute myocardial infarction and of unrecognized healed myocardial infarction in elderly patients. Am J Cardiol 1987; 60:1182.

19. Brush JE, Cabin HS, Wohlgelernter D, Hammond GL, Cohen LS. Ventricular septal rupture following a clinically unrecognized myocardial infarction. Am Heart J 1985; 110:667.

20. Raper AJ, Hastillo A, Paulsen WJ. The syndrome of sudden severe painless myocardial ischemia. Am Heart J 1984; 107:813.

21. Sigurdsson E, Thorgeirsson G, Sigvaldason H, Sigfusson N. Unrecognized myocardial infarction: epidemiology, clinical characteristics, and the prognostic role of angina pectoris. Ann Intern Med 1995; 112:96–102.

22. Jonsdottir LS, Sigfusson N, Sigvaldason H, Thorgeirson G. Incidence and prevalence of recognized and unrecognized myocardial infarction in women. Eur Heart J 1998; 19:1011–1018.

23. Cabin HS, Roberts WC. Quantitative comparison of extent of coronary narrowing and size of healed myocardial infarct in 33 necropsy patients with clinically recognized and in 28 with clinically unrecognized ("silent") previous acute myocardial infarction. Am J Cardiol 1982; 50:677.

24. Procacci P, Zoppi M, Padeletti L, Maresca M. Myocardial infarction without pain. A study of the sensory function of the upper limbs. Pain 1976; 2:309.

25. Bradley RF, Schonfeld A. Diminished pain in diabetic patients with myocardial infarction. Geriatrics 1962; 17:322.

26. Faerman I, Faccio E, Milei J, Nunez R, Jadzinsky M, Fox D, Rapaport M. Autonomic neuropathy and painless myocardial infarction in diabetic patients: Histologic evidence of their relationship. Diabetes 1977; 26:1147.

27. Ranjadayalan K, Umachandran V, Ambepityia G, Kopelman PG, Mills PG, Timmis AD. Prolonged anginal perceptual threshold in diabetes: Effects on exercise capacity and myocardial ischemia. J Am Coll Cardiol 1990; 16:1120.

28. Nesto RW, Phillips RT, Kett KG, Hill T, Perper E, Young E, Leland OS. Angina and exertional myocardial ischemia in diabetic and nondiabetic patients: Assessment by exercise thallium scintigraphy. Ann Intern Med 1988; 108:170.

29. Nesto RW, Watson FS, Kowalchuk GJ, Zarich SW, Hill T, Lewis SM, Lane SE. Silent myocardial ischemia and infarction in diabetics with peripheral vascular disease: Assessment by dipyridamole thallium-201 scintigraphy. Am Heart J 1990; 120:1073.

30. Koistinen MJ, Kuikuri HV, Pirttiaho H, Linnaluoto MK, Takkunen JT. Evaluation of exercise electrocardiography and thallium tomographic imaging in detecting asymptomatic coronary artery disease in diabetic patients. Br Heart J 1990; 63:7.

31. Holley JL, Fenton RA, Arthur RS. Thallium stress testing does not predict cardiovascular risk in diabetic patients with end-stage renal disease undergoing cadaveric renal transplantation. Am J Med 1991; 90:563.

32. Aronow WS, Mercando AD, Epstein S. Prevalence of silent myocardial ischemia detected by 24-hour ambulatory electrocardiography, and its association with new coronary events at 40-month follow-up in elderly diabetic and nondiabetic patients with coronary artery disease. Am J Cardiol 1992; 69:555.

III

DETECTION OF ASYMPTOMATIC CORONARY ARTERY DISEASE

7
What Can Be Learned from Standard Diagnostic Procedures?

Considerable controversy surrounds the use of screening procedures for detecting coronary artery disease in asymptomatic populations [1–4]. The controversy concerns not only which procedures are most reliable, but also whether screening is even appropriate in the general population. We begin our review with a consideration of the more "routine" tests.

Standard diagnostic procedures for evaluating suspected coronary artery disease in persons *with* chest pain include history taking, physical examination, blood lipid and glucose determinations, the resting ECG, and chest X-rays and related procedures. Exercise testing—with or without associated radioisotopic procedures—is usually the next step after these standard procedures and is discussed in subsequent chapters. Obviously, screening asymptomatic populations for the presence of coronary artery disease is a more difficult undertaking and in this regard not all of the above-mentioned procedures have the same value as they do in patients with chest pain syndromes.

I. HISTORY TAKING

This is of limited value since, by definition, the individual to be screened has no symptoms. (This, of course, does not include patients now asymptomatic who have experienced a prior infarction.) At times, cardiologists will clearly recognize anginal equivalents that have been misdiagnosed by the patients (or their physicians) as gastrointestinal or neuromuscular complaints. Some complaints may or may not reflect underlying heart disease. "Breathlessness" is one such symptom that must be carefully considered as having a cardiac basis, since true dyspnea can be a sign of left ventricular failure due to ischemia [5]. Perhaps the most important information that truly asymptomatic individuals can provide, however, relates to their family history and/or their own known coronary risk factors.

As Sharp et al. [6] have noted, if a member of the individual's immediately family (i.e., parents, grandparents, aunts, uncles) died of cardiac (or unknown) causes or developed a myocardial infarction or angina before the age of 55, this should alert the cardiologist or internist to the possibility of latent coronary atherosclerosis. Since much of a "positive family history" is due to the prevalence of the three most important genetically determined risk factors (hypertension, diabetes mellitus, hypercholesterolemia), patients should then be queried directly about the presence of these factors in their relatives—and themselves. Although cigarette smoking is not an inherited problem, smoking is another risk factor that can be part of a positive family history since patients who smoke encourage their children to do likewise merely by setting an example. Smoking can increase the risk of silent ischemia [7].

II. PHYSICAL EXAMINATION

Unless the patient has experienced a prior myocardial infarction with resulting left ventricular asynergy and its characteristic cardiac findings, the physical examination is usually negative. A fourth heart sound may be present even in individuals without prior infarctions, but this is too nonspecific a finding to be used by itself to diagnose coronary artery disease. The reliability of the "ear lobe crease" sign is also uncertain.

III. BLOOD TESTS

Abnormal blood glucose of lipid levels are recognized risk factors for the development of coronary artery disease. Whether they can be used as *indicators* of asymptomatic coronary artery disease is less clear.

   Epidemiological studies—such as that in Framingham, Massachusetts— have clearly shown the increased risk associated with increasing levels of serum cholesterol [8]. Other studies have examined the ratio of total cholesterol to high-density lipoprotein (HDL) cholesterol. Williams et al. [9] studied 2568 asymptomatic men and found that a ratio of 4.0 or less identified a group with a very low prevalence of disease, whereas a ratio of 8.0 or above identified a very high-risk group in relation to future cardiac events. Serum lipid levels have also been used to aid in the selection of subjects for coronary arteriography. Uhl et al. [10] found a ratio greater than 6.0 generated an odds ratio of 172/1 based on coronary angiographic results in 132 asymptomatic airmen with a positive exercise test. Only 2 of the 16 with coronary artery disease had a ratio less than 6.0, whereas only 4/102 persons with normal coronary angiographic findings had a ratio greater than 6.0. The ratio was a better discriminator than total cholesterol or HDL cholesterol levels (Figs. 1 and 2). The value of this ratio was recently confirmed in a preliminary report by Houck [11] in screening over 11,000 Air Force personnel. In another preliminary report, Kwiterovich et al. [12] investigated the elevated apoprotein levels of coronary artery disease in an asymptomatic population. Apoproteins are associated with cholesterol transport, and the major apoprotein B of low-density lipoproteins has previously been shown to be elevated in symptomatic individuals. In their report, Kwiterovich et al. studied plasma levels of various types of cholesterol and apoproteins in 68 asymptomatic siblings of 40 patients with premature coronary artery disease. Of the 19 siblings with a positive stress-thallium test, 10 had elevated apoprotein B levels. Bivariate analysis showed that apoprotein B was significantly more sensitive in this regard than other cholesterol and apoprotein measurements. As this study suggests, the presence of single or multiple risk factors combined with abnormal exercise responses can also improve predictive value for coronary artery disease. This is discussed at greater length in Chapters 9 and 10. As noted in Chapter 5, a new approach to

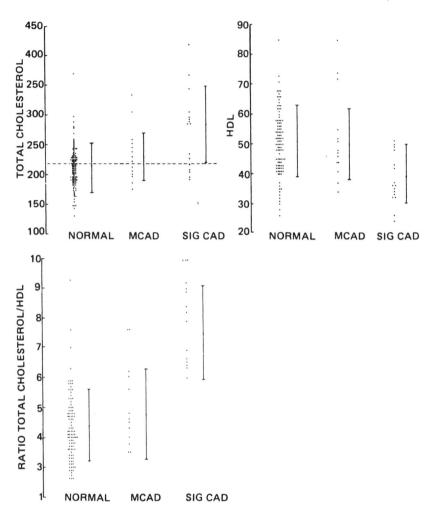

Figure 1   Values for total cholesterol, HDL cholesterol, and cholesterol/HDL cholesterol ratio in each of the patients plotted according to angiographic classification [normal, minimal coronary artery disease (MCAD) and significant coronary artery disease (SIG CAD)]. An arbitrary cutoff value for total cholesterol of 220 mg/100 mL is represented by the dotted line. Total cholesterol and HDL cholesterol levels did not discriminate between those with significant coronary artery disease and those with normal coronary angiograms. A cholesterol/HDL cholesterol ratio greater than 6.0 was the best discriminator. (From Uhl GS, Troxler RG, Hickman JR, Jr., Clark D. Am J Cardiol 1981; 48:903.)

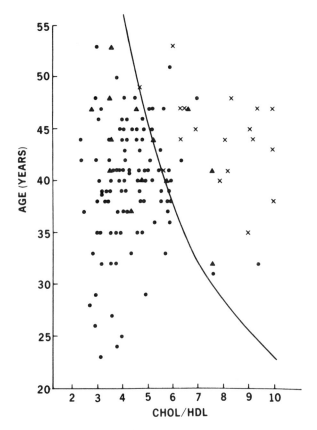

Figure 2 Graph plotting the cholesterol (CHOL)/HDL cholesterol ratio versus age for each patient who underwent cardiac catheterization. The ratio and age appear to be independent risk factors. The solid line plots the equation: age × (total cholesterol/HDL cholesterol) = 230. It demonstrates that a simple equation can separate normal subjects from patients with significant coronary artery disease (CAD). ● = normal; ▲ = minimal CAD; x = significant CAD. (From Uhl GS, Troxler RG, Hickman JR, Jr., Clark D. Am J Cardiol 1981; 48:903.)

the diagnosis of asymptomatic coronary artery disease in individuals with familial hypercholesterolemia is with ultrafast CT scanning, also referred to as electron beam tomography. Coronary calcification identified by this technique was found in 7 of 29 subjects aged 11 to 23, a decidedly uncommon occurrence in persons so young [13]. (See also p. 132.)

IV. THE RESTING ELECTROCARDIOGRAM

The standard baseline ECG obtained at rest is of value if it shows unequivocal evidence of new or old myocardial infarction. In totally asymptomatic individuals, one assumes the infarct was either silent, or painless enough not to warrant concern by the patient and/or his physician at the time. The finding of ST abnormalities alone suggests that underlying coronary artery disease will be found in a relatively small number of subjects, but when combined with a positive exercise test, the predictive value increases to nearly 50%, which is higher than that observed with T-wave changes alone (Table 1) [14]. Resting ECG changes in an asymptomatic diabetic population are important clues to underlying coronary artery disease, and also have prognostic implications [15]. Joy and Trump [16] concluded from their study of 103 asymptomatic men with minor ST segment abnormalities that the predictive value for coronary artery disease for these changes alone was about 8%, whereas it was 44% when combined with a positive exercise test. Changes with hyperventilation were not as

Table 1 Angiographic Findings in 111 Air Crewmen with an Abnormal Exercise Electrocardiogram Grouped According to Annual Rest Electrocardiographic (ECG) Findings

Annual rest ECG	n	Mean age (%)	Significant angiographic coronary disease (%)
Normal	34	44	23.5
Previous ST-T change but current ECG normal	21	43	23.8
Low-amplitude T waves	24	42	25.0
ST segment abnormal	32	44	46.9

Source: Froelicher V, Thompson AJ, Wolthius R, et al. Am J Cardiol 1977; 23:32.

impressive and these could not be used to separate presumably normal persons from those with coronary artery disease. This was also true of the U.S. Air Force studies [14]. In other Air Force patients, the prevalence rate of coronary artery disease was 22% in asymptomatic airmen with new left bundle branch block and 18% in right bundle branch block [14].

The Reykjavik study in Iceland (cited in Chap. 6) is the most recent example of correlating prognosis with "silent" ST-T abnormalities on the resting ECG. In this study, 9139 men born in the years 1907 to 1934 without overt coronary artery disease were followed for 4 to 24 years. The prevalence of the ECG abnormalities was strongly affected by increasing age (2% at age 40 vs. 30% at age 80). Other risk factors for coronary artery disease were usually present, but even *after* adjustment for these factors patients with resting ECG abnormalities had elevated risk ratios for development of angina, myocardial infarction, or death [17]. In another recent report concerning ST abnormalities on the resting ECG, Davislus et al. [18] also found increased risk (Table 2) and DeBacquer et al. linked parental history of premature coronary artery disease to these ECG abnormalities [19]. Ventricular premature beats—either on resting ECGs or on Holter monitors—are not in themselves regarded as indicators, or predictors, of coronary artery disease if other evidence of organic heart dis-

Table 2 Age- and Multivariate-Adjusted Relative Risks of Death During 29 Years with Presence of Any Minor ST-T Abnormalities in 5 Annual Examinations[a]

Cause of death	Any ST-T abnormalities	
	Age-adjusted	Multivariate-adjusted[b]
Myocardial infarction	1.85 (1.30–2.64)[c]	1.58 (1.09–2.28)[d]
Coronary heart disease	2.00 (1.50–2.65)[c]	1.67 (1.25–2.25)[c]
Cardiovascular diseases	1.73 (1.33–2.24)[c]	1.38 (1.05–1.80)[d]
All causes	1.46 (1.19–1.77)[a]	1.28 (1.04–1.58)[d]

[a] Compared with men with no minor ST-T abnormalities. All data are presented as relative risk (95% confidence interval).
[b] Adjustment variables in the Cox multivariate proportional hazards model were age in year 5, education at baseline, family history of cardiovascular disease, and average of first 5 examinations, 1957 to 1958 through 1961 to 1962, systolic blood pressure, number of cigarettes smoked per day, serum cholesterol level, body mass index, and body mass index squared.
[c] $p < 0.001$.
[d] $p < 0.05$.
Source: Daviglus ML, Liao Y, Greenland P, Dyer AR, Liu K, Xie X, Huang CF, Prineas RJ, Stamler J. JAMA 1999; 281:530–536.

ease is lacking [20]. If ST depression is also present, however, risk of future events is increased [21].

V. CHEST X-RAYS AND RELATED PROCEDURES

The chest x-ray is usually normal in this type of patient unless a prior infarction has occurred, or an ischemic cardiomyopathy has developed. Fluoroscopic screening for coronary artery disease (via detection of coronary artery calcification) is simple, rapid, and inexpensive, but its reliability has been questioned, especially in older patients. Loecker et al. [22] screened 1466 men, 613 of whom subsequently underwent coronary angiography. Detection of coronary artery calcification substantially increased the likelihood of angiographically demonstrable coronary artery disease, whether minimal or severe (over 50% reduction in luminal diameter) (Table 3). Probably the most exciting development in this area has been the introduction of ultrafast CT scanning (also called electron beam tomography), which has been discussed earlier. There are now a host of studies in which symptomatic and asymptomatic persons [13,23–25] have been studied with this technique and the results correlated with coronary arteriography. Many patients have other coronary artery disease risk factors in addition to coronary calcifications. The cost effectiveness of this procedure versus coronary angiography has been demonstrated by Rumberger et al. [25]. Some groups have used the combination of calcified coronary arteries and exercise testing as screening markers in asymptomatic populations. We will consider this in Chapter 10. Echocardiograms and radionuclide ventriculography are also considered in Chapter 10 as adjuncts to the exercise test, since stress-related abnormalities of left ventricular wall motion are much more common than resting abnormalities in asymptomatic persons.

Table 3 Coronary Artery Fluoroscopy (Fluoro) Versus Arteriographic Coronary Artery Disease

	Disease ≥10%		Disease ≥50%	
	Yes	No	Yes	No
Fluoro positive	126	57	69	114
Fluoro negative	82	348	35	395

Source: Loecker TH, Schwartz RS, Cotta CW, Hickman JR, Jr. J Am Coll Cardiol 1992; 19:1167. Reproduced with permission.

VI. CONCLUSIONS

Standard clinical procedures are of limited value as indicators of asymptomatic coronary artery disease, though coronary risk factors can help predict who will *subsequently* develop coronary artery disease. However, the modern approach to the diagnosis of coronary artery disease recognizes the importance of asymptomatic disease and utilizes all available strategies—including standard diagnostic procedures—to aid in its detection [26].

REFERENCES

1. Uhl GS, Froelicher V. Screening for asymptomatic coronary artery disease. J Am Coll Cardiol 1983; 1:946.
2. Detrano R, Froelicher V. A logical approach to screening for coronary artery disease. Ann Intern Med 1987; 106:846.
3. Berman DS, Rozanski A, Knoebel SB. The detection of silent ischemia: Cautions and precautions. Circulation 1987; 75:101.
4. Helfant RH, Klein LW, Agarwal JB. Role of cardiac testing in an era of proliferating technology and cost containment. J Am Coll Cardiol 1987; 9:1194.
5. Nixon PGF, Freeman LJ. What is the meaning of angina pectoris today? Am Heart J 1987; 114:1542.
6. Sharp SD, Williams RR, Hunt SC, Schumacher MC. Coronary risk factors and the severity of angiographic coronary artery disease in members of high-risk pedigrees. Am Heart J 1992; 123:279.
7. Deedwania PC, Jamner L, Carbajal E. Cigarette smoking increases risk of silent ischemia and alters cardiovascular reactivity during exercise (abstr.). Circulation 1991; 84:(suppl II) II-538.
8. Kannell WB, Castelli WP, Gordon T. Cholesterol in the prediction of atherosclerotic disease: New perspective based on the Framingham study. Ann Intern Med 1979; 90:85.
9. Williams P, Robinson D, Bailey A. High density lipoprotein and coronary risk factors in normal men. Lancet. 1979; 1:72.
10. Uhl GS, Troxler RG, Hickman JR, Jr., Clark D. Angiographic correlation of coronary artery disease with high density lipoprotein cholesterol in asymptomatic men. Am J Cardiol 1981; 48:903.
11. Houck PD. Epidemiology of total-cholesterol-to-HDL (ratio) in 11,669 Air Force personnel and coronary artery anatomy in 305 healthy aviators. J Am Coll Cardiol 1988; 11:222A.
12. Kwiterovich PO, Becker DM, Pearson T, Fintel DJ, Bachorik P, Sniderman A. HyperapoB is a potent predictor of occult coronary artery disease in asymptomatic relatives (abstr). Circulation 1984; 70 (suppl 11):313.

13. Gidding SS, Brookstein LC, Chomka EV. Usefulness of electron beam tomography in adolescents and young adults with heterozygous familial hypercholesterolemia. Circulation 1998; 98:2580–2583.

14. Froelicher V, Thompson AJ, Wolthuis R, et al. Angiographic findings in asymptomatic aircrewmen with electrocardiographic abnormalities. Am J Cardiol 1977; 39:32.

15. Scheidt-Nave C, Barrett-Connor E, Wingard DL. Resting electrocardiographic abnormalities suggestive of asymptomatic ischemic heart disease associated with non-insulin-dependent diabetes mellitus in a defined population. Circulation 1990; 81:899.

16. Joy M, Trump DW. Significance of minor ST segment and T wave changes in the resting electrocardiogram of asymptomatic subjects. Br Heart J 1981; 45:48.

17. Sigurdsson E, Sigfusson N, Sigvaldason H, Thorgeirsson G. Silent ST-T changes in an epidemiologic cohort study—a marker of hypertension or coronary heart disease, or both: the Reykjavik study. J Am Coll Cardiol 1996; 27:1140–1147.

18. Daviglus ML, Liao Y, Greenland P, Dyer AR, Liu K, Xie X, Huang CF, Prineas RJ, Stamler J. Association of nonspecific minor ST-T abnormalities with cardiovascular mortality. JAMA 1999; 281:530–536.

19. De Bacquer D, De Backer G, Kornitzer M, Blackburn H. Parental history of premature coronary heart disease mortality and signs of ischemia on the resting electrocardiogram. J Am Coll Cardiol 1999; 33:1491–1499.

21. Moss AJ. Clinical significance of ventricular arrhythmias in patients with and without coronary artery disease. Prog Cardiovasc Dis 1980; 23:33.

21. Hedblad B, Janzon L, Johanssont BS, Juul-Mollert S. Survival in men with ambulatory ECG-detected ventricular arrhythmias. Eur Heart J 1997; 18:1787–1795.

22. Loecker TH, Schwartz RS, Cotta CW, Hickman JR, Jr. Fluoroscopic coronary artery calcification and associated coronary disease in asymptomatic young men. J Am Coll Cardiol 1992; 19:1167.

23. Janowitz WR, Agatston AS, Kaplan G, Viamonte M. Differences in prevalence and extent of coronary artery calcium detected by ultrafast computed tomography in asymptomatic men and women. Am J Cardiol 1993; 72:247–254.

24. Detrano RC, Wong ND, French WJ, Tang W, Georgiou D, Young E, Brezden OS, Doherty T, Brundage. Prevalence of fluoroscopic coronary calcific deposits in high-risk asymptomatic persons. Am Heart J 1994; 127:1526–1532.

25. Rumberger JA, Behrenbeck T, Breen JF, Sheedy PF. Coronary calcification by electron beam computed tomography and obstructive coronary artery disease: A model for costs and effectiveness of diagnosis as compared with conventional cardiac testing methods. J Am Coll Cardiol 1999; 33:453–463.

26. Anderson HV, King SB, III. Modern approaches to the diagnosis of coronary artery disease. Am Heart J 1992; 123:1312.

8
Ambulatory Electrocardiography (Holter Monitoring)

Along with the exercise test, the 24- to 48-h ambulatory electrocardiogram (popularly known as the Holter monitor after its inventor) has become closely identified with the documentation of silent myocardial ischemia. In 1991, Corday provided a fascinating historical vignette celebrating Holter's achievement [1]. It is well worth reading. No longer is this device used only for the detection of arrhythmias, but as Holter noted in his initial report [2], it is the best way of detecting transient myocardial ischemia during daily activities. The validity of this approach has been confirmed in a host of studies.

I. TECHNICAL CONSIDERATIONS

The issue of whether or not ST segment changes recorded on Holter monitors are reliable indicators of myocardial ischemia is no longer controversial. There are still problem areas, however. Whatever the ECG recording procedure employed—Holter, exercise tests, etc.—it is well known that ST segments are labile and notoriously susceptible to hyperventilation, electrolyte abnormalities, drugs, etc., but there have also been specific criticisms concerning the ambulatory ECG. Some of these involve technical considerations in recording of the electrocardiographic signal. The American Heart Association [3] has recommended a flat amplitude signal for frequency responses between 0.1 and 80 Hz, but many of the amplitude-modulated (AM) ambulatory ECG monitoring systems amplify low-frequency information normally present in the ST segment. This can have the effect of overestimating the degree of ST segment depression relative to the height of the R wave. In addition to the concerns with frequency response curves, there is also the specific monitor to consider. Different systems will record standardized ST segment signals with different wave forms (Fig. 1). Analysis of Holter types can also present difficulties. Computer programs for detecting transient ST changes appear to offer the best ways of analyzing the Holter tapes [4] (Fig. 2). Whether three-channel monitoring offers advantages over the standard two-channel approach is unclear [5,6]—as are the location of such leads [7]—but there is no question that competence in interpreting standard ECGs is essential to analyzing ambulatory Holter reports no matter what techniques are used [8].

Since most of the equipment in use at hospitals and diagnostic laboratories is of the AM type, it is important that physicians have assurances that the report they receive is accurate. Lambert et al. [9] have provided such assurances for the reliability of AM devices in their study of low-frequency requirements for recording ischemic ST segment abnormalities. Their conclusion—that current AM models are as reliable as the "gold standard" frequency-modulated (FM) systems—has been confirmed by Shook et al. [10] in a different study protocol (Fig. 3 and 4). Ironically, as this issue appears to be resolved, another has emerged. A new type of Holter monitor using real-time analysis has been developed. This has presented a new set of problems, as discussed by Kennedy and Wiens [11], but validation studies comparing the devices with conventional AM and FM monitors, have been done with several systems [12,13]. Three-dimensional graphs constructed from real-time 12-lead monitors are also in use [14].

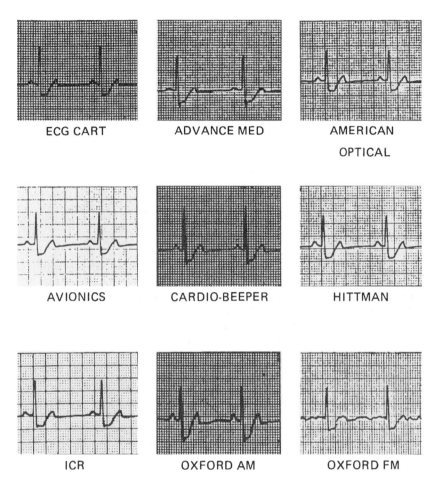

Figure 1 The representative output from one record/transmitter and one scanner/receiver of the input of the modified ECG stimulator with 4-mm flatline ST segment depression of 80-ms duration. Note the output from an HP 12-lead ECG cart (model 1541A) used as the standard. Note that the American Optical, Avionics, and ICR systems gave good reproduction of the signal. Although the Hittman system reproduced the ST segment, there was some attenuation of the terminal S wave. The Oxford AM gave considerably more than 4.0-mm ST segment depression. Advance Med and Cardio-Beeper had slightly upsloping ST segments. Note the baseline noise present on Oxford FM which limits clinical interpretation. (From Bragg-Remschel DA, Anderson CM, Winkle RA. Am Heart J 1982; 103:20.)

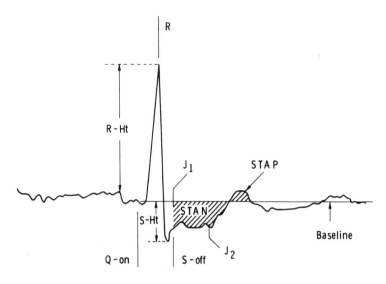

Figure 2 Diagram showing the variables identified and measured for each cardiac cycle by a computer system. J_1 = J joint; J_2 = level of the ST segment 60 ms after the J point; R = R wave; R-Ht = R-wave amplitude; S-Ht = S-wave amplitude; Q-on = onset on Q wave; S-off = end of S wave; STAN = ST segment negative area; STAP = ST segment positive area. Heart rate is calculated from the RR interval. (From Gallino A, Chierchia S, Smith G, Croom M, Morgan M, Marchesi C, Maseri A. J Am Coll Cardiol 1984; 4:245.)

II. CORRELATION BETWEEN HOLTER STUDIES AND CORONARY ARTERIOGRAPHY: HISTORICAL PERSPECTIVE

Stern and Tzivoni [15] were the first to demonstrate ST segment abnormalities on Holter monitoring in a series of 80 patients with chest pain syndromes, normal resting electrocardiograms, and normal exercise tests. Thirty-seven of the eighty patients had ischemic ST segment abnormalities (either elevation or depression) on their ambulatory recordings. Many of these episodes were unaccompanied by pain (Fig. 5). In the initial 12-month follow-up period, 1 of these 37 patients developed a myocardial infarction; 23 others developed increasing chest pain or further ECG changes suggestive of coronary artery disease. Coronary arteriography was not performed in any of these patients. In another study, Stern and Tzivoni [16] studied 140 patients with chronic ischemic heart disease documented by anginal histories or myocardial infarc-

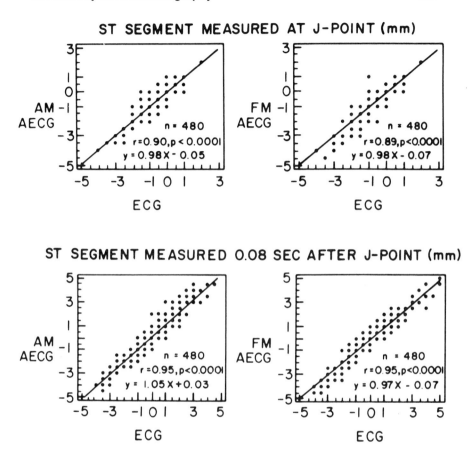

Figure 3 Reproduction of the ST segment measured at the J point and 0.08 s after the J point by amplitude-modulated (AM) and frequency-modulated (FM) systems, compared with the standard direct-writing electrocardiogram (1 mV = 10 mm). Note: Each point may represent more than one determination. AECG = ambulatory electrocardiogram. (From Shook TL, Balke CW, Kotilainen PW, Hubelbank M, Selwyn AP, Stone PH. Am J Cardiol 1987; 60:895.)

tions. Ninety-seven of the 140 patients had ST segment abnormalities during their daily activities. Some individuals (24%) had more ischemic episodes during sleep, while others (38%) had less episodes. In yet another of their early studies [17], this group correlated the results of ambulatory monitoring with coronary arteriography: ambulatory ECGs identified nearly 80% of patients with angiographically documented coronary artery disease. The false-positive

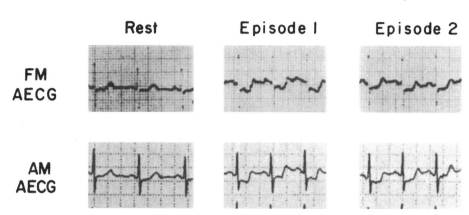

Figure 4 Representative simultaneous frequency-modulated (FM) and amplitude-modulated (AM) Holter recording during episodes of out-of-hospital ischemic ST segment change. AECG = ambulatory electrocardiogram. (From Shook TL, Balke CW, Kotilainen PW, Hubelbank M, Selwyn AP, Stone PH. Am J Cardiol 1987; 60:895.)

rate (abnormal Holter findings with normal coronary arteriograms) was only 13%.

III. HOLTER MONITORING AND SILENT MYOCARDIAL ISCHEMIA

Following the landmark studies of Stern and Tzivoni [15–17] the first Holter study to specifically evaluate the significance of asymptomatic episodes was that of Schang and Pepine [18]. Twenty patients with angiographically confirmed coronary artery disease and positive exercise tests were each monitored for several 10-h periods over the course of 16 months. In the total of 2826 h of technically adequate recordings, 411 episodes of transient ST segment abnormalities were documented (Fig. 6). Of the 411 episodes, 308 (or 75%) were asymptomatic. Most of these occurred during sleep, sitting, or periods of slow walking and at heart rates very much less than those at which patients complained of angina during their stress tests. Schang and Pepine indirectly "proved" that the silent ST segment episodes were truly ischemic by markedly reducing their occurrence with the frequent, prophylactic use of nitrate preparations. This was an important feature of their study, since, as noted previously, considerable criticism had been directed toward the use of the ST segment as a marker of ischemia.

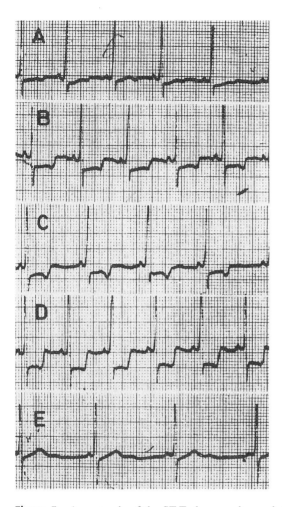

Figure 5 An example of the ST-T changes observed during 24-h ambulatory ECG monitoring in a 56-year-old man. Slight ST-T abnormalities were noted during most of the day (panel A); increasing degrees of ST segment depression were observed after meals (panel B), at rest (panel C), and during walking (panel D). Only during sleep at night (panel E) was the ECG normal. Although the patient had apparent evidence of myocardial ischemia as shown in panels B, C, and D, he only experienced pain during walking (panel D). (From Stern S, Tzivoni D. Am Heart J 1976; 91:820.)

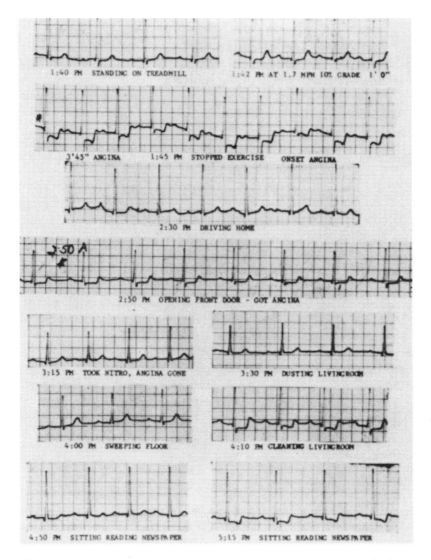

Figure 6   Another example of ST-T changes observed on ambulatory monitoring in a building manager. ECG changes occurred on an exercise test, during work, and at rest, but were not always accompanied by pain. (From Schang SJ, Pepine CJ. Am J Cardiol 1977; 39:396.)

However, it was not until the study published by Deanfield and coworkers [19] appeared that this criticism abated. This study and its successor [20] succeeded in refuting much of the skepticism concerning the occurrence and significance of symptomatic versus asymptomatic episodes. In 30 patients with stable angina and positive exercise tests, ambulatory ST segment monitoring was used to record episodes of transient ischemia during daily life. All patients had four consecutive days of monitoring, and in 20 patients long-term variability was evaluated by repeated 48-h monitoring and exercise testing over an 18-month period. Of the 1934 episodes of horizontal or downsloping ST segment depression, only 470 (or 24%) were accompanied by angina—a figure almost identical to that of Schang and Pepine in their study published 6 years earlier. Physiological validation of the ST segment change was an especially important part of their second study [20], which included 34 patients. Ischemia without angina was documented by positron tomography (see Figs. 16 and 17 in Chap. 4) with the occurrence of ST segment depression being consistently underestimated by symptoms. Heart rate increase was not common (Fig. 7), suggesting that transient increases in coronary vasomotor tone were a major

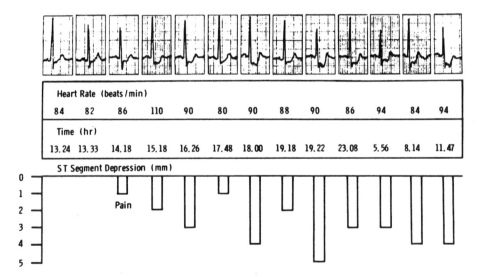

Figure 7 Typical 24-h ambulatory electrocardiographic recording showing 11 episodes of ST depression, only one of which was accompanied by angina. The episodes occurred throughout day and night and lasted for up to 40 min. (From Deanfield JE, Ribiero P, Oakley K, Krikler S, Selwyn AP. Am J Cardiol 1984; 54: 1195.)

contributor to myocardial ischemia—with or without symptoms—during daily activities. As noted previously in Chapter 3, more recent work has moderated this view. It is now clear that increased myocardial demand *does* play an important role in many episodes of myocardial ischemia during daily activity even though frank tachycardia is not present. Small, but significant, increases in heart rate and/or blood pressure are often recorded in the 15–30 min preceding the ischemic episode (Fig. 8) [21,22] and this can affect choice of therapeutic agents [23].

Many studies have confirmed the frequency of silent ischemic episodes in patients with classic exertion-induced angina pectoris. Cecci and colleagues [24] were among the first to find that the number of silent episodes outnumbered the symptomatic ones. In their study of 39 patients with exertion-induced angina, they performed 24-h Holter monitoring in addition to exercise testing. Coronary artery disease was confirmed by coronary arteriography in 31 patients, and 16 patients had a prior myocardial infarction. Of the 39 patients, 32 had ST depression during ambulatory monitoring (Table 1). Fifteen of the thirty-two patients had both symptomatic and asymptomatic episodes (with

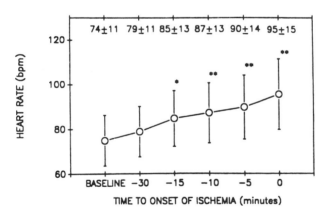

Figure 8 Plot of mean heart rate (shown in graph and numerical form) plus standard deviations during the nonischemic portion of the day (baseline) and at 30, 15, 10, 5, and 0 (onset) min before ischemia. Analysis of variance demonstrated a highly significant change over time ($p < 0.001$). Comparison of each time point with baseline heart rate showed that this rise first became significant 15 min before the onset of ischemia. $*p < 0.01$ and $**p < 0.001$, difference from baseline nonischemic heart rate. (From McLenachan JM, Weidinger FF, Barry J, Yeung A, Nabel EG, Rocco MB, Selwyn AP. Circulation 1991; 83:1263. Reproduced with permission of American Heart Association.)

Table 1 Ischemic Episodes During Holter Monitoring (39 patients)

| Patients (no.) | Total | Episodes (no.) | |
		Symptomatic	Asymptomatic
	7 —	0	—
8	25	25	—
15	105	29	76
9	40	—	40
Total	170	54	116

Source: Cecci AC, Dovellini EV, Marchi F, Pucci P, Santoro CM, Fazzini PF. J Am Coll Cardiol 1983; 1:934.

symptomatic episodes being three times as frequent); in this study, the duration and degree of ST segment depression were greater during the asymptomatic episodes (Table 2). Deanfield et al. [19] noted that most of the asymptomatic episodes were short, while the symptomatic ones were just as likely to be long as short. The myocardial perfusion defects appeared similar, however as noted in Chapter 4, Cecci et al. [24] also reported that patients who took longer to register chest pain during treadmill stress testing had a greater ratio of symptomatic to painless episodes of myocardial ischemia on 24-h monitoring (Table 3). Their studies suggested that the severity of the ischemic episode (i.e., the amount of myocardium at jeopardy) is an important factor in determining whether a specific ischemic episode would be symptomatic or not (see also Chap. 4). By contrast, Kunkes et al. [25] reported that patients with multivessel disease (and presumably *more* myocardium at jeopardy) had a higher frequency of silent ischemic episodes than did patients with one-vessel disease.

As more and more studies using the Holter monitor have been published, it is apparent that episodes involving ST elevation often have similar characteristics to episodes involving ST depression in regard to heart rate, duration of ischemia, etc. [26]; that there is a circadian variation in these episodes, with most coming after arousal in the morning [27] or waking and rising at night [28] (Fig. 9), perhaps related to enhanced platelet aggregation [29] or variations in vascular tone [30]. This circadian variation is the same in both men and women [31] (Fig. 10). What triggers myocardial ischemia during certain activities and not during others? This is a question to which ambulatory ECG monitoring has helped provide answers by correlating ECG data to diaries of daily events, concurrent drawing of blood catecholamines, etc. The importance of physical exertion, anger, smoking, and mental stress have all been well docu-

Table 2 24-Hour Holter Monitoring: Duration of Ischemia Attacks and Magnitude of Maximal ST Depression

	Patients (no.)	Episodes (no.)	Type of episodes	Duration of episodes	Mean magnitude of maximal ST depression
All patients	32	54	Symptomatic	$7' \pm 5'42''$	3.3 ± 1.7 mm
		116	Asymptomatic	$4'12'' \pm 2'30''$	2.5 ± 1 mm
		Total 170		$(p < 0.001)$	$(p < 0.001)$
Patients who experienced only symptomatic	8	25	Symptomatic	$5'12'' \pm 3'50''$	2.3 ± 0.9 mm
or asymptomatic episodes	9	40	Asymptomatic	$4'33'' \pm 3'r$	2.7 ± 1.2 mm
		Total 65		$(p > 0.05)$	$(p > 0.05)$
Patients who exhibited both symptomatic and	15	29	Symptomatic	$8'36'' \pm 6'35''$	4.3 ± 1.7 mm
asymptomatic episodes		76	Asymptomatic	$4'06'' \pm 2'15''$	2.4 ± 1.0 mm
		Total 105		$(p < 0.001)$	$(p < 0.001)$

Source: Cecci AC, Dovellini EV, Marchi F, Pucci P, Santoro CM, Fazzini PF. J Am Coll Cardiol 1983; 1:934.

Table 3 Results of Stress Testing and Holter Monitoring

| Stress testing | | Holter monitoring | | |
| Patients (no.) | Finding | Patients (no.) | Episodes (no.) | | |
			Symptomatic	Asymptomatic	Ratio between symptomatic and asymptomatic episodes
11	Angina precedes or coincides with ST depression	11	27	17	1:0.62
10	ST depression precedes angina by 10 to 60 s	8	11	12	1:1.09
18	ST depression precedes angina by more than 60s	13	16	87	1:5.43

Source: Cecci AC, Dovellini EV, Marchi F, Pucci P, Santoro CM, Fazzini PF. J Am Coll Cardiol 1983; 1: 934.

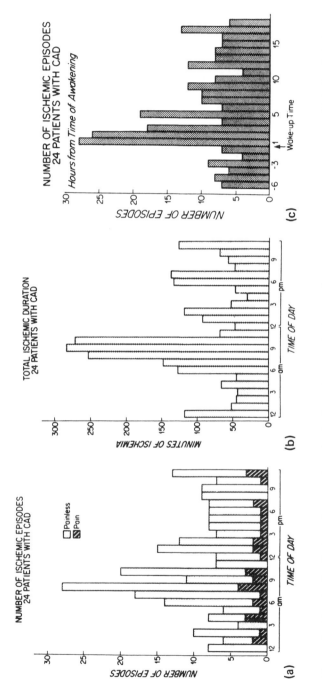

Figure 9 Hourly distribution of (a) number of episodes and (b) total minutes of ischemic duration in 24 patients with ischemic ST segment depression. There is a significant peak of ischemic activity between 6 A.M. and 12 noon. When the number of episodes is corrected for the (c) time of waking the peak density of ischemic activity occurs immediately upon rising. (From Rocco MB, Barry J, Campbell S, Nabel E, Cook EF, Goldman L, Selwyn AP. Circulation 1987; 75:392.)

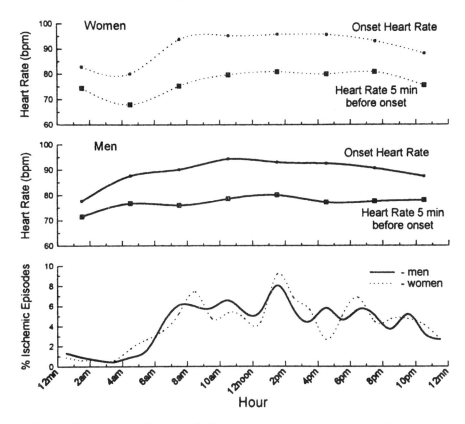

Figure 10   Relation of heart rate 5 min before ischemia onset (squares) and heart rate at onset of ischemia (circles) on a 3-h basis in women (⋯⋯) and men (——) and corresponding 24-h patterns of ischemic activity in both men and women. (Reproduced with permission from Mulcahy D, Dakak N, Zalos G, Andrews NP, Proschan M, Waclawin MA, Schenke WH, Quyyum AA. J Am Coll Cardiol 1996; 27:1629–1636.)

mented [32–34]. Of these factors, probably none has received greater study than the influence of mental stress in precipitations of ischemia. An increased heart rate response has been noted [35] as well as other hemodynamic abnormalities [36], and feelings of "tension, frustration, and sadness" (Fig. 11) can more than double the risk of myocardial ischemia in the subsequent hour of monitoring [37]. Even high-risk asymptomatic populations can have exaggerated reactivity to mental stress [38]. ST segment depression during mental

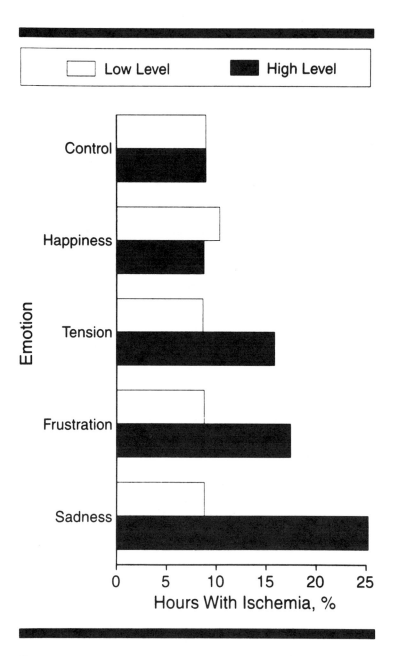

Figure 11 Percentage of hours with low and high ratings of feeling in control, happiness, tension, frustration, and sadness. The percentage of ischemic hours was greater during higher levels of the negative emotions associated with mental stress. (Reproduced with permission from Gullette ECD, Blumenthal JA, Babyak M, Jiang W, Waugh RA, Frid DJ, O'Connor CM, Morris JJ Krantz DS. JAMA 1997; 277:1521–1526.)

stress is more predictive of ST depression during routine daily activities than other laboratory-based ischemic markers [39].

Silent ischemic events are not only common in patients with unstable angina but help to provide risk-stratification data after treatment [41] as they do in postinfarction ischemia [42]. Marchant et al. [43] found a difference in pathophysiological mechanisms when patients with predominantly silent ischemia in the postinfarction period are compared to patients with chronic angina, (i.e., more supply-driven ischemia is present in the former than the latter). We have also learned that silent ischemia is more common in patients with positive rather than negative exercise tests [44] (Fig. 12) and is also common in patients with nondiagnostic exercise tests compared to regular tests [45]. Holter monitoring is also useful in assessing success of coronary angioplasty [46,47]. The day-to-day variability in these events must be considered [48,49], however (Table 4). This will be discussed further when therapy is discussed in subsequent chapters. At that time we will also consider the use of Holter monitoring in multicenter trials. [50,51] When considering the effects of therapy in any of the trials cited, we must always bear in mind the possibility that myocardial preconditioning exists, as indicated by the attenuation of the severity of the Holter episodes when there are repeated daily events [52] (Fig. 13).

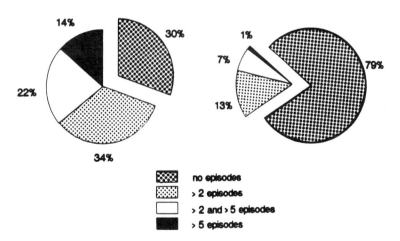

no episodes
> 2 episodes
> 2 and > 5 episodes
> 5 episodes

Figure 12 Frequency distribution of total ischemic episodes/24 h on ambulatory ECG monitoring in 187 patients with a positive exercise test (left) and 90 patients with a negative test (right). (From Mulcahy D, Keegan J, Sparrow J, Park A, Wright C, Fox K. J Am Coll Cardiol 1989; 14:1166. Reproduced with permission.)

The use of ambulatory monitoring for detecting silent ischemia via ST segment abnormalities in *asymptomatic persons* without coronary arteriographic evidence of coronary artery disease has been questioned very strenuously. When Armstrong and Morris [53] evaluated 50 asymptomatic middle-aged men with treadmill exercise tests and ambulatory ECG monitoring and found evidence of "ischemic" ST segment changes in 15 of the 50 men (30%), they concluded that these were false-positive responses, similar to those

Table 4   Results in All Patients and Day-to-Day Variations

	Results of 3 monitoring days				% Maximal day-to-day variations			
Pt.	No. of episodes	Total duration of ST↓ (min)	Maximal ST↓ (min)	HR at beginning of ST↓ (beats/min)	No. of episodes (%)	Duration of ST↓ (%)	Maximal ST↓ (%)	HR at beginning of ST↓ (%)
1	28	121	1.5	75	36	78	0	16.7
2	12	280	2	87	60	48	0	3.3
3	16	132	3.5	85	43	25	43	13.3
4	23	609	6	85	33	75	17	10.5
5	13	673	6	85	20	90	17	10.5
6	12	147	2	85	60	58	25	15
7	7	136	3	90	33	48	50	14.3
8	9	60	4	85	50	56	62	7.6
9	22	52	6	95	44	83	75	5
10	18	44	1.5	93	17	29	33	7
11	25	190	3	95	22	43	33	0
12	16	159	3	100	43	62	25	4.8
13	12	126	2	90	40	30	38	8.2
14	29	329	4	77	10	39	33	8.3
15	12	78	1.5	75	40	57	37	8.5
16	31	268	4	78	25	48	14	13.3
17	38	390	3.5	75	26	23	33	8.5
18	19	212	4.5	90	29	23	22	5.3
19	29	366	3.5	88	27	66	30	12
20	18	200	3.5	80	56	39	29	8.1
Mean	19.5	228.6	3.4	81.4	35.9	51.1	30.8	9

HR = heart rate; ↓ = depression.
Source: Tzivoni D, Gavish A, Benhorin J, Banai S, Keren A, Stern S. Am J Cardiol 1987; 60: 1003.

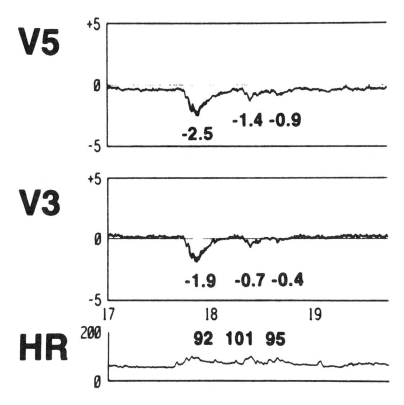

Figure 13 ST segment and heart rate (HR) histogram. During the 3 walks, there was a similar increase in heart rate (92,101 and 95 beats/min, respectively), but the degree of ST depression in leads V5 and V3 decreased markedly. (Reproduced with permission from Tzvoni D, Maybaum S. J Am Cardiol 1997; 30:119–124.)

observed in cases of mitral valve prolapse or neurocirculatory asthenia or in any condition where the autonomic nervous system can be overactive. Others [54,55] have also reported ST segment changes in presumably healthy men, but Deanfield et al. [56] found significant depression only rarely. Certainly from a prognostic point of view the Swedish study of men born in 1914 has documented that ischemic episodes during daily life carry an increased risk for morbidity and mortality in otherwise apparently healthy individuals [57]. When asymptomatic patients with known coronary artery disease are studied, Holter monitoring commonly detects episodes of silent ischemia [40–42]. In some of the patients, the disease is quite extensive. Diabetics appear especially prone to silent ischemia [43], presumably as a reflection of their high incidence of coronary artery disease and visceral neuropathy.

IV. CONCLUSIONS

Holter monitoring is used to document silent myocardial ischemia in coronary patients experiencing both symptomatic and asymptomatic episodes. Still uncertain, however, is whether ST changes seen in otherwise healthy individuals (who have not undergone coronary arteriography) has the same connotation. Consequently, the role of routine Holter monitoring in detecting coronary artery disease in a totally asymptomatic population remains unclear [62]. What has become clear, however, is an emerging consensus for what constitutes an ischemic episode on the Holter recording: ST segment depression of at least 1.0 mm (0.1 mV) lasting 1 min and separated from other episodes by at least 1 min [63]. This "$1 \times 1 \times 1$" rule or some variation should serve as a helpful guideline in defining myocardial schemia on Holter monitoring especially in research studies. It is also apparent that 24 h may not be the optimum time period for monitoring events; 48 h is probably more appropriate.

REFERENCES

1. Corday E. Historical vignette celebrating the 30th anniversary of diagnostic ambulatory electrocardiographic monitoring and data reduction systems. J Am Coll Cardiol 1991; 17:286.
2. Holter NJ. New methods for heart studies. Science 1961; 134:1214.
3. Pipberg HV, Arzbaecher RC, Berson AS, Briller SA, Brody DA, Flowers NC, Geselowitz DB, Lepeschkin E, Oliver CG, Schmitt OH, Spach M. Recommendations for standardization of leads and of specifications for instruments in electrocardiography and vectorcardiography: Report of the Committee on Electrocardiography, American Heart Association. Circulation 1975; 52:11.
4. Gallino A, Chierchia S, Smith G, Croom M, Morgan M, Marchesi C, Maseri A. Computer system for analysis of ST segment changes on 24 hour Holter monitor tapes: Comparison with other available systems. J Am Coll Cardiol 1984; 4:245.
5. Shandling AH, Bernstein SB, Kennedy HL, Ellestad MH. Efficacy of three-channel ambulatory electrocardiographic monitoring for the detection of myocardial ischemia. Am Heart J 1992; 123:310.
6. Lanza GA, Mascellanti M, Placentino M, Lucente M, Crea F, Maseri A. Usefulness of a third Holter lead for detection of myocardial ischemia. Am J Cardiol 1994; 74:1216–1219.

7. Jiang W, Blumenthal JA, Hanson MW, Coleman RE, O'Connor CM, Frid D, Morris JJ, Waugh RA. Relative importance of electrode placement over number of channels in transient myocardial ischemia detection by Holter monitoring. Am J Cardiol 1995; 76:350–354.

8. Kennedy HI. Importance of the standard electrocardiogram in ambulatory (Holter) electrocardiography. Am Heart J 1992; 123:1660.

9. Lambert CR, Imperi GA, Pepine CJ. Low-frequency requirements for recording ischemic ST-segment abnormalities in coronary artery disease. Am J Cardiol 1986; 58:225.

10. Shook TL, Balke W, Kotilainen PW, Hubelbank M, Selwyn AP, Stone PH. Comparison of amplitude-modulated (direct) and frequency-modulated ambulatory techniques for recording ischemic electrocardiographic changes. Am J Cardiol 1987; 60:895.

11. Kennedy HL, Wiens RD. Ambulatory (Holter) electrocardiography using real-time analysis. Am J Cardiol 1987; 59:1190.

12. Jamal SM, Mitra-Duncan L, Kelly DT, Breedman SB. Validation of a real-time electrocardiographic monitor for detection of myocardial ischemia secondary to coronary artery disease. Am J Cardiol 1987; 60:525.

13. Barry J, Campbell S, Nabel EG, Mead K, Selwyn AP. Ambulatory monitoring of the digitized electrocardiogram for detection and early warning of transient myocardial ischemia in angina pectoris. Am J Cardiol 1987; 60:483.

14. Krucoff MW, Wagner NB, Pope JE, Mortara DM, Jackson YR, Bottner RK, Wagner GS, Kent KM. The portable programmable microprocessor-driven real-time 12-lead electrocardiographic monitor: A preliminary report of a new device for the noninvasive detection of successful reperfusion or silent coronary reocclusion. Am J Cardiol 1990; 65:143.

15. Stern S, Tzivoni D. Early detection of silent ischaemic heart disease by 24-hour ECG monitoring during normal daily activity. Br Heart J 1974; 36:481.

16. Stern S, Tzivoni D. Dynamic changes in the ST-T segment during sleep in ischemic heart disease. Am J Cardiol 1973; 32:17.

17. Stern S, Tzivoni D, Stern Z. Diagnostic accuracy of ambulatory ECG monitoring in ischemic heart disease. Circulation 1975; 52:1045.

18. Schang SJ, Pepine CJ. Transient asymptomatic S-T segment depression during daily activity. Am J Cardiol 1977; 39:396.

19. Deanfield JE, Maseri A, Selwyn AP, Chierchia S, Ribiero P, Krikler S, Morgan M. Myocardial ischemia during daily life in patients with stable angina: Its relation to symptoms and heart rate changes. Lancet 1983; 2:753.

20. Deanfield JE, Shea M, Ribiero P, deLandsheere CM, Wilson RA, Horlock P, Selwyn AP. Transient ST segment depression as a marker of myocardial ischemia during daily life. Am J Cardiol 1984; 54:1195.

21. Deedwania PC, Nelson JR. Pathophysiology of silent myocardial ischemia during daily life: Hemodynamic evaluation by simultaneous electrocardiographic and blood pressure monitoring. Circulation 1990; 82:1296.

22. Hinderliter A, Miller P, Bragdon E, Ballenger M, Sheps D. Myocardial ischemia during daily activities: The importance of increased myocardial oxygen demand. J Am Coll Cardiol 1991; 18:405.

23. Andrews TC, Fenton T, Toyosaki N, Glasser SP, Young PM, MacCallum G, Gibson RS, Shook TL, Stone PH, for the Angina and Silent Ischemia Study Group (ASIS). Subsets of ambulatory myocardial ischemia based on heart rate activity. Circulation 1993; 88:92–100.

24. Cecchi AC, Dovellini EV, Marchi F, Pucci P, Santoro CM, Fazzini PF. Silent myocardial ischemia during ambulatory electrocardiographic monitoring in patients with effort angina. J Am Coll Cardiol 1983; 1:934.

25. Kunkes SH, Prichard AD, Smith H, Jr., Gorlin R, Herman MV, Kupersmith J. Silent ST segment deviations and extent of coronary artery disease. Am Heart J 1980; 100:813.

26. vonArnim T, Hofling B, Schreiber M. Characteristics of episodes of ST elevation or ST depression during ambulatory monitoring in patients subsequently undergoing coronary angiography. Br Heart J 1985; 54:484.

27. Rocco MB, Barry J, Campbell S, Nabel E, Cook EF, Goldman L, Selwyn AP. Circadian variation of transient myocardial ischemia in patients with coronary artery disease. Circulation 1987; 75:395.

28. Barry J, Campbell S, Yeung AC, Raby KE, Selwyn AP. Waking and rising at night as a trigger of myocardial ischemia. Am J Cardiol 1991; 67:1067.

29. Brezinski DA, Tofler GH, Muller JE, Pohjola-Sintonen S, Willich SN, Schafer AI, Czeisler CA, Williams GH. Morning increase in platelet aggregability: Association with assumption of the upright posture. Circulation 1988; 78:35.

30. Panza JA, Epstein SE, Quyyumi AA. Circadian variation in vascular tone and its relation to alpha-sympathetic vasoconstrictor activity. N Engl J Med 1991; 325:986.

31. Mulcahy D, Dakak N, Zalos G, Andrews NP, Proschan M, Waclawin MA, Schenke WH, Quyyumi AA. Patterns and behavior of transient myocardial ischemia in stable coronary disease are the same in both men and women: A comparative study. J Am Coll Cardiol 1996; 27:1629–1636.

32. Gottdiener JS, Krantz DS, Howell RH, Hecht GM, Klein J, Falconer JJ, Rozanski A. Induction of silent myocardial ischemia with mental stress testing: relation to the triggers of ischemia during daily life activities and to ischemic functional severity. J Am Coll Cardiol 1994; 24:1645–1651.

33. Krantz DS, Kop WJ, Gabbay FH, Rozanski A, Barnard M, Klein J, Pardo Y, Gottdiener JS. Circadian variation of ambulatory myocardial ischemia. Circulation 1996; 93:1364–1371.

34. Gabbay FH, Krantz DS, Kopo WJ, Hedges SM, Klein J, Gottdiener JS, Rozanski A. Triggers of myocardial ischemia during daily life in patients with coronary artery disease: Physical and mental activities, anger and smoking. J Am Coll Cardiol 1996; 27:585–592.

35. Krittayaphong R, Light KC, Biles PL, Ballenger MN, Sheps DS. Increased heart rate response to laboratory-induced mental stress predicts frequency and duration

of daily life ambulatory myocardial ischemia in patients with coronary artery disease. Am J Cardiol 1995; 76:657–660.

36. Blumenthal JA, Jiang W, Waugh RA, Frid DJ, Morris JJ, Coleman E, Hanson M, Babyak M, Thyrum E T, Krantz DS, O'Connor C. Mental stress-induced ischemia in the laboratory and ambulatory ischemia during daily life. Circulation 1995; 92:2102–2108.

37. Gullette ECD, Blumenthal JA, Babyak M, Jiang W, Waugh RA, Frid DJ, O'Connor CM, Morris JJ, Krantz DS. Effects of mental stress on myocardial ischemia during daily life. JAMA 1997; 277:1521–1526.

38. Kral BG, Becker LC, Blumenthal RS, Aversano T, Fleisher LA, Yook RM, Becker DM. Exaggerated reactivity to mental stress is associated with exercise-induced myocardial ischemia in an asymptomatic high-risk population. Circulation 1997; 96:4246–4253.

39. Stone PH, Krantz DS, McMahon RP, Goldberg AD, Becker LC, Chaitman BR, Taylor HA, Cohen JD, Freedland KE, Bertolet BD, Coughlan C, Pepine CJ, Kaufman PG, Sheps DS for the PIMI Study Group. Relationship among mental stress-induced ischemia and ischemia during daily life and during exercise: The psychophysiologic investigation of myocardial ischemia (PIMI) study. J Am Coll Cardiol 1999; 33:1476–1484.

40. Gottlieb SO, Weisfeldt ML, Ouyang P, Mellits ED, Gerstenblith G. Silent ischemia as a marker for early unfavorable outcomes in patients with unstable angina. N Engl J Med 1986; 314:1214.

41. Holmvang L, Andersen K, Dellborg M, Clemmensen P, Wagner G, Grande P, Abrahamsson P. Relative contributions of a single-admission 12-lead electrocardiogram and early 24-hour continuous electrocardiographic monitoring for early risk stratification in patients with unstable coronary artery disease. Am J Cardiol 1999; 83:667–674.

42. Gurfinkel E, Altman R, Scazziota A, Rouvier J, Mautner B. Importance of thrombosis and thrombolysis in silent ischaemia: comparison of patients with acute myocardial infarction and unstable angina. Br Heart J 1994; 71:151–155.

43. Marchant B, Stevenson R, Vaishnav S, Ranjadayalan K, Timmis AD. Myocardial ischaemia and angina in the early post-infarction period: a comparison with patients with stable coronary artery disease. Br Heart J 1993; 70:438–442.

44. Mulcahy D, Keegan J, Sparrow J, Park A, Wright C, Fox K. Ischemia in the ambulatory setting—the total ischemic burden: Relation to exercise testing and investigative and therapeutic implications. J Am Coll Cardiol 1989; 14:1166.

45. Raby KE, Barry J, Treasure CB, Hirsowitz G, Fantasia G, Selwyn AP. Usefulness of Holter monitoring for detecting myocardial ischemia in patients with nondiagnostic exercise treadmill test. Am J Cardiol 1993; 72:889–893.

46. Josephson MA, Nademanee K, Intarachot V, Lewis HS, Singh BN. Abolition of Holter-detected silent myocardial ischemia following percutaneous transluminal coronary angioplasty. J Am Coll Cardiol 1987; 10:499.

47. Mulcahy D, Keegan J, Phadke K, Wright C, Sparrow J, Purcell H, Fox K. Effects

of coronary artery bypass surgery and angioplasty on the total ischemic burden: A study of exercise testing and ambulatory ST segment monitoring. Am Heart J 1992; 123:597.

48. Tzivoni D, Gavish A, Benhorin J, Banai S, Keren A, Stern S. Day-to-day variability of myocardial ischemic episodes in coronary artery disease. Am J Cardiol 1987; 60:1003.

49. Nabel EG, Barry J, Rocco MB, Campbell S, Mead K, Fenton T, Orav EJ, Selwyn AP. Variability of transient myocardial ischemia in ambulatory patients with coronary artery disease. Circulation 1988; 78:60.

50. Cohn PF, Vetrovec GW, Nesto R, Gerber FR, the Total Ischemia Awareness Program Investigators. The Nifedipine-Total Ischemia Awareness Program: A national survey of painful and painless myocardial ischemia including results of antiischemic therapy. Am J Cardiol 1989; 63:534.

51. Sharaf BL, Williams DO, Miele NJ, McMahon RP, Stone PH, Bjerregaard P, Davies R, Goldberg AD, Parks M, Pepine CJ, Sopko G, Conti R for the ACIP Investigators. A detailed angiographic analysis of patients with ambulatory electrocardiographic ischemia: results from the asymptomatic cardiac ischemia pilot, (ACIP) study angiographic core laboratory. J Am Cardiol 1997; 29:78–84.

52. Tzivoni D, Maybaum S. Attenuation of severity of myocardial ischemia during repeated daily ischemic episodes. J Am Cardiol 1997; 30:119–24.

53. Armstrong WF, Morris SN. The ST segment during ambulatory electrocardiographic monitoring. Ann Intern Med 1983; 98:249.

54. Quyumi AA, Wright C, Fox K. Ambulatory electrocardiographic ST segment changes in healthy volunteers. Br Heart J 1983; 50:460.

55. Kohli RS, Cashman PMM, Lahiri A, Raftery EB. The ST segment of the ambulatory electrocardiogram in a normal population. Br Heart J 1988; 60:4.

56. Deanfield JE, Ribiero P, Oakley K, Krikler S, Selwyn AP. Analysis of ST segment changes in normal subjects: Implications for ambulatory monitoring in angina pectoris. Am J Cardiol 1984; 54:1321.

57. Hedblad B, Juul-Moller S, Svensson K: Increased mortality in men with ST segment depression during 24hr ambulatory long-term ECG recordings. Eur Heart J 1989; 10:149–58.

58. Campbell S, Barry J, Rebecca GS, Rocco MB, Nabel EG, Wayne RR, Selwyn AP. Active transient myocardial ischemia during daily life in asymptomatic patients with positive exercise tests and coronary artery disease. Am J Cardiol 1986; 57:1010.

59. Coy KM, Imperi GA, Lambert CR, Pepine CJ. Silent myocardial ischemia during daily activities in asymptomatic men with positive exercise test responses. Am J Cardiol 1987; 59:45.

60. Cohn PF, Lawson WE. Characteristics of silent myocardial ischemia during out-of-hospital activities in asymptomatic angiographically documented coronary artery disease. Am J Cardiol 1987; 59:746.

61. Chiariello M, Indolfi C, Cotecchia MR, Sifola C, Romano M, Condorelli M. Asymptomatic transient ST changes during ambulatory ECG monitoring in diabetic patients. Am Heart J 1985; 110:529.

62. DiMarco JP, Philbrick JT. Use of ambulatory electrocardiographic (Holter) monitoring. Ann Intern Med 1990; 113:53.

63. Cohn PF, Kannel WB, eds. Recognition, pathogenesis, and management options in silent coronary artery disease. Circulation 1987; 75(suppl II):1–54.

9
Exercise Testing

While the Holter monitor is being used with increasing frequency to evaluate silent myocardial ischemia, it still must share center stage with the exercise test. The latter is an established procedure for assessing ischemic responses, arrhythmias and cardiac performance in persons with known or suspected heart disease. In addition, many epidemiological studies have been performed to evaluate the accuracy of exercise electrocardiographic testing in predicting the occurrence of overt cardiac events in asymptomatic populations. The exercise test has also been used as a procedure to screen asymptomatic individuals in order to identify those persons who warrant further noninvasive or invasive testing because of an abnormal exercise response. The latter approach considers the exercise electrocardiogram as an *indicator* of myocardial ischemia, rather than as only a risk factor for the development of coronary artery disease.

I. EXERCISE TESTS AS PREDICTORS OF FUTURE CARDIAC EVENTS

One of the earliest and largest of the epidemiological studies was that initiated in 1971 by Bruce and colleagues (the Seattle Heart Watch Study). In this prospective community study of symptom-limited maximal exercise testing, more than 4000 persons clinically free of heart disease were registered between 1971 and 1974. Annual follow-up surveillance of subsequent primary coronary artery disease (defined as admission to a hospital for evaluation or treatment) was continued until the beginning of 1981. A 1983 report [1] provides a unique 10-year experience for evaluating the interactive value of exercise test predictors combined with the usual coronary risk factors (hypertension, hyperlipidemia, diabetes, cigarette smoking) and a family history of premature coronary artery disease, in the 3611 men and 547 women enrolled in this study. Mean age of the men was 45.5 ± 8.4 (SD) years; for the women it was 49.1 ± 9.0 years. The standard Bruce protocol for symptom-limited maximal exercise, using progressive increments in speed and gradient on a motor-driven treadmill, was employed. The most common cause for stopping the tests was fatigue. Patients were divided into subgroups based on presence of conventional risk factors and four abnormal exercise predictors. These included (1) chest pain during the test; (2) inability to complete stage 2 of the protocol; (3) maximal heart rate less than 90% of age-predicted normal value [based on the formulae $y = 227 - 1.067$ (age in years for men) and $y = 206 - 0.597$ (age in years for women)]; and (4) development of 1 mm or more of horizontal or downsloping ST depression for at least 1 min into the recovery period. Event rates for cardiac events per 1000 person-years of follow-up were calculated. Prior to applying the results of exercise testing, the annual incidence rate of total cardiac events was 0.35% in asymptomatic healthy men and 0.31% in women. When the interaction of any conventional risk factor and two or more of the exercise predictors were considered, the annual risk of cardiac death (for men and women combined) increased from 0.12% to 9.61% ($p < 0.05$). Six-year survival rates decreased from $97.8 \pm 0.4\%$ to 75.7 ± 7.1 ($p < 0.001$) in this subgroup when life-table analysis was performed (Fig. 1).

Other studies have used ST segment depression alone as a predictor of future cardiac events. For example, Ellestad and Wan [2] collected follow-up data on 2700 patients, including 323 who had previous infarcts. They found that

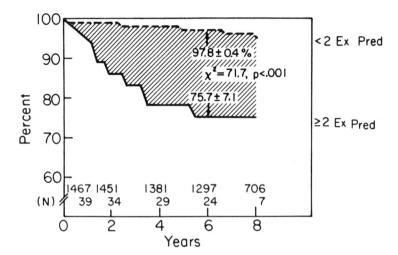

Figure 1 Stepwise assessment of survival without any primary coronary heart disease events in three groups of middle-aged men and women initially free of coronary heart disease manifestations. Shaded areas represent differences in survival rates attributable to the detection of less than two or more than two exercise predictors. (From Bruce RA, Hossack KF, DeRouen TA, Hofer V. J Am Coll Cardiol 1983; 2:565.)

by using a 1.5-mm criterion for ST segment depression, they could demonstrate a significant difference between positive and negative responders in terms of future cardiac events such as death, myocardial infarction, or progressive angina (9.5%/year vs. 1.7%/year). The adverse prognosis seen with a positive stress test was especially marked in those individuals who had experienced a prior myocardial infarction. Allen et al. [3] studied 888 clinically normal men and women. They did not evaluate conventional risk factors but did assess multiple exercise predictors, including ST segment depression, abnormal R-wave response, and exercise duration of 5 min or less. All three factors were present in five men aged 40 or over; all subsequently developed cardiac events (Table 1). Similarly, absence of all three factors provided 94% predictive accuracy for absence of cardiac events in the 206 men who were aged 40 and over. These predictive values were not reliable, however, in men under 40 or in women.

Another study of this type was performed in Italy by Giagnoni et al. [4]. These investigators controlled their study for the effect of conventional risk factors so that they could isolate the ST segment response as a predictor of ischemic events. Between 1971 and 1974, they identified 10,723 subjects (8866

Table 1 Correlation of Combining All Three Positive Criteria (ST, R-Wave and Exercise Duration) vs. Absence of Criteria with Development of Coronary Heart Disease Within 5 Years in Men Older Than 40 Years

	ST positive and increase or no change in R-wave and duration $\leq$ 5 min	ST negative and decrease in R-wave and duration > 5 min
CHD	5[a]	12
	(100%)	(5.8%)
No CHD	0	194
	(0%)	(94.2%)

Sensitivity 29.4%; specificity 100%; predictive value of a positive test 100%; risk ratio 17.2.
[a] $p < 0.001$.
CHD = coronary heart disease
Source: Allen WH, Aronow WS, Goodman P, Stinson P. Circulation 1980; 62:522.

men and 1857 women) who were apparently free of heart disease and hypertension; 135 persons had bicycle ergometer exercise-induced ST depression of 1 mm or more on two exercise electrocardiograms. For each person, two or three controls with negative exercise tests were selected after being matched for age, sex, occupation, and conventional heart risk factors. Follow-up for cardiac events (angina, myocardial infarction, sudden death) was conducted for a period of 6 years (Table 2). The incidence of coronary events was very low in the controls (0.8% for the first 5 years) as compared to 10.37% in the study group (Fig. 2). This difference was higher than that observed in the second 5 years. Although, as expected, the conventional risk factors were also prognos-

Table 2 Occurrence of Coronary Events in 135 Cases and 379 Controls

	Cases	Controls	Total
	no. (%)	no. (%)	no. (%)
Coronary events			
Present	21 (15.55)	13 (3.43)	34 (6.61)
Absent	114 (84.45)	336 (96.57)	480 (93.39)
Total	135 (100)	379 (100)	514 (100)
Relative risk	4.53		

Source: Giagnoni E, Secchi MB, Wu SC, Morabito A, Oltrona L, Mancarella S, Volpin N, Fossa L, Bettazzi L, Arangio G, Sachero A, Folli G. N Engl J Med 1983; 309:1085.

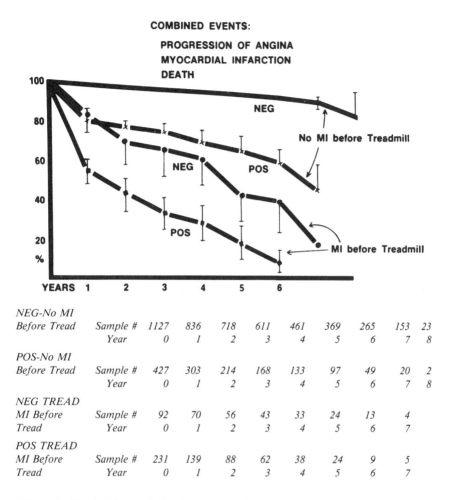

NEG-No MI									
Before Tread	Sample #	1127	836	718	611	461	369	265	153	23
	Year	0	1	2	3	4	5	6	7	8
POS-No MI									
Before Tread	Sample #	427	303	214	168	133	97	49	20	2
	Year	0	1	2	3	4	5	6	7	8
NEG TREAD									
MI Before	Sample #	92	70	56	43	33	24	13	4
Tread	Year	0	1	2	3	4	5	6	7
POS TREAD									
MI Before	Sample #	231	139	88	62	38	24	9	5
Tread	Year	0	1	2	3	4	5	6	7

Figure 2   The incidence of all coronary events in the negative and positive ST responders who had not had a previous infarction is compared with the negative and positive responders who had a previous myocardial infarction. (From Ellestad MH, Wan MKC. Circulation 1975; 51:363, with permission from the American Heart Association.)

tic indicators in this study, the authors concluded that the positive exercise electrocardiogram was an *independent* risk predictor. In a subsequent letter to the editor of the *New England Journal of Medicine* [5], these results were criticized on a cost-benefit basis since it required exercise testing in over 10,000 healthy individuals to produce 135 persons (1.2%) with a positive test, of whom only 21 or (19%) had coronary events over a 5-year period. In their reply, Giagnoni et al. drew attention to the fact that they were not advocating mass screening but rather suggested confining exercise testing to males over 45 with "high levels" of conventional risk factors. This is also my approach. The two most recent studies of this type are the MRFIT study [6] and the Lipid Research Clinics Mortality Follow-Up Study [7]. In the former, involving over 6000 men, a positive exercise test was associated with nearly a fourfold (3.80) risk of death for coronary heart disease (Table 3) during a 7-year follow-up period. In the latter, involving over 3000 men, a positive exercise test was associated with a cumulative mortality of 11.9% over 8.1 years mean follow-up time, versus 1.2% over 8.6 years for men with a negative test. This occurred despite similar levels of serum cholesterol in both groups (Fig. 3). In contrast to these studies, McHenry et al. [8] have reported that ST segment depression in asymptomatic policemen predicts an increased incidence of angina as the initial coronary event, but not infarction or death. A more recent study of police officers by Camp et al. [9] found *all* cardiac events to be increased in positive responders. The importance of serial exercise testing has been nicely demonstrated by Josephson et al. [10] in their asymptomatic cohort from the Baltimore Longitudinal Aging Study. Conversion from a normal to an abnormal ST segment response carried the same risk of future cardiac events as an initially abnormal response did (Fig. 4). Central to all these studies is the importance of the study population. When the clinical yield is contrasted to the cost of exercise testing in low-risk asymptomatic adults, the "survival benefit" (i.e., those patients referred for coronary bypass surgery on the basis of screening) is low and it is also a costly screening procedure, according to a recent Canadian study [11].

Exercise-induced ventricular premature beats, as opposed to ST segment depression or duration of exercise, do not appear to be reliable predictors of cardiac events in asymptomatic persons.

II. EXERCISE TESTS AS INDICATORS OF ASYMPTOMATIC CORONARY ARTERY DISEASE

In my opinion, what is overlooked in the epidemiological studies cited is that the abnormal ST segment response may be more than merely a risk factor that *predicts* disease. An abnormal response may instead be an *indicator* that latent

Table 3 Number and Rate of Coronary Heart Disease Deaths (per 1000 person-years of risk), Crude Relative Risk, and Cox Adjusted Relative Risk[a] by the Presence of Exercise Electrocardiographic Abnormalities for Multiple Risk Factor Intervention Trial Usual Care Men

| | Exercise ECG | | | | | |
| | Normal | | Abnormal | | | Cox adjusted relative risk |
Endpoint	No.	Rate/ 1000	No.	Rate/ 1000	Relative risk	
CHD death	73	2.0	38	7.61	3.80**	3.45*
CVD death	90	2.48	40	8.02	3.25**	2.99**
Non-CVD death	101	2.78	5	1.00	0.36*	0.35*
All deaths	191	5.25	45	9.02	1.72**	1.61**
Angina	632	18.34	132	28.26	1.55**	1.58**
Nonfatal MI by serial ECG change	129	3.53	18	3.54	1.04	0.93
Definite clinical MI	183	5.03	31	6.21	1.25	1.17
CHD death, serial ECG change or definite clinical MI	356	9.79	85	17.04	1.76**	1.67**

*$p < 0.05$.
**$p < 0.01$.
[a] Adjusted for age, diastolic pressure, serum cholesterol, and number of cigarettes smoked daily.
CHD = coronary heart disease; CVD = cardiovascular disease; ECG = electrocardiogram; MI = myocardial infarction.
Source: Rautaharju PM, Prineas RJ, Eifler WJ, Furberg CD, Neaton JF, Crow RS, Stamler J, Cutler JA. J Am Coll Cardiol 1986; 8:1.

disease is already present. To confirm this hypothesis, it would be necessary to submit positive responders to coronary arteriography (i.e., "case finding"). However, the frequency of false-positive responses in an asymptomatic population is high, based on low disease prevalence (i.e., Bayes' theorem) [12], discussed at length in Chapter 10. For example, Erikssen et al. [13], in their studies of Norwegian factory workers, selected 115 men out of a cohort of 2014 presumably healthy men based on a positive exercise test. Of the 115, 105 underwent coronary angiography but only 69 had significant disease (75% stenosis). In Froelicher's study of U.S. Air Force personnel [14], 1390 men were exercised and 135 had abnormal tests. Only 35 (25.4%) had significant coronary artery disease. When Hopkirk et al. [15] added more study subjects to Froelicher's original group and then investigated the predictive value of exer-

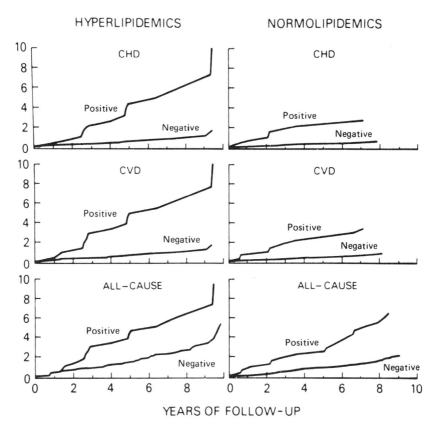

Figure 3 Age-adjusted life table curves for men with positive and negative exercise tests within the hyperlipidemic (left) and normolipidemic (right) subpopulations. These six pairs of curves were generated from six separate proportional-hazards models, each containing age as a continuous variable and exercise test outcome as a categorical variable. (From Gordon DJ, Ekelund LG, Karon JM, Probstfield JL, Rubenstein C, Sheffield LT, Weissfeld L. Circulation 1986; 74:252.)

cise duration plus persistence of ST depression plus the depth of ST depression, they achieved almost 90% predictive accuracy for coronary artery disease, and a predictive value only slightly less than that for multivessel disease (84%). The three test variables (i.e., those with the highest "likelihood ratio") were 3 mm or more of ST segment depression, persistence of ST depression 5 min after exercise, and total duration of exercise of less than 10 min. The combination of

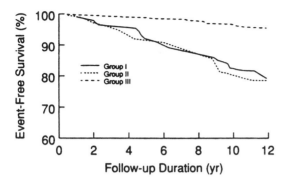

Figure 4 Graphic actuarial analysis of event-free survival comparing groups 1, 2, and 3 using Cox's proportional hazards model to adjust for standard coronary risk factors. Survival curves for groups 1 (abnormal response) and 2 (normal converting to abnormal response) are similar but lie significantly below that of group 3 (normal response) ($n = 726$, $z = 5.78$; $p = <0.0001$). (From Josephson RA, Shefrin E, Lakatta EG, Brant LJ, Fleg JL. Circulation 1990; 81:20. Reproduced with permission of American Heart Association.)

any two of these three exercise risk predictors plus one of the conventional risk factors yielded the predictive value noted earlier.

Other investigators [16–18] have also examined the degree of ST depression and its persistence into the recovery period with or without hypotension. They agree that the greater the ischemic change, the more likely asymptomatic or minimally symptomatic patients will have severe disease. For example, in the study by Hamby et al. [18] (Table 4), 27 patients had positive exercise tests. Of the six with an abnormal blood pressure response, five (or 83%) had left main or triple-vessel disease. By contrast, only 9 of the 21 persons (43%) with a normal blood pressure response had this finding on coronary angiography.

Changes in the R wave on the electrocardiogram have also been looked at specifically in studies of U.S. Air Force personnel; 65 men with coronary artery disease and 190 normal subjects formed the study population [19] (Table 5). R-wave amplitude changes were evaluated in bipolar leads X, Y, and Z. Exercise-induced changes in R-wave height (diminution or no change) increased the specificity of detecting coronary artery disease in asymptomatic men over ST segment criteria alone, but the sensitivity was poor and the overall predictive value not enhanced. These results differ from those of Yiannikas et al. [20], who have found that the R-wave response was more helpful than ST segment responses. As noted earlier, Allen et al. [3] also used the R-wave

Table 4   Relation of Exercise Blood Pressure Response to Main Left or Triple-Vessel Coronary Disease, or Both

	Patient group			
	A ($n = 27$)	B ($n = 36$)	C ($n = 57$)	Total ($n = 120$)
Abnormal blood pressure response	6	9	21	36[a]
Left main or triple vessel coronary disease (%)	5 (83%)	8 (89%[a])	17 (81%)	30 (83%)
Normal blood pressure response	21	27	36	84[a]
Main left or triple-vessel coronary disease, or both (%)	9 (43%)	8 (30%[a])	25 (69%)	42 (50%)

[a] $p < 0.01$ (comparison of percent of patients in group B with left main or triple-vessel coronary disease, or both, in the subgroups with abnormal and normal blood pressure responses).
Group A = no angina; Group B = mild angina; Group C = moderate angina.
Source: Hamby RI, Davison ET, Hilsenrath J, Shanies S, Young M, Murphy DH, Hoffman I. J Am Coll Cardiol 1984; 3:1375.

Table 5   Diagnostic Accuracy of Different Criteria in Detecting Different Angiographic Definitions of Coronary Artery Disease [50 or 70% Reduction (R) in Luminal Diameter or Multivessel Disease (MVD[a])]

	Sensitivity (%)			Specificity (%)			Predictive value (%)		
	50 R	70 R	MVD	50 R	70 R	MVD	50 R	70 R	MVD
ST depression R-wave amplitude at stress	—	—	—	—	—	—	25	18	14
↑X	28	28	31	87	86	86	42	30	28
↑Y	32	33	32	81	80	81	37	26	32
↑ΣXY	22	24	26	88	88	88	38	30	34
↓Z	82	97	95	20	5	16	26	2	16

[a] Multivessel disease = coronary disease, defined as 50% reduction of luminal diameter, in two or three major vessels. ↑ = increase; ↓ = decrease. X, Y, and Z refer to X, Y, and Z bipolar leads.
Source: Hopkirk JAC, Uhl CS, Hickman JR, Jr., Fischer J. J Am Coll Cardiol 1984; 3:821.

response in combination with other ECG measurements to improve diagnostic accuracy in asymptomatic men. Heart-rate adjusted indices of ST depression are also being employed for increased accuracy [21].

There are two other settings in which exercise test results are of importance. The first is in detecting silent coronary artery disease in diabetic populations [22–24], and the second is in combination with Holter monitoring. In the latter instance, the exercise test can be used to "calibrate" the Holter [25] and to indicate which patients are most likely to develop out-of-hospital ischemic events [26] (i.e., those with exercise-induced ischemia at less than 6 min of exercise duration) (Fig. 5). Excerise testing results also include other parameters (such as time-to-onset of ST depression, maximal ST depression, etc.) that are useful in predicting presence and duration of ambulatory ischemia in patients with proven coronary artery disease [26,27]. By contrast, a recent Swedish study reported that ischemia on exercise correlated to ambulatory ischemia in males *only* [28], perhaps due to catecholamine responses. A similarity in ischemic threshhold between Holter monitoring and exercise testing was noted by some groups [29], but not all studies report such clear-cut correlations [30]. The Asymptomatic Cardiac Ischemic Pilot (ACIP) Study is one such example where correlation coefficients between the two techniques were not impressive but "odds ratios" for different scenarios could be established (Fig. 6) [31]. A clue to identifying many patients with silent ischemia may be the cutaneous thermal pain threshold which correlates with time-to-exercise–induced angina, according to a recent report [32]. The type of exercise protocol (i.e., gradual onset vs. Bruce) is also important in comparing exercise responses to the results of Holter monitoring [33]. With the Bruce protocol, the severity of myocardial ischemia on the exercise ECG cannot predict the severity of ischemia on the ambulatory ECG during daily activities [34]. Prognostic risk stratification is also enhanced when both procedures are combined (see Chap. 12).

III. CONCLUSIONS

Abnormal exercise test responses in asymptomatic populations not only appear to be reliable *predictors* of future cardiac events, but they also are valuable as *indicators* of occult coronary artery disease. Because of the problem of false-positive responses in an asymptomatic population, stress tests should be considered as screening procedures for coronary artery disease only in those individuals with multiple risk factors and/or family histories of premature coronary

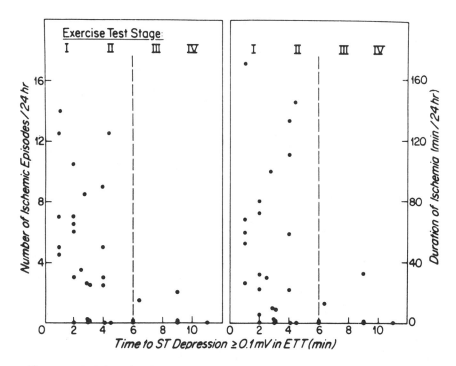

Figure 5   Relationship of time in minutes to onset of significant ST depression (≥0.1 mV) during the Bruce protocol exercise test to degree of ischemic activity out of hospital as detected by ambulatory monitoring, expressed as number of ischemic episodes per 24 h (left) and total duration of ischemia in minutes per 24 h (right) in patients with electrocardiographically positive exercise tests (group I). Stages of the Bruce protocol are listed at the top of each panel. Note that the frequency and duration of ischemia out of hospital declines as the time to ischemia during exercise increases, especially after 6 or more min (end of stage II). (From Campbell S, Barry J, Rocco MB, Nable EG, Mead-Walters K, Rebecca GS, Selwyn AP. Circulation 1986; 74:72.)

artery disease [35]. The abnormal test is more likely to be a "true-positive" response when other abnormalities besides ST changes are present. Despite the impressive results of exercise testing in predicting future cardiac events, its limitations in regard to "false-negative" responders must also be noted. As Coplan and Fuster [36] (among others), have pointed out, in large-scale surveys the *absolute* numbers of persons experiencing subsequent cardiac events is larger in

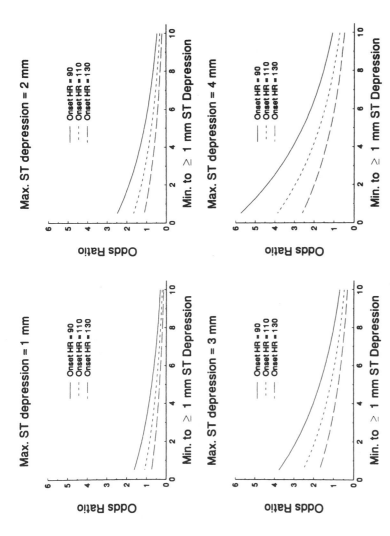

Figure 6 Odds ratios (OR) for ambulatory ECG ischemia are predicted in four different scenarios (i.e., when maximal ST depression on the exercise test is 1, 2, 3, or 4 min). The OR increases in each scenario when the HR at onset of the ST depression is lowest and the time (in min) to initial ST depression the least. (Reproduced with permission from Stone PH, Chaitman BR, McMahon RP, Andrews TC, MacCallum G, Sharaf B, Frishman W, Deanfield JE, Sopko G, Pratt C, Goldberg D, Rogers WJ, Jill J, Proschan M, Pepine CJ, Bourassa MG, Conti R, for the ACIP Investigators. Circulation 1996; 94:1537–1554.

the negative-responder group than in the positive-responder group, even though the event *rate* is higher in the latter group. This is, in part, explained by the larger number of individuals in the negative-response group, some of whom may have noncritical stenoses (at the time of exercise testing) that will be acutely transformed (by plaque rupture, hemorrhages, etc.) into total occlusions [36].

REFERENCES

1. Bruce RA, Hossack KF, DeRouen TA, Hofer V. Enhanced risk assessment for primary coronary heart disease events by maximal exercise testing: 10 years' experience of Seattle Heart Watch. J Am Coll Cardiol 1983; 2:565.
2. Ellestad MH, Wan MKC. Predictive implications of stress testing: Follow-up of 2700 subjects after maximum treadmill stress testing. Circulation 1975; 51:363.
3. Allen WH, Aronow WS, Goodman P, Stinson P. Five-year follow-up of maximal treadmill stress test in asymptomatic men and women. Circulation 1980; 62:522.
4. Giagnoni E, Secchi MB, Wu SC, Morabito A, Oltrona L, Mancarella S, Volpin N, Fossa L, Bettazzi L, Arangio G, Sachero A, Folli G. Prognostic value of exercise EKG testing in asymptomatic normotensive subjects: A prospective matched study. N Engl J Med 1983; 309:1085.
5. Nicklin D, Balaban DJ. Exercise EKG in asymptomatic normotensive subjects. N Engl J Med 1984; 310:853.
6. Rautaharju PM, Prineas RJ, Eifler WJ, Furberg CD, Neaton JD, Crow RS, Stamler J, Cutler JS. Prognostic value of exercise electrocardiogram in men at high risk of future coronary heart disease: Multiple Risk Factor Intervention Trial Experience. J Am Coll Cardiol 1986; 8:1.
7. Gordon DJ, Elelund L-G, Karon JM, Probstfield JL, Rubenstein C, Sheffield LT, Weissfeld L. Predictive value of the exercise test for mortality in North American men: The Lipid Research Clinics Mortality Follow-Up Study. Circulation 1986; 2:252.
8. McHenry PL, O'Donnell J, Norris SN, Jordon JJ. The abnormal exercise electrocardiogram in apparently healthy men: A predictor of angina pectoris as an initial coronary event during long-term follow-up. Circulation 1984; 70:547.
9. Camp AD, Sullivan NA, Vandeevan EA, Kichura GM, Thoma GE, Chaitman BR. Assessment of ACC exercise test guidelines for screening asymptomatic subjects: Experience with police officers (abstr). J Am Coll Cardiol 1991; 17:236A.
10. Josephson RA, Shefrin E, Lakatta EG, Brant LJ, Fleg JL. Can serial exercise testing improve the prediction of coronary events in asymptomatic individuals? Circulation 1990; 81:20.
11. Pilote L, Pashlow F, Thomas JD, Snader CE, Harvey SA, Marwick TH, Lauer MS. Clinical yield and cost of exercise treadmill testing to screen for coronary artery disease in asymptomatic adults. Am J Cardiol 1998; 81:219–224.

12. Detrano R, Yiannikas J, Salcedo EE, Rincon G, Go RT, Williams G, Leatherman J. Bayesian probability analysis: A prospective demonstration of its clinical utility in diagnosing coronary disease. Circulation 1984; 69:541.

13. Erikssen J, Enge I, Forfang R, Storstein D. False positive diagnostic tests of coronary angiographic findings in 105 presumably healthy males. Circulation 1976; 54:371.

14. Froelicher VF, Thompson AJ, Longo MR, Jr., Triebwasser JH, Lancaster MC. Value of exercise testing for screening asymptomatic men for latent coronary artery disease. Prog Cardiovasc Dis 1976; 18:265.

15. Hopkirk JAC, Uhl GS, Hickman JR, Jr., Fischer J, Medina A. Discriminant value of clinical and exercise variables in detecting significant coronary artery disease in asymptomatic men. J Am Coll Cardiol 1984; 3:887.

16. Blumenthal DS, Weiss JL, Mellits ED, Gerstenblith G. The predictive value of a strongly positive stress test in patients with minimal symptoms. Am J Med 1981; 70:1005.

17. Lozner EC, Morganroth J. New criteria to enhance the predictability of coronary artery disease by exercise testing in asymptomatic subjects. Circulation 1977; 56:799.

18. Hamby RI, Dvison ET, Hilsenrath J, Shanies S, Young M, Murphy DH, Hoffman I. Functional and anatomic correlates of markedly abnormal stress tests. J Am Coll Cardiol 1984; 3:1375.

19. Hopkirk JAC, Uhl GS, Hickman JR, Jr., Fischer J. Limitation of exercise-induced R wave amplitude changes in detecting coronary artery disease in asymptomatic men. J Am Coll Cardiol 1984; 3:821.

20. Yiannikas J, Marcomichelakis J, Taggart P, Keely BH, Emanuel R. Analysis of exercise-induced changes in R-wave amplitude in asymptomatic men with electrocardiographic ST-T changes at rest. Am J Cardiol 1981; 47:238.

21. Okin PM, Anderson KM, Levy D, Kligfield P. Heart rate adjustment of exercise-induced ST segment depression: Improved risk stratification in the Framingham Offspring Study. Circulation 1991; 83:866.

22. Chipkin SR, Frid D, Alpert JS, Baker SP, Dalen JE, Aronin N. Frequency of painless myocardial ischemia during exercise tolerance testing in patients with and without diabetes mellitus. Am J Cardiol 1987; 59:61.

23. Rubler S, Gerber D, Reitano J, Chokshi V, Fisher VJ. Predictive value of clinical and exercise variables for detection of coronary artery disease in men with diabetes mellitus. Am J Cardiol 1987; 59:1310.

24. Caracciolo EA, Chaitman BR, Forman SA, Stone PH, Bourassa MG, Sopko G, Geller NL, Conti CR, for the ACIP Investigators. Diabetics with coronary disease have a prevalence of asymptomatic ischemia during exercise treadmill monitoring similar to that of nondiabetic patients. Circulation 1996; 93:2097–2105.

25. Tzivoni D, Benhorin J, Gavish A, Stern S. Holter recording during treadmill testing in assessing myocardial ischemic changes. Am J Cardiol. 1985; 55:1200.

26. Campbell S, Barry J, Rocco MB, Nabel EG, Mead-Walters K, Rebecca GS, Sel-

wyn AP. Features of the exercise test that reflect the activity of ischemic heart disease out of hospital. Circulation 1986; 1:72.

27. Paul SD, Orav EJ, Gleason RE, Nesto RW. Use of exercise test parameters to predict presence and duration of ambulatory ischemia in patients with coronary artery disease. Am J Cardiol 1994; 74:991–996.

28. Forslund L, Hjemdahl P, Held C, Bjorkander I, Eriksson SV, Rehnqvist N. Ischaemia during exercise and ambulatory monitoring in patients with stable angina pectoris and healthy controls. Eur Heart J 1998; 19:578–587.

29. Krittayaphong R, Biles PL, Christy CG, Sheps DS. Association between angina pectoris and ischemic indexes during exercise testing and ambulatory monitoring. Am J Cardiol 1996; 78:266–270.

30. Benhorin J, Pinsker G, Moriel M, Gavish A, Tzivoni D, Stern S. Ischemic threshold during two exercise testing protocols and during ambulatory electrocardiographic monitoring. J Am Cardiol 1993; 22:671–677.

31. Stone PH, Chaitman BR, McMahon RP, Andrews TC, MacCallum G, Sharaf B, Frishman W, Deanfield JE, Sopko G, Pratt C, Goldberg D, Rogers WJ, Jill J, Proschan M, Pepine CJ, Bourassa MG, Conti R, for the ACIP Investigators. Asymptomatic Cardiac Ischemia Pilot (ACIP) Study. Relationship between exercise-induced and ambulatory ischemia in patients with stable coronary disease. Circulation 1996; 94:1537–1554.

32. Sheps DS, McMahon RP, Light KC, Maixner W, Pepine CJ, Cohen JD, Goldberg AD, Bonsall R, Carney R, Stone PH, Sheffield D, Kaufmann PG and the PIMI Investigators. Low hot pain threshold predicts shorter time to exercise-induced angina: results from the psychophysiological investigations of myocardial ischemia (PIMI) Study. J Am Coll Cardiol 1999; 33:1855–1862.

33. Panza JA, Quyyumi AA, Diodati JG, Callahan TS, Epstein SE. Prediction of the frequency and duration of ambulatory myocardial ischemia in patients with stable coronary artery disease by determination of the ischemic threshold from exercise testing: Importance of the exercise protocol. J Am Coll Cardiol 1991; 17:657.

34. Benhorin J, Moriel M, Gavish A, Medina A, Banai S, Shapira M, Stern S, Tzivoni D. Usefulness of severity of myocardial ischemia on exercise testing in predicting the severity of myocardial ischemia during daily activities. Am J Cardiol 1991; 68:176.

35. Sox HC, Littenberg B, Garber AM. The role of exercise testing in screening for coronary artery disease. Ann Intern Med 1989; 110:456.

36. Coplan NL, Fuster V. Limitations of the exercise test as a screen for acute cardiac events in asymptomatic patients. Am Heart J 1990; 119:987.

10
Combining the Exercise Test with Other Procedures

In patients with angina or prior myocardial infarctions, the positive but painless exercise test can often stand alone as a true marker of silent ischemia. But this is not true in asymptomatic populations that are the individuals this chapter is most concerned with. In these persons we usually combine the exercise test with other procedures in order to increase the reliability of detecting occult coronary artery disease. This is necessary because of the frequency of false-positive test responses, which is a function of Bayes' theorem. This theorem was alluded to in Chapter 9, but several points deserve further emphasis.

I. BAYES' THEOREM

Bayes' theorem states that test results cannot be adequately interpreted without knowing the prevalence of the disease in the population under study. This is called the pretest likelihood (or prior probability) of disease, as opposed to the post-test likelihood (or posterior probability). Definitions and equations for these terms are as follows:

Pretest likelihood (prior probability) is defined as the probability of disease in a subject to be tested

$$= \frac{\text{number of patients with disease in the test population}}{\text{total number of patients in the test population}} \quad (1)$$

Post-test likelihood (posterior probability) is defined as the probability of disease in a subject showing a given test result

$$= \frac{\text{number of patients with disease showing a given test result}}{\text{total number of subjects showing the test result}} \quad (2)$$

Bayes' theorem helps to explain the well-known observation that a small proportion of normal persons will have a "false-positive" response (i.e., they will have an abnormal test response but will prove to be normal on more exact study). A good example is an abnormal exercise test response that is suggestive of coronary artery disease in a person who subsequently undergoes coronary angiography and is found to have normal coronary arteries. In short, the predictive value of any less-than-perfect test, such as the exercise stress test, is reduced to an extent that is related in part to the fraction of normal persons in the study population [1].

Epstein [2] gives two examples to illustrate this point. Key terms are sensitivity, specificity, and predictive value. These are defined as follows with appropriate equations also provided:

Sensitivity is defined as the probability a patient with disease will have a given test result

$$= \frac{\text{number of patients with disease with a given test result}}{\text{total number of diseased subjects tested}} \quad (3)$$

Specificity is defined as the probability a patient with disease will have a given test result

$$= \frac{\text{number of patients without disease without a given test result}}{\text{total number of disease-free subjects tested}} \quad (4)$$

Predictive value of a positive test is defined as the probability that a patient has disease, given a positive test outcome

$$= \frac{\text{number of patients with disease}}{\text{total number of patients with a positive test}} \qquad (5)$$

Predictive value of a negative test is defined as the probability that a patient does not have disease, given a negative test outcome

$$= \frac{\text{number of subjects without disease}}{\text{total number of subjects with a negative test}} \qquad (6)$$

Assuming exercise tests have a sensitivity of 75% and a specificity of 85%, what are the chances that a positive test in any *asymptomatic* person (with a 3% pretest likelihood of coronary artery disease) truly indicates coronary artery disease? The answer is that the positive test's predictive value (or post-test likelihood) of disease being present is 14%. By contrast, the same positive test result in a person *with angina* (and thus a 90% pretest likelihood of coronary artery disease) yields a 98% post-test likelihood. The predictive value of a negative test is inverse to that of a positive test. The complete spectrum of pre- and post-test likelihoods of the exercise test predicting coronary artery disease is depicted in Figure 1. The post-test likelihoods are highest in those individuals with a high pretest likelihood and vice versa. The low predictive value in asymptomatic subjects had led investigators to search for other ways of increasing the post-test likelihood. One way is to construct a "family" of ST segment depression curves as in Figure 2. We now no longer look upon the exercise test as merely providing a "yes or no" statement regarding the presence of coronary artery disease, but as providing a continuum of risk based on different probability estimates. A "very positive" test (i.e., one with more than 2.5 mm of ST depression) greatly increases the post-test likelihood of coronary artery disease.

II. ADDING OTHER PROCEDURES INCREASES POST-TEST LIKELIHOOD

When *conventional risk factors* are taken into consideration, a high-risk subgroup can be identified in which a positive exercise test has more validity than in a low-risk group. Several groups have used data from the *Coronary Risk Handbook* based on the Framingham Study to provide relevant data. As seen in Figure 3, a 55-year-old man with a cholesterol level of 350 mg% and a systolic blood pressure of 195 mmHg would have a 20% pretest risk of coronary artery

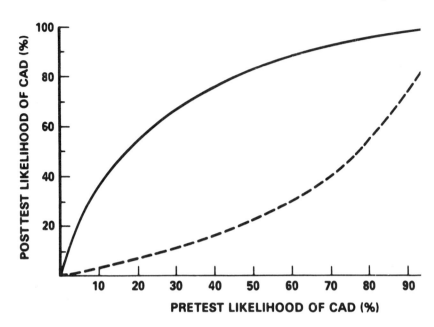

Figure 1 Influence of pretest likelihood of coronary artery disease (CAD) on the post-test likelihood of coronary artery disease. ———— = positive test (sensitivity 75%); – – – = negative test (specificity 85%). (From Epstein SE. Am J Cardiol 1980; 46:491.)

disease. With a positive exercise test, post-test likelihood could increase to 50 to 90% depending on the degree of ST segment depression.

When a second independent test is employed, the post-test likelihood from the exercise test becomes the pretest likelihood for the second test. An example is the demonstration of *coronary artery calcification* by fluoroscopy, as depicted by Diamond and Forrester [3] in Figure 4. This particular observation is based partly on the work of Langou et al. [4], who have shown that the presence of coronary artery calcification is a powerful predictor of coronary artery disease in asymptomatic men with a positive exercise test. Langou et al. [4] screened 120 middle-aged males free of clinical heart disease. Of the original group, 108 completed the submaximal exercise protocol by achieving at least 90% of their age-predicted maximal heart rate; these subjects made up the study population. Sixteen subjects had a positive exercise test; 13 (81%) also had at least one calcified artery on fluoroscopy. By contrast, only 13 (35%) of the 37 subjects with coronary artery calcification had a positive exercise test. Cardiac catheterization was performed in the 13 men with both a positive exercise test and coronary calcification. As depicted in Table 1, one subject had

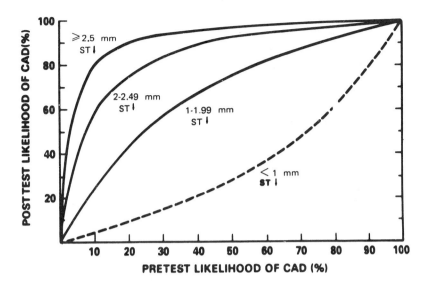

Figure 2 Family of ST segment depression curves (based on data derived from Ref. 3 and likelihood of coronary artery disease (CAD). ST↓ segment depression. (From Epstein SE. Am J Cardiol 1980; 46:491.)

<50% luminal stenosis; all the rest had at least 75% luminal stenosis in one vessel with five persons having two-vessel disease and three having three-vessel disease. Thus, the predictive accuracy obtained by combining both noninvasive tests was 92%. (Data on combining ultrafast CT scanning and exercise testing is still limited.)

The influence of other serial tests besides cardiac fluoroscopy on posttest likelihood has also been studied. Diamond et al. [5] evaluated other noninvasive tests including stress thallium-201 scintigraphy, used for assessment of exercise-induced regional myocardial hypoperfusion. The greater the number of abnormal responses observed in a given patient, the greater the predictive accuracy for coronary artery disease and especially multivessel disease. Of the 974 patients studied in this manner, 278 (29%) were asymptomatic.

Epstein [2] also considered serial testing with radionuclide procedures since they have a higher predictive value than the exercise ECG alone. He reasoned that the combination of a positive exercise ECG and either an abnormal thallium perfusion scan or radionuclide ventriculogram would markedly increase the predictive value of the exercise test (Fig. 5), although he cautioned that sensitivity and specificity of these tests in asymptomatic persons might well be different from that in symptomatic patients. (In his more recent com-

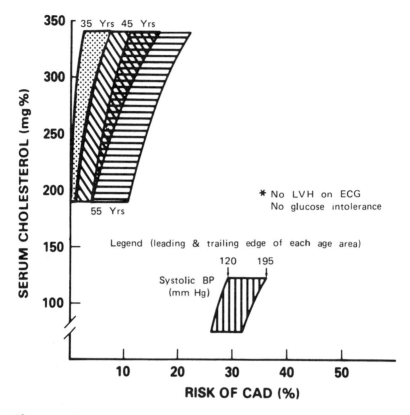

Figure 3 Effect of age, serum cholesterol, and blood pressure (BP) on risk of coronary artery disease (CAD) in nonsmoking men 35 to 55 years of age. (The graph is based on data derived from the Framingham study, in which the cholesterol values were obtained using the Abell–Kendall method. Most direct and automated cholesterol determinations give values 5 to 15% above that given in this graph.) ECG = electrocardiogram; LVH = left ventricular hypertrophy. (From Epstein SE. Am J Cardiol 1980; 46:491.)

munications, he continues to be cautious about the value of screening protocols in asymptomatic populations [6,7].) The attractiveness of the radionuclide procedures has been reviewed by Rozanski and Berman [8] and is based on several studies of asymptomatic persons. For example, Caralis et al. [9] found that 22 persons out of 3496 developed 2 mm or more ST segment depression on exercise testing. Of the 22 persons, 15 agreed to undergo thallium-201 exercise scintigrams: 10 were abnormal. Nolewaijka et al. [10] found less promising

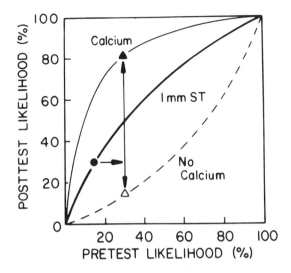

Figure 4 Influence of serial tests on post-test likelihood. The closed circle represents a patient with a pretest likelihood of 15% (*x* axis) and a 1.0-mm depression of the ST segment after a stress test (heavy solid line). The resultant post-test likelihood is 27% (*y* axis). If cardiac fluoroscopy showed calcification of one coronary vessel (light solid line), the resultant post-test likelihood would rise (↑) to 79% (▲). If no calcification was observed (dashed line), the likelihood would fall (↓) to 14% (△). Note that the post-test likelihood from the first test becomes the pretest likelihood of the second test (horizontal arrow). (From Diamond GA, Forrester JS. N Engl J Med 1979; 300:1350.)

Table 1 Predictive Accuracy of Coronary Artery Calcification at Fluoroscopy and Abnormal Exercise Stress Test

	No. pts.	Significant CAD	CAD
Coronary calcification			
+			
abnormal exercise test	13	12	13
Predictive accuracy		92%	100%

Source: Langou RA, Huang EK, Kelley MJ, Cohen LS. Circulation 1980; 62:1196.

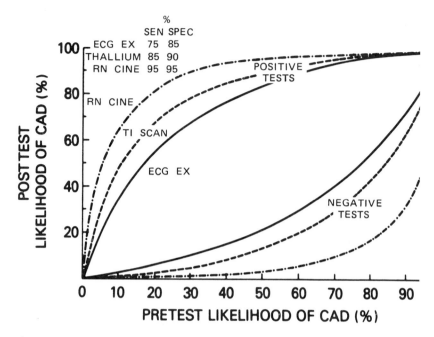

Figure 5 Probability of coronary artery disease (CAD). Comparison of electrocardiographic exercise testing (ECG EX), thallium perfusion scanning (TI SCAN), and radionuclide cineangiography (RN CINE). [Sensitivity (SEN) and specificity (SPEC) values are approximations derived from published series.] (From Epstein SE. Am J Cardiol 1980; 46:491.

results in their study of 58 asymptomatic men studied. Of the five men with abnormal thallium scans, subsequent coronary arteriography in three was normal. Guiney et al. [11] had similar results in their study of 35 patients. Uhl et al. [12] studied 191 airmen with abnormal exercise ECGs. Predictive value of the ECG was 21%, compared to 75% on scintigraphy. They felt the thallium test was a good second-line screening procedure. They also compared the thallium-201 myocardial scintigram to the radionuclide ventriculogram; 32 airmen with abnormal exercise ECGs had both thallium scintigrams and radionuclide ventriculograms. Thirteen patients had angiographically documented coronary artery disease; 12 had abnormal thallium scans; 11 had reduced ejection fractions at maximal exercise. Table 2 compares the sensitivity and specificity of the two procedures.

Table 2 Comparison of Thallium Scintigraphy and Radionuclide Angiography

	Thallium 201		Ejection fraction		Wall motion		Ejection fraction + wall motion
	Normal	Abnormal	Normal	Abnormal	Normal	Abnormal	Abnormal
Normal	18	1	16	3	18	1	1
Coronary artery disease	1	12	2	11	5	8	7
Sensitivity	92%		85%		62%		
Specificity	95%		85%		95%		

Source: Uhl GG, Kay TN, Hickman JR. Jr. J Cardiac Rehabil 1982; 2:118.

On the basis of these observations, serial testing procedures have been advocated for use in U.S. Air Force personnel, as described by Uhl and Froelicher [13] and recently updated by Schwartz et al. [14]. After initial history, physical examination, and resting ECG are performed, a fasting biochemical profile is obtained, and a risk factor index calculated based on Framingham data. Men with positive exercise tests then undergo cardiac fluoroscopy and thallium perfusion scintigraphy before being considered for cardiac catheterization. These authors have stressed the importance of lipid screening, citing the U.S. Air Force studies described in Chapter 7, in which the ratio of total cholesterol to high-density lipoprotein (HDL) cholesterol was a useful predictor of disease. Only 42 (9.5%) of 440 men with abnormal exercise test had a ratio greater than 6.0; by contrast, 87% of those with coronary artery disease had this finding for an odds ratio of 172 to 1 [15]. The U.S. Army also has a similar cardiovascular screening program [16] (Table 3).

At the Johns Hopkins Hospital, serial testing procedures are used to identify high-risk subgroups in families with premature coronary artery disease. Hypertension and hyperlipidemia in asymptomatic siblings were strongly correlated with positive stress thallium tests. In one subgroup, for example, men over the age of 40 with a systolic blood pressure greater than 150 mmHg had an 82% prevalence of positive stress tests [17]. In this preliminary report, coronary arteriographic findings were not presented, but 2-year follow-up has shown a 6% frequency of subsequent myocardial infarction [18]. In another study (the Baltimore Longitudinal Aging Study) from that same institution,

Table 3   Criteria for Primary Cardiovascular Screen Failure
in the U.S. Army Over-Forty Program[a]

Framingham risk index of 5% or greater
Abnormal cardiovascular history or examination
Electrocardiogram abnormality
(LVH, interventricular conduction defects, ST-T wave
changes. etc.)
Fasting blood sugar ≥ 115 mg/dL

[a] Any one abnormality requires secondary screening.
LVH = left ventricular hypertrophy.
Source: Zoltick JM, McAllister HA, Bedynek JL, Jr. J Cardiac Rehabil
1984; 4:530.

Fleg et al. [19] have demonstrated the value of combined exercise-ECG abnormalities and exercise-thallium scintigraphic defects in diagnosing silent
ischemia in asymptomatic populations as well as in determining prognosis (see
Chap. 12). Using the same protocol, Blumenthal et al. [20] continued their evaluation of siblings of patients with premature coronary artery disease cited earlier [17,18]. The percentage of clinical abnormalities in different age groups
according to gender is depicted in Figure 6 and the prognostic implications of
these findings in Figure 7. In an unrelated study in a group of asymptomatic
high-risk men with normal stress tests, positron emission tomography allowed
early detection of abnormal coronary flow reserve [21]. It should also be noted
that even though exercise was the main "stressor" in these randomized studies,
several investigators have assessed the value of comparing or adding mental
(psychological) stress to their exercise protocols with interesting results (e.g.,
not only is there a heterogeneity of responses with different stresses [22], but
combing the two tests leads to more marked ischemia [23].)

The radionuclide ventriculogram can also be used to detect silent
ischemia, although as noted earlier in this chapter (and discussed in more detail
in Chaps. 4 and 5) radionuclide ventriculography has been used mostly in
symptomatic populations, as in the study by Quyyumi et al. comparing it to
ambulatory electrocardiography [24].

As noted in preceding chapters, diabetic populations show an especially
high prevalence of exercise-induced silent ischemia. This is true not only for
ECG findings, but also thallium defects [25]. Other studies involving thallium
scintigraphy have been reported in asymptomatic postinfarction patients; this
avoids problems in interpreting ST depression which may be artificial ("recip-

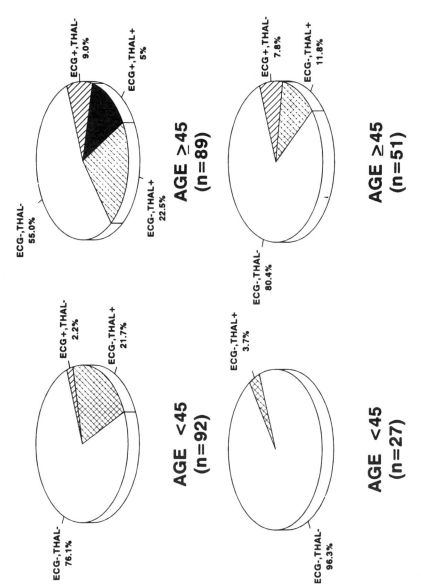

Figure 6 Exercise ECG and thallium results for male siblings (upper graphs) and female siblings (lower graphs) categorized by age. (Reproduced with permission from Blumenthal RS, Becker DM, Moy TF, Coresh J, Wilder LB, Becker LC. Circulation 1996; 93:915–923.)

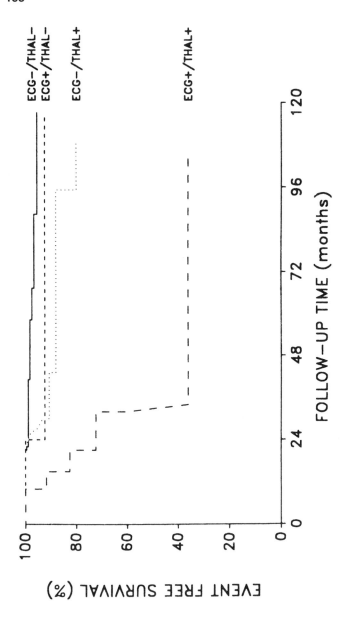

Figure 7 Kaplan–Meier survival curves for each combination of exercise test results (normal ECG and thallium scan, only ECG abnormal, only thallium scan abnormal, or both ECG and thallium scan abnormal). Curves are drawn until the end of follow-up for each group. (Reproduced with permission from Blumenthal RS, Becker DM, May TF, Coresh J, Wilder LB, Becker LC. Circulation 1996; 93:915–923.)

rocal changes"). Patients who demonstrate *both* silent and painful myocardial ischemia also are evaluated with radionuclide exercise tests. These can be performed with either thallium or the newest radionuclide, sestamibi. The results of these tests provide data for and against the argument that silent ischemia is—or is not—as "severe" as painful ischemia [26–28] discussed in Chapter 4. The correlation between ambulatory ECG monitoring and nuclear stress tests such as those cited above is often not as striking as one might have theorized [29].

III. PHARMACOLOGICAL STRESS TESTS

It is not always possible to perform exercise testing. Because of peripheral vascular disease or other problems, some individuals are unable to do treadmill or bicycle tests. The intravenous administration of dipyridamole, adenosine, or dobutamine has been used in such individuals both to detect ischemic heart disease (via perfusion defects) and obtain prognostic information, such as in the study by Younis et al. [30] and others noted in Chapters 4 and 5. Asymptomatic diabetic subjects with peripheral vascular disease are especially apt to be studied with these techniques, particularly when they are about to undergo surgical procedures [31] (Fig. 8). In most instances, however, pharmacological stress tests are employed in symptomatic patients, whether diabetic or not. Stress echocardiography using either dipyridamole [32] or dobutamine [33] is a relatively new technique that has shown promise in identifying myocardial regions with reduced coronary blood flow in patients with silent ischemia.

IV. CONCLUSIONS

In asymptomatic patients with no prior history of coronary artery disease, non-invasive detection of coronary artery disease is best approached with a variety of procedures that can confirm an abnormal stress test, since the next step—usually cardiac catheterization—should only be performed when there is a very high suspicion that latent coronary atherosclerosis is present. No one—not even master athletes—are above suspicion for this phenomenon, especially those individuals with risk factors [34].

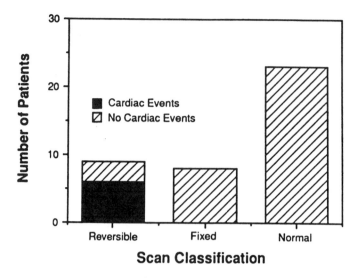

Figure 8 Among 40 diabetic patients undergoing evaluation for renal transplantation, preoperative and postoperative cardiac events occurred only in those with reversible defects on dipyridamole thallium testing. (From Camp AD, Garvin PJ, Hoff JJ, Marsh J, Byers SL, Chaitman BR. Am J Cardiol 1990; 65:1459. Reproduced with permission.)

REFERENCES

1. Rifkin RD, Hood WB, Jr. Bayesian analysis of electrocardiographic exercise stress testing. N Engl J Med 1977; 297:681.
2. Epstein SE. Implications of probability analysis on the strategy used for noninvasive detection of coronary artery disease: Role of single or combined use of exercise electrocardiographic testing, radionuclide cineangiography and myocardial perfusion imaging. Am J Cardiol 1980; 46:491.
3. Diamond GA, Forrester JS. Analysis of probability as an aid in the clinical diagnosis of coronary artery disease. N Engl J Med 1979; 300:1350.
4. Langou RA, Huang EK, Keeley MJ, Cohen LS. Predictive accuracy of coronary artery disease in asymptomatic men. Circulation 1980; 62:1196.
5. Diamond GA, Staniloff HM, Forrester JS, Pollack BH, Swan HJC. Computer-assisted diagnosis in the noninvasive evaluation of patients with suspected coronary artery disease. J Am Coll Cardiol 1983; 1:444.
6. Epstein SE, Quyyumi AA, Bonow RO. Myocardial ischemia—silent or symptomatic. N Engl J Med 1988; 318:1038.

7. Epstein SE, Quyyumi AA, Bonow RO. Sudden cardiac death without warning: Possible mechanisms and implications for screening asymptomatic populations. N Engl J Med 1989; 321:320.

8. Rozanski A, Berman DS. Silent myocardial ischemia. I. Pathophysiology, frequency of occurrence, and approaches toward detection. Am Heart J 1987; 114:615.

9. Caralis DG, Bailey I, Kennedy HL, Pitt B. Thallium-201 myocardial imaging in evaluation of asymptomatic individuals with ischaemic ST segment depression on exercise electrocardiogram. Br Heart J 1979; 42:452.

10. Nolewaijka AJ, Kostuk WJ, Howard J, et al. Thallium stress myocardial imaging: An evaluation of fifty-eight asymptomatic males. Clin Cardiol 1981; 4:135.

11. Guiney TE, Pohost GM, McKusick KA, Beller GA. Differentiation of false- from true-positive ECG responses to exercise stress by thallium-201 perfusion imaging. Chest 1981; 80:1.

12. Uhl GS, Kay TN, Hickman JR, Jr. Comparison of exercise radionuclide angiography and thallium perfusion imaging in detecting coronary artery disease in asymptomatic men. J Cardiac Rehabil 1982; 2:118.

13. Uhl GS, Froelicher V. Screening for asymptomatic coronary artery disease. J Am Coll Cardiol 1983; 1:946.

14. Schwartz RS, Jackson WG, Cello PV, Hickman JR. Exercise thallium-201 scintigraphy for detecting coronary artery disease in asymptomatic young men (abstr). J Am Coll Cardiol 1988; 11:80A.

15. Uhl GS, Troxler RG, Hickman JR, Jr., Clark D. Relation between high density lipoprotein cholesterol and coronary artery disease in asymptomatic men. Am J Cardiol 1981; 48:903.

16. Zoltick JM, McAllister HA, Bedynek JL, Jr. The United States Army Cardiovascular Screening Program. J Cardiac Rehabil 1984; 4:530.

17. Becker DM, Pearson T, Fintel DJ, Levine DM, Becker LC. Risk factors identify high risk subgroups in families with early coronary heart disease (CHD) (abstr). Circulation 1984; 70(suppl II):127.

18. Becker LC, Becker DM, Pearson TA, Fintel DJ, Links J, Frank TL. Screening of asymptomatic siblings of patients with premature coronary artery disease. Circulation 1987; 75(suppl II):14.

19. Fleg JL, Gerstenblith G, Zonderman AB, et al. Prevalence and prognostic significance of exercise-induced silent myocardial ischemia detected by thallium scintigraphy and electrocardiography in asymptomatic volunteers. Circulation 1990; 81:428.

20. Blumenthal RS, Becker DM, Moy TF, Coresh J, Wilder LB, Becker LC. Exercise thallium tomography predicts future clinically manifest coronary heart disease in a high-risk asymptomatic population. Circulation 1996; 93:915–923.

21. Dayanikli F, Grambow D, Muzik O, Mosca L, Rubenfire M, Schwaiger M. Early detection of abnormal coronary flow reserve in asymptomatic men at high risk for coronary artery disease using positron emission tomography. Circulation 1994; 90:808–817.

22. Sheps DS, McMahon RP, Pepine CJ, Stone PH, Goldberg AD, Taylor H, Cohen JD, Becker LC, Chaitman B, Knatterud GL, Kaufman PG. Heterogeneity among cardiac ischemic and anginal responses to exercise, mental stress, and daily life. Am J Cardiol 1998; 21:1–6.

23. Hunziker PR, Gradel C, Muller-Brand J, Buser P, Pfisterer M. Improved myocardial ischemia detection by combined physical and mental stress testing. Am J Cardiol 1998; 82:109–112.

24. Quyyumi AA, Panza JA, Diodati JG, Dilsizian V, Callahan TS, Bonow RO. Relation between left ventricular function at rest and with exercise and silent myocardial ischemia. J Am Coll Cardiol 1992; 19:962.

25. Nesto RW, Phillips RT, Kett KG, Hill T, Perper E, Young E, Leland OS, Jr. Angina and exertional myocardial ischemia in diabetic and nondiabetic patients: Assessment by exercise thallium scintigraphy. Ann Intern Med 1988; 108:170.

26. Klein J, Chao SY, Serman DS, Rozanski A. Is "silent" myocardial ischemia really as severe as symptomatic ischemia? Circulation 1994; 89:1959–1966.

27. Marcassa C, Galli M, Baroffio C, Campini R Pantaleo G. Ischemic burden in silent and painful myocardial ischemia: a quantitative exercise sestamibi tomographic study. J Am Coll Cardiol 1997; 29:948–954.

28. Narins CR, Zareba W, Moss AJ, Goldstein RE, Hall AJ. Clinical implications of silent versus symptomatic exercise-induced myocardial ischemia in patients with stable coronary disease. J Am Coll Cardiol 1997; 29:756–763.

29. Mahmarian JJ, Steingard RM, Forman S, Sharaf BL, Coglianese ME, Miller DD, Pepine CJ, Goldberg AD, Bloom MF, Byers S, Dvorak L, Pratt CM. Relation between ambulatory electrocardiographic monitoring and myocardial perfusion imaging to detect coronary artery disease and myocardial ischemia: An ACIP Ancillary Study. J Am Cardiol 1997; 29:764–769.

30. Younis LT, Byers S, Shaw L, Barth G, Goodgold H, Chaitman BR. Prognostic importance of silent myocardial ischemia detected by intravenous dipyridamole thallium myocardial imaging in asymptomatic patients with coronary artery disease. J Am Coll Cardiol 1989; 14:1635.

31. Camp AD, Garvin PJ, Hoff J, Marsh J, Byers SL, Chaitman BR. Prognostic value of intravenous dipyridamole thallium imaging in patients with diabetes mellitus considered for renal transplantation. Am J Cardiol 1990; 65:1459.

32. Bjoernstad KN, Aakhus S, Lundborn J, Bolz KD, Rokseth R, Skjaerpe T, Hatle L. Digital dipridamole stress echocardiography in silent ischemia after coronary artery bypass grafting and/or after healing of acute myocardial infarction. Am J Cardiol 1993; 72:640–646.

33. Elhendy A, Geleijnse ML, Roelandt JRTC, Cornel JH, van Domburg RT, Fioretti P M. Stress-induced left ventricular dysfunction in silent and symptomatic myocardial ischemia during dobutamine stress test. Am J Cardiol 1995; 75:1112–1115.

34. Katzel LI, Fleg JL, Busby-Whitehead J, Sorkin JD, Becker LC, Lakatta EG, Goldberg AP. Exercise-induced silent myocardial ischemia in master athletes. Am J Cardiol 1998; 81:261–265.

11
Cardiac Catheterization

Despite considerable advances in noninvasive imaging technology, cardiac catheterization (including coronary arteriography and usually left ventriculography) is still the accepted standard for the in vivo diagnosis of coronary artery disease. Indications for performing the procedure are still not uniformly agreed upon [1]. Because of this uncertainty, there is considerable controversy when asymptomatic coronary artery disease is detected in a patient via the noninvasive procedures discussed in Chapters 7 through 10, and coronary arteriography is considered to confirm the diagnosis. This controversy is most marked in totally asymptomatic persons and less so in those who are asymptomatic following a myocardial infarction. In those individuals with episodes of both symptomatic and asymptomatic myocardial ischemia, there is the least amount of controversy.

I.   INDICATIONS FOR CARDIAC CATHETERIZATION IN TOTALLY ASYMPTOMATIC PERSONS

Ambrose [1] concluded that coronary arteriography "appears warranted in patients with objective evidence of significant ischemia at low work loads even though they are asymptomatic or minimally symptomatic. The purpose of catheterization is to identify those patients with significant coronary artery disease, so that appropriate therapy can be instituted if considered necessary." Before proceeding to catheterization, Ambrose emphasizes the need for a confirmatory radionuclide procedure in addition to a positive exercise test. This is in keeping with Conti's philosophy [2], among others, and it is certainly with which I concur. The flow diagram that Conti uses to illustrate the subsequent evaluation of asymptomatic patients with a positive exercise test is depicted in Figure 1. In summary, these authors and myself feel that a positive exercise test should be followed by another independent demonstration of ischemia, such as an abnormal thallium-201 scintigram or radionuclide ventriculogram, or demonstration of coronary artery calcification on fluoroscopy before proceeding to cardiac catheterization, an invasive procedure with small, but definite, associated morbidity and mortality.

Of course, not all physicians agree with this approach. Some "question the justification for the wide case-finding effort of subjective asymptomatic persons to coronary arteriography . . . unless unusual findings suggest an especially poor prognosis" [3]. Others share this reluctance for an aggressive workup [4], while some take a middle-of-the-road position that appears to leave open the possibility of coronary arteriographic study in appropriate patients with abnormal noninvasive tests [5].

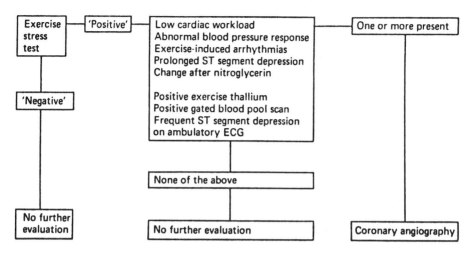

Figure 1 Flow diagram to illustrate one approach to evaluation of asymptomatic patients with a positive stress test. (From Conti CR. Adv Cardiol 1980; 27:181.)

II. INDICATIONS FOR CARDIAC CATHETERIZATION AFTER A MYOCARDIAL INFARCTION

Epstein et al. [7] have proposed a schema to identify patients who should undergo cardiac catheterization after a myocardial infarction (Fig. 2). In addition to patients who are symptomatic with angina or congestive heart failure, they also recommend coronary arteriography in uncomplicated patients with adequate left ventricular function and inducible ischemia (i.e., ST segment depression and/or a fall in radionuclide ejection fraction). This recommendation is based on the adverse short-term prognosis associated with these findings. Veenbrink et al. [8] also used the exercise test response as a guide in their asymptomatic patients.

Mautner and Phillips [9] have a similar approach. They studied 31 patients, none (29%) of whom were found to have triple-vessel disease (Table 1). Chaitman et al. [10] found triple-vessel disease in 8 of 37 patients (22%), while Miller et al. [11] found this degree of obstruction in 38 to 84 patients (45%). Turner et al. [12] studied 117 patients with angiography—61 of whom were asymptomatic (i.e., uncomplicated)—and found triple-vessel disease in

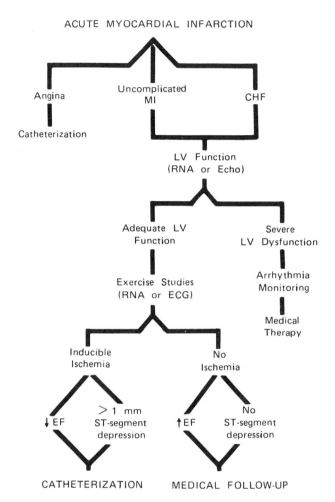

Figure 2 Strategy for identifying patients who should undergo cardiac catheterization after acute myocardial infarction. The strategy is based on clinical assessment, evaluation of left ventricular (LV) function by radionuclide angiography (RNA) or echocardiography, arrhythmia analysis, and stress testing. MI denotes acute myocardial infarction; CHF overt congestive heart failure; and EF ejection fraction. (From Epstein SE, Palmeri ST, Patterson RE. N Engl J Med 1982; 307:1487.)

Table 1 Coronary Arteriographic Findings

Left main disease	0
Left main equivalent	2 (6%)
Left anterior descending stenosis	22 (71%)
Inferior MI[a]	11
Anterior MI	11
Three-vessel disease	9 (29%)
Two-vessel disease	10 (32%)
Single-vessel disease	10 (32%)
Normal	2 (6%)
Coronary artery aneurysms	1
Anomalous circumflex from right coronary artery	1
Absent collateral vessels	10 (32%)

[a] One proximal and nine distal to the first septal perforator.
Source: Mautner RK, Phillips JH. Cardiovasc Diag 1981; 7:1.

14 (29%), but also found left main disease in four (7%). Despite this high frequency of severe disease (36%), Turner et al. did *not* recommend routine coronary arteriography after a myocardial infarction because of the "uncertainty of bypass surgery in prolonging life" in this subgroup of patients.

III. INDICATIONS FOR CARDIAC CATHETERIZATION IN PATIENTS WITH BOTH SYMPTOMATIC AND ASYMPTOMATIC EPISODES OF MYOCARDIAL ISCHEMIA

The prevalence of this type of mixed picture varies from series to series but probably includes most anginal patients. In these patients, the factors that normally determine the decision to perform or not to perform coronary arteriography—refractoriness of symptoms, degree of abnormality of noninvasive tests—continue to be of prime importance. It is my belief, however, that we are rapidly reaching the point where consideration of the *total* number of ischemic episodes (symptomatic and silent) as documented by Holter monitoring will also be a determining factor in recommending both coronary arteriography and more aggressive management.

IV. CORONARY ARTERY DISEASE WITH AND WITHOUT SYMPTOMS: ARE THERE DISTINCTIVE ARTERIOGRAPHIC FEATURES?

One of the more intriguing questions concerning the pathophysiology of silent myocardial ischemia is whether there are any distinctive arteriographic features that help to identify patients with this phenomenon, or with silent myocardial infarction. Accordingly, pertinent data acquired in a number of studies will be reviewed.

Comparisons between *totally asymptomatic* Air Force personnel and angiographically normal persons are provided by Uhl and Froelicher [13]. The distribution of vessel disease in these patients is usually similar to that found in the symptomatic population. For example, Uhl reported that of the 65 men in his study, 32 had one-vessel disease, 17 had two-vessel disease, and 16 had three-vessel disease. In a series of 89 patients with significant left main coronary artery disease, Shawl et al. [14] reported that 10 (11%) were completely asymptomatic. Their clinical characteristics were very similar to the 79 patients with symptomatic disease (Table 2).

What of patients who are *asymptomatic following a myocardial infarction?* The study from the Duke–Harvard Collaborative Coronary Artery Disease Data Bank [15] can be used as a model for this kind of study since most of the patients had experienced a myocardial infarction. The clinical and angiographic findings in the 171 study patients (127 with and 44 without angina) were comparable. As we noted earlier in this chapter, Turner et al. [16], in a study of 92 asymptomatic postmyocardial infarction patients, found a 35% frequency of triple-vessel disease, 31.5% two-vessel disease, and 23% one-vessel disease. Mautner and Phillips [9] found a similar distribution (Table 1). When silent ischemia is clearly diagnosed on the basis of exercise testing, such as in the CASS registry, Weiner et al. [16] have shown no significant differences in prevalence of multivessel disease. Asymptomatic left main disease was present in 1477 of 20,137 (3.6%) of CASS Registry patients [17].

The final group to consider is patients with episodes of *both symptomatic and asymptomatic myocardial ischemia*. In one of the earliest studies, Lindsey and I [18] found multivessel disease in 75% of our patients. This compared to 83% (pNS) in patients who were symptomatic during a positive test. The prevalence of collateralization and low ejection fractions was also similar (Fig. 3). Samek et al. [19] studied 102 patients with anginal histories but without angina on positive exercise test. Thirty-five percent had one-vessel disease, 32% two-vessel disease, and 43% three-vessel disease. Ouyang et al. [20] performed an

Table 2 Clinical Characteristics of Patients with Asymptomatic (ALMD) and Symptomatic (SLMD) Left Main Disease

	ALMD	SLMD
Total group		
Number	10	79
Age (yr)		
Mean	53	52
Range	40–65	32–62
Male/female	10/0	74/5
Risk factors		
Family history of CAD	7	31 (39%)
Hypertension	5	37 (46%)
Smoking[a]	4	69 (81%)
Serum cholesterol (>250 mg/dL)	3	32 (40%)
Diabetes mellitus	0	14 (17%)
Laboratory data		
ECG		
Normal	4	21 (26%)
Abnormal	6	58 (73%)
PVCs	3	1 (1%)
ST-T changes	2	26 (44%)
RBBB	1	1 (1%)
MI	0	28 (48%)
LVH	0	2 (1%)
Chest x-ray		
Cardiomegaly	0	22 (27%)

CAD, coronary artery disease; LVH, left ventricular hypertrophy; MI, myocardial infarction; PVCs, premature ventricular contractions; RBBB, right bundle branch block.
[a] $p < 0.05$.
Source: Shawl FA, Chun PKC, Mutter ML, Slama RD, Donohue DJ, Zajtchuk R, Davis JE. Am Heart J 1989; 117:537.

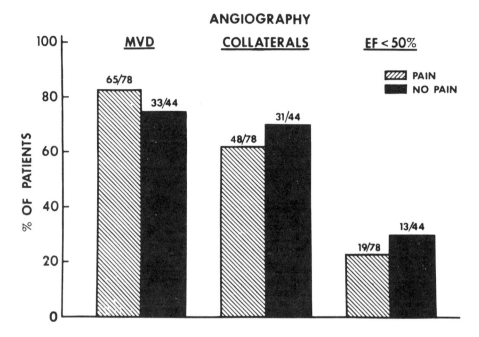

Figure 3   Frequency of multivessel disease (MVD), collateral vessels, and poor ventricular function in patients with and without angina pain. EF = ejection fraction. (From Lindsey HE, Jr, Cohn PF. Am Heart J 1978; 94:441.)

angiographic comparison early after myocardial infarction in 60 consecutive patients with positive exercise tests (38, or 63%, had no pain and 22 had pain). No differences were found (Table 3). This is also the conclusion of a similar study by Falcone et al. and others [21–22]. The ACIP study has observed a high frequency of multivessel coronary disease, severe proximal stenoses, and complex plaques in patients exhibiting asymptomatic ischemia on Holter monitoring [23] (Fig. 4).

Finally, let us consider patients with *silent myocardial infarctions*. Compared to patients with recognized myocardial infarctions, patients with clinically unrecognized myocardial infarctions have a similar extent of coronary artery disease, as determined by Gohlke et al. [24]. This is the same conclusion that Cabin and Roberts [25] reached in their autopsy study, which was discussed at greater length in Chapter 6.

Table 3 Angiographic Characteristics in 60 Patients with Positive Early Post-infarction Exercise Tests[a]

	Silent treadmill ischemia (n = 38)	Symptomatic treadmill ischemia (n = 22)
	n (%)	n (%)
Left main disease	4 (11)	1 (6)
No. of CAs with ≥70% stenosis		
0	1 (3.6)	0 (0)
1	9 (24)	6 (27)
2	17 (45)	6 (27)
3	11 (29)	10 (45)
Totally occluded infarct artery	25 (66)	12 (55)
Coronary thrombus	28 (74)	12 (55)

[a] There is no significant difference between the two groups for any characteristic listed.
CAs = coronary arteries.
Source: Ouyang P, Shapiro EP, Chandra NC, Gottlieb SH, Chew PH, Gottlieb SO. Am J Cardiol 1987; 59:730.

In conclusion, it appears that there are no striking arteriographic differences between coronary artery disease patients with and without angina.

V. CORONARY ARTERIOGRAPHIC ASSESSMENT OF DIABETICS BEING EVALUATED FOR RENAL TRANSPLANTATION

Because atherosclerotic cardiovascular disease is the most common cause of death in diabetic patients with severe renal disease, it has become accepted policy in many hospitals to clarify surgical risk by "screening" diabetic patients with noninvasive tests (see Chaps. 9 and 10) and/or cardiac catheterization. The latter findings are often quite dramatic. For example, Bennett et al. found severe coronary artery disease in all such patients in their study [26], while Weinrauch et al. [27] found severe coronary artery disease in 9 of 21 patients. A simple test—determination of microalbuminuria—may help identify silent ischemia in asymptomatic diabetics [28].

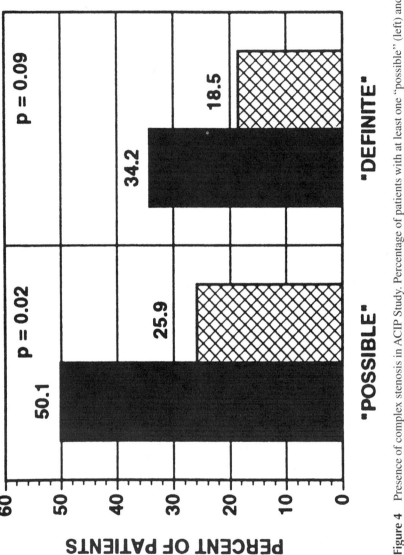

Figure 4 Presence of complex stenosis in ACIP Study. Percentage of patients with at least one "possible" (left) and one "definite" (right) complex plaque for patients with (solid bars) and without (crosshatched bars) AECG ischemia. Reproduced with permission from Sharaf BL, Williams DO, Miele NJ, McMahon RP, Stone PH, Bjerregard P, Davies R, Goldberg AD, Parks M, Pepine CJ, Sopko G, Conti CR. J Am Coll Cardiol 1997; 39:396–402.

VI. CONCLUSIONS

Aside from treatment of asymptomatic persons, there is probably no more controversial area than indications for cardiac catheterization in totally asymptomatic individuals. Patients with positive exercise tests—generally those with early onset of ST changes and hypotension, or those who also have abnormal radionuclide studies—deserve aggressive follow-up with cardiac catheterization. Asymptomatic postinfarction patients with similar findings merit an equally aggressive approach, but this is less of an issue. Results of cardiac catheterization studies do not seem to indicate any particular angiographic patterns in any of the three types of silent ischemia patients when compared to symptomatic persons.

REFERENCES

1. Ambrose JA. Unsettled indications for coronary angiography. J Am Coll Cardiol 1984; 3:1575.
2. Conti CR. Detection and management of the asymptomatic patient with coronary artery disease. Adv Cardiol 1980; 27:181.
3. Selzer A, Cohn K. Asymptomatic coronary artery disease and coronary bypass surgery. Am J Cardiol 1977; 39:614.
4. Rozanski A, Berman DS. Silent myocardial ischemia: II. Prognosis and implications for the clinical assessment of patients with coronary artery disease. Am Heart J 1987; 114:627.
5. Epstein SE, Quyyumi AA, Bonow RO. Myocardial ischemia—Silent or symptomatic. N Engl J Med 1988; 318:1039.
6. Scanlon PJ, Faxon DP, Audet AM, Carabello B, Dehmer GJ, Eagle KA, Legako RD, Leon DF, Murray FA, Nissen SE, Pepine CJ, Watson RM. ACC/AHA Guidelines for Coronary Angiography: A report of the American College of Cardiology/American Heart Association Task Force on Practice Guidelines (Committee on Coronary Angiography) Circulation 1999; 99:2345–2357.
7. Epstein SE, Palmeri ST, Patterson RE. Evaluation of patients after acute myocardial infarction. N Engl J Med 1982; 307:1487.
8. Veenbrink Th WG, Van Der Werf T, Westerhof PW, Robles EO, Meijler FL. Is there an indication for coronary angiography in patients under 60 years of age with no or minimal angina pectoris after a first myocardial infarction? Br Heart J 1985; 53:30.
9. Mautner RK, Phillips JH. Coronary angiography post first myocardial infarction in the asymptomatic or mildly symptomatic patient: Clinical, angiographic, and prospective observations. Cath Cardiovasc Diag 1981; 7:1.

10. Chaitman BR, Waters D, Corbara F, Bourassa M. Predictors of multivessel disease after inferior myocardial infarction. Circulation 1978; 57:1085.
11. Miller R, DeMaria AN, Vismara LA, et al. Chronic stable inferior myocardial infarction: Unsuspected harbinger of high risk proximal left coronary arterial obstruction amenable to surgical revascularization. Am J Cardiol 1977; 39:953.
12. Turner JD, Rogers WJ, Mantle JA, Rackley CE, Russell RO, Jr. Coronary angiography soon after myocardial infarction. Chest 1980; 77:58.
13. Uhl GS, Froelicher V. Screening for asymptomatic coronary artery disease. J Am Coll Cardiol 1983; 1:946.
14. Shawl FA, Chun PKC, Mutter ML, Slama RD, Donohue DJ, Zajtchuk R, Davia JE. Asymptomatic left main coronary artery disease and silent myocardial ischemia. Am Heart J 1989; 117:537.
15. Cohn PF, Harris P, Barry WH, Rosati RA, Rosenbaum P, Waternaux C. Prognostic importance of anginal symptoms in angiographically defined coronary artery disease. Am J Cardiol 1981; 47:233.
16. Weiner DA, Ryan TJ, McCabe CH, Luk S, Chaitman BR, Sheffield LT, Tristani F, Fisher LD. Significance of silent myocardial ischemia during exercise testing in patients with coronary artery disease. Am J Cardiol 1987; 49:725.
17. Taylor HA, Deumite J, Chaitman BR, Davis KB, Killip T, Rogers WJ. Asymptomatic left main coronary artery disease in the Coronary Artery Surgery Study (CASS) Registry. Circulation 1989; 79:1171.
18. Lindsey HE, Cohn PF. "Silent" myocardial ischemia during and after exercise testing in patients with coronary artery disease. Am Heart J 1978; 94:441.
19. Samek L, Beta P, Roskamm H. ST-segment depression during exercise without angina pectoris in postinfarction patients: Angiographic findings and prognostic relevance. In: Rutishauser W, Roskamm H, eds. Silent Myocardial Ischemia. Berlin: Springer-Verlag, 1984:170–175.
20. Ouyang P, Shapiro EP, Chandra NC, Gottlieb SH, Chew PH, Gottlieb SO. An angiographic and functional comparison of patients with silent and symptomatic treadmill ischemia early after myocardial infarction. Am J Cardiol 1987; 59:730.
21. Falcone C, DeServi S, Pom E, Campana C, Scire A, Montemartini C, Specchia G. Clinical significance of exercise-induced silent myocardial ischemia in patients with coronary artery disease. J Am Coll Cardiol 1987; 9:295.
22. Deedwania PC, Carbajal EV. Silent ischemia during daily life is an independent predictor of mortality in stable angina. Circulation 1990; 81:748.
23. Sharaf BL, Williams DO, Miele NJ, McMahon RP, Stone PH, Bjerregaard P, Davies R, Goldberg AD, Parks M, Pepine CJ, Sopko G, Conti CR. A detailed angiographic analysis of patients with ambulatory electrocardiographic ischemia: results from the asymptomatic cardiac ischemia pilot (ACIP) study angiographic core laboratory. J Am Coll Cardiol 1997; 39:396–402.
24. Gohlke H, Peters K, Betz P, Sturzenhofecker P, Steinmann E, Vellguth T, Roskamm H. Angiography in patients with silent myocardial infarction. In: Rutishauser W, Roskamm H, eds. Silent Myocardial Ischemia. Berlin: Springer-Verlag, 1984:138–143.

25. Cabin HS, Roberts WC. Quantitative comparison of extent of coronary narrowing and size of healed myocardial infarct in 33 necropsy patients with clinically unrecognized ("silent") previous acute myocardial infarction. Am J Cardiol 1982; 50:677.

26. Bennett WM, Kloster F, Rosch J, Barry J, Porter GA. Natural history of asymptomatic coronary arteriographic lesions in diabetic patients with end-stage renal disease. Am J Med 1978; 65:779.

27. Weinrauch T, D'Elia JA, Healy RW, Gleason RE, Christlieb AR, Leland OS, Jr. Asymptomatic coronary artery disease: Angiographic assessment of diabetics evaluated for renal transplantation. Circulation 1978; 58:1184.

28. Rutter MK, McComb JM, Brady S, Marshall SM. Silent myocardial ischemia and microalbuminuria in asymptomatic subjects with non-insulin-dependent diabetes mellitus. Am J Cardiol 1999; 83:27–31.

IV

PROGNOSIS IN ASYMPTOMATIC CORONARY ARTERY DISEASE

12
Prognosis in Patients with Silent Myocardial Ischemia

By its very nature, silent myocardial ischemia is a ubiquitous phenomenon; therefore, any discussion of prognosis quickly becomes mired down in confusion if groups of patients are not clearly differentiated. As noted earlier in this book, since 1981 we consider this phenomenon in three types of patients. One group consists of individuals who have never had symptoms (type 1), the second group consists of individuals who are asymptomatic following a myocardial infarction but still manifest ischemia (type 2), and the third group includes individuals who are symptomatic with some of their ischemic episodes but not with others and who may or may not have had a prior infarction (type 3). Type 3 patients can be further divided into patients with chronic versus unstable angina pectoris.

I. PROGNOSIS IN TOTALLY ASYMPTOMATIC INDIVIDUALS

Data in individuals of this type who also have angiographically confirmed disease are especially hard to come by, since physicians are naturally reluctant to submit asymptomatic individuals to a potentially dangerous invasive procedure. One of the few surveys that have provided a large series of subjects is that conducted by the U.S. Air Force School of Aerospace Medicine in San Antonio, Texas. The Air Force survey, commented on earlier in this book, was begun by Froelicher and colleagues in the mid-1970s [1]. Cardiac catheterization was performed on asymptomatic airmen with abnormal treadmill tests, as described in Chapters 5, 9, and 10. Subsequent treadmill or radionuclide studies, or both, performed by Uhl and Froelicher [2] and later by Uhl et al. [3] resulted in a total of 78 asymptomatic airmen with significant coronary artery disease being detected. Along with 12 other airmen with minimal coronary artery disease, this group was followed for several years to evaluate those factors influencing prognosis.

In their 1980 report from the San Antonio survey, Hickman et al. [4] noted that 22 of the 78 airmen with significant disease (more than 50% luminal stenosis) developed overt signs of coronary artery disease (i.e., angina, myocardial infarction, death within a 4 to 90-month follow-up period). The mean time was 57 months and the men ranged in age from 47 to 54 years. Of the 22 with significant coronary artery disease, 16 developed angina at a mean duration of 31.5 months, four sustained a myocardial infarction, and two died suddenly. In addition to the 22, six other men developed symptoms at a later time (mean age 46 months). Of these six, five developed angina and one died suddenly. The authors investigated the influence of the four standard coronary risk factors (cigarette smoking, hyperlipidemia, diabetes, and hypertension) and found that at least three of these risk factors were present in nearly half of the men who had subsequent cardiac events. These provocative findings highlight the importance of risk factors in prognosis of asymptomatic men, as well as in the screening of such populations, as discussed in Part III.

In the smaller series reported by Langou et al. [5] from Yale University, the authors followed their 12 subjects with significant coronary artery disease for 3 years. In that period of time, three men developed angina and one a myocardial infarction, though none died.

The most ambitious of all of these studies was the one performed in Norway by Erikssen and colleagues [6,7]. From a large cohort of men aged 40 to 50 years who underwent a comprehensive cardiovascular screening in 1972 to 1975, 69 were identified as having significant coronary artery disease, 18 with one-vessel disease, 25 with two-vessel disease, and 26 with three-vessel disease. Fifty of the 69 men were unequivocally felt to have asymptomatic coronary artery disease; in the other 19, it was questionable whether mild symptoms were present. After an 8- to 10-year period of following the 50 asymptomatic men (15 of whom had one-vessel disease, 18 two-vessel, and 17 three-vessel), the authors found that three died from cardiac disease and seven had a myocardial infarction (five of which were silent). In addition, as depicted in Figure 1, 16 other men developed angina pectoris. Twenty-four patients had repeat angiograms; 23 of the 24 had progression (56%) (Fig. 2) and 11 underwent coronary bypass surgery. Thus, a total of 28 (56%) of the 50 men either died, had a myocardial infarction, developed angina, or had progression on coronary angiography. (Men with and without these events were of similar age, had similar heart rates and blood pressure.) The total mortality was less than 1%/year, but this may be skewed by the 11 men sent for bypass surgery. Clinical events

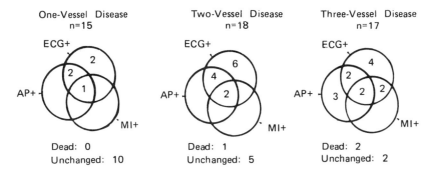

Figure 1 Venn diagrams showing the relation between baseline angiographic findings and coronary artery disease (CAD) events during a mean follow-up of 8½ years in 50 men with asymptomatic CAD. AP = angina pectoris. (From Erikssen J, Thaulow E. In: Rutishauser W, Roskamm H, eds. Silent Myocardial Ischemia. Berlin: Springer-Verlag, 1984:156–164.)

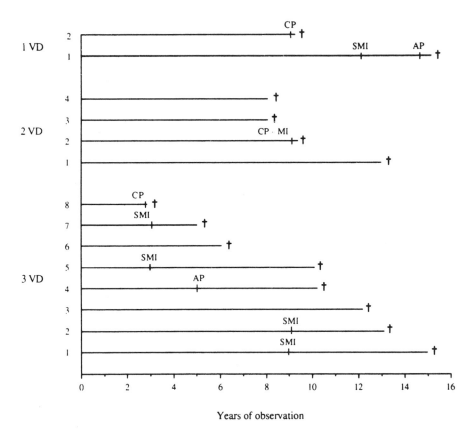

Figure 2 Lifetime curves after first identification of a significant exercise-induced ST depression in 14 asymptomatic men with angiographically proven coronary artery disease who died during the first 15 years of follow-up. AP = clinical angina pectoris; CP = atypical chest pain; MI = clinically evident myocardial infarction; SMI = silent myocardial infarction; 1 VD = 1-vessel disease; 2 VD = 2-vessel disease; 3 VD = 3-vessel disease; + = death. (Reproduced with permission from Thaulow E, Erikssen J, Sandvik L, Erikssen G, Jorgensen L, Cohn PF. Am J Cardiol 1993; 72:629–633.)

were observed mostly in men with multivessel disease. The authors concluded that once they are diagnosed, subjects with asymptomatic coronary artery disease should be followed yearly. In that manner, rapid detection of clinical events is possible and appropriate therapy can be initiated. This is usually conservative, though the authors infer that patients with left main disease—like their symptomatic counterparts—should be offered aggressive management in light of the "malignant" course of the five patients in the study—two dead and three others with angiographic or clinical progression. The importance of close follow-up is emphasized by the most recent report from the Norwegian survey. At the 15-year mark, there were now two deaths in the one-vessel disease subgroup, four in the two-vessel disease subgroup, and eight in the three-vessel disease subgroup [8]. Thus, yearly 3-year mortality was 3% in the latter group—more than that of the other two subgroups combined. As indicated in Figure 2, warning signs such as typical angina often were not present before death [9]. The clinical course of the *surviving* men is depicted in Figures 3, 4, and 5. Again, typical angina was uncommon.

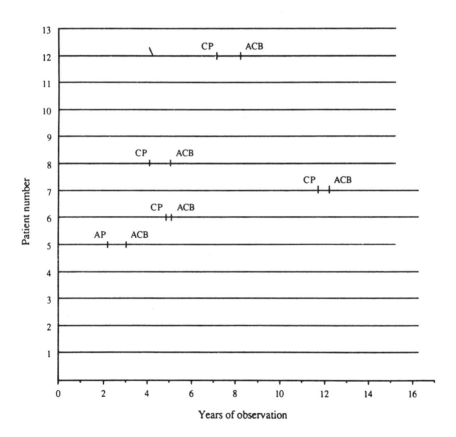

Figure 3 Clinical course in 13 men with one-vessel disease surviving 15-year follow-up after first angiographic confirmation of coronary artery disease. ACB = aortocoronary bypass surgery; other abbreviations same as Figure 2. (Reproduced with permission from Thaulow E, Erikssen J, Sandvik L, Erikssen G, Jorgensen L, Cohn PF. Am J Cardiol 1993; 72:629–633.)

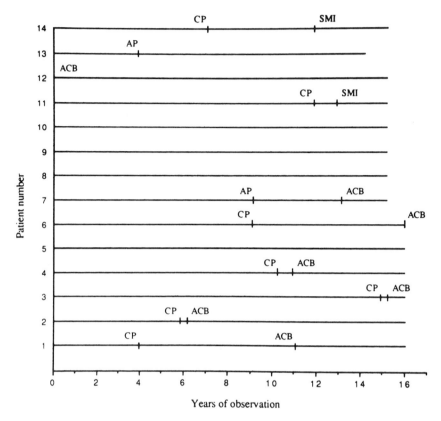

Figure 4   Clinical course in 14 men with two-vessel disease surviving 15-year follow-up after first angiographic confirmation of coronary artery disease. Abbreviations as in Figures 2 and 3. (Reproduced with permission from Thaulow E, Erikssen J, Sandvik L, Erikksen G, Jorgensen L, Cohn PF. Am J Cardiol 1993; 72:629–633.)

In individuals without angiographically defined coronary artery disease, several epidemiological surveys have called attention to the increased mortality associated with positive exercise tests in asymptomatic persons. These have been discussed in Chapters 9 and 10, but it is again worth commenting on the most recent of these, the Baltimore Longitudinal Aging Study (BLAS). Fleg et al. [9] evaluated the prognostic value of a combination of an abnormal exercise electrocardiogram and exercise thallium scintigram. Subsequent cardiac events

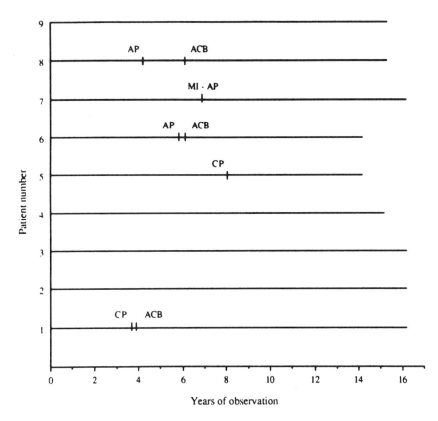

Figure 5   Clinical course in nine men with three-vessel disease surviving 15-year follow-up after first angiographic confirmation of coronary artery disease. Abbreviations as in Figures 2 and 3. (Reproduced with permission from Thaulow E, Erikssen J, Sandvik L, Erikssen G, Jorgensen L, Cohn PF. Am J Cardiol 1993; 72:629–633.)

occurred in 48% of those individuals with both abnormalities, compared with 7% of those with both tests normal ($p < 0.001$) (Fig. 6). In a 1998 report from the BLAS, Rywik et al. assessed the predictive value of ST depression in the postexercise recovery period [10] in 828 healthy volunteers aged 22 to 89. They compared prognosis in 151 individuals with ST segment depression that began in the exercise period with 63 patients whose changes were limited to the recovery period. Risk of coronary events was similar in both groups but significantly higher than in the 611 patients without *any* ST changes at all (i.e., the negative responders). Even more recently, the BLAS investigators reported that

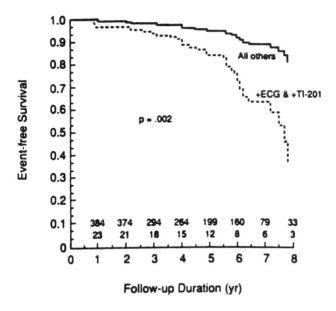

Figure 6   Plot of event-free survival in subjects with concordant positive exercise ECG and thallium-201 results versus all others. Numbers along the *x* axis indicate the number of individuals at risk each year. (From Fleg JL, Gerstenblith G, Zonderman AB, Becker LC, Weisfeldt ML, Costa PT, Jr., Lakatta EG. Circulation 1990; 81: 428. Reproduced with permission of American Heart Association.)

normalization of a previously abnormal study improved prognosis [11]. As discussed in Chapter 7, another current approach to diagnosing asymptomatic coronary artery disease is with cardiac electron beam CT scanning. The validity of this procedure can be traced back to the original fluoroscopic studies of Langou et al. [5] and the more recent ones by Detrano et al. [12] using cardiac cinefluoroscopy. In their study of 1461 high-risk but asymptomatic adults, Detrano et al. reported the coronary event rate to be high in patients with coronary calcification independent of other risk factors. In an even more recent study using CT scanning, however, Detrano et al. followed 1196 asymptomatic high coronary risk factor subjects but found that this procedure did *not* add prognostic data to that obtained with conventional risk factors [13].

Another interesting group of asymptomatic patients are those with diabetes mellitus. As discussed earlier in this book, exercise tests (with or without thallium scintigraphy) and dipyridamole-thallium scintigraphy have been used not only to detect underlying coronary artery disease, but also to predict prognosis and assess risk for various surgical procedures [14] (see Fig. 8 in Chap. 10).

In addition to exercise studies, there are now two reports of Holter monitoring studies in asymptomatic populations. In 1989, Hedblad et al. reported the results of their "Men born in 1914" study from Sweden [15]. Of the 394 men who had ST-segment analysis after 24 h of Holter monitoring, 341 had no prior history of coronary artery disease. Of these 341 men, 70 had at least one episode of ST segment depression and 12 (14%) died over the course of the 43-month follow-up. This incidence was twice as high as that observed in the 262 men without ST segment depression (19 deaths or 7%; $p < 0.005$) when frequent or complex ventricular arrhythmias were also present, prognosis was even less favorable [16]. Fleg et al. have also used Holter monitoring in their volunteers in the Baltimore Longitudinal Aging Study [17]. ST depression was seen in only 5 of 98 subjects, but cardiac events occurred in 2 of these (40%) over the course of the 10-year follow-up, compared with 8 of 93 (8%) subjects without changes.

One of the most fascinating aspects of both the epidemiological and clinical studies concerns the initial presentation of coronary artery disease. Based on data from the Framingham study and other surveys of apparently healthy individuals, it is apparent that angina is the initial presentation in only about half of these individuals [18]. Myocardial infarction or sudden death are the other common presentations. Similar data have been reported by Erikssen et al., in angiographically documented coronary artery disease [8], and Fleg et al. [9]. The Framingham investigators found no difference in prognosis between patients who presented first with myocardial infarctions versus those who presented with angina pectoris [19].

II. PROGNOSIS IN PATIENTS WHO ARE ASYMPTOMATIC FOLLOWING A MYOCARDIAL INFARCTION

These studies usually have heterogeneous populations. For example, an investigation at the National Institutes of Health (NIH) followed 20 patients who were asymptomatic after an infarction but included five other totally asymptomatic persons and 122 mildly asymptomatic persons (61 of whom had prior infarctions) in their study group [20]. As expected, there was a high frequency of coronary risk factors in this group. Thus, 90 patients were (or had been) cigarette smokers, 33 had hypertension, 22 had hypercholesterolemia, and 48 had either clinical diabetes or an abnormal glucose tolerance test. Forty-one of the patients had single-vessel coronary artery disease (28%), 45 had double-vessel disease (31%), and 61 had triple-vessel disease (41%). In the entire group, the authors could not find any combination of *clinical* risk factors that identified a high-risk subgroup, and the entire group mortality was 3%/year, a figure lower than reported for symptomatic groups. The life-table analysis of the entire cohort of 147 patients is depicted in Figure 7. In the 4 years of follow-up, eight deaths occurred. The triple-vessel group was studied separately. Figure 8 shows that patients with good exercise capacity had an annual mortality of 4%, while those with poor exercise capacity had an annual mortality of 9%; total mortality was 6%. (This compared to 3% in the Norwegian survey of asymptomatic patients without prior infarctions [8].) In a follow-up study at the NIH, the authors evaluated only patients with resting ejection fractions >0.40 (new patients with ejection fractions >0.40 were also added). The purpose of the new study of 117 patients was "to test the hypothesis that in patients with preserved left ventricular function at rest, the presence and severity of reversible ischemia (measured by both radionuclide angiography and exercise electrocardiogra-

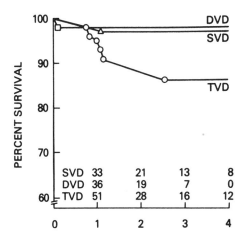

Figure 7 Life-table analysis of 147 patients with single- (SVD), double-(DVD), and triple-vessel (TVD) coronary artery disease for up to 4 years after entry into the study. Eight deaths occurred during the follow-up period at which time the probability data were generated. The line is extended to 4 years in each group after the last death occurred, although this is an extrapolation and not based on another set of probability data. The number of patients in the study at each yearly interval in each subgroup is shown at bottom. (From Kent KM, Rosing DR, Ewels CJ, Lipson L, Bonow R, Epstein SE. Am J Cardiol 1982; 49:1823.)

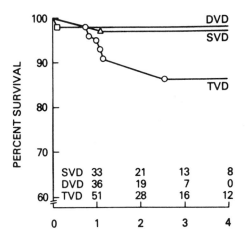

Figure 8 Life-table analysis comparing patients with triple-vessel disease who were able to achieve 100 or more watts on the bicycle ergometer and patients who had poor exercise capacity (less than 100 watts). In this comparison between two groups, probability data are calculated for both groups when an event occurs in either group. (From Kent KM, Rosing DR, Ewels CJ, Lipson L, Bonow R, Epstein SE. Am J Cardiol 1982; 49:1823.)

phy) may be a more specific predictor of prognosis during medical therapy." The authors found that patients with three-vessel disease, positive ST segment response to exercise, exercise capacity less than 120 watts, and an exercise-induced fall in ejection fraction had an annual mortality rate of 7% [21], confirming their hypotheses. In their most recent series of 131 patients with ejection fractions >0.40 (53 of whom had prior infarctions), they concentrated on patients with left main and triple-vessel disease [22]. They found that, in patients with both a decrease in radionuclide ejection fraction during exercise and ST depression, there was a similar percentage of left main and triple-vessel disease in both the angina and nonangina groups (Fig. 9); the death rate in these patients was also similar. The authors concluded that "Once inducible ischemia is demonstrated, the symptomatic response to exercise, by itself, appears irrelevant for risk stratification considerations." These conclusions are confirmed by the experience from the Coronary Artery Surgery Study (CASS) registry, which consists largely of asymptomatic or mildly symptomatic postinfarction patients. In a 1987 report, Weiner et al. [23] found painless exercise-induced ischemia to carry the same prognosis as painful ischemia (Fig. 10). When the severity of coronary artery disease is considered, the group with

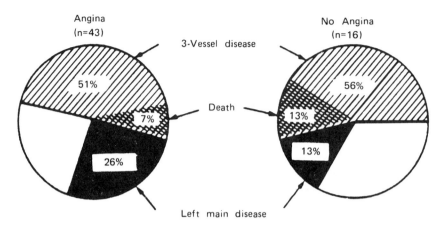

Figure 9 Prevalence of left main and three-vessel disease among patients with both a decrease in ejection fraction (EF) and a positive ST segment response. Patients are subdivided on the basis of symptomatic vs. silent ischemia during exercise. Patients with these ischemic responses had a similar likelihood of three-vessel disease, left main disease, and death during medical therapy, regardless of the presence or absence of angina during exercise. (From Bonow RO, Bacharach SL, Green MV, LaFreniere RL, Epstein SE. Am J Cardiol 1987; 60:778.)

three-vessel disease had a 6% yearly mortality (Fig. 11), similar to the prior figures from the NIH group.

Another study that arrived at a similar percentage was reported several years earlier by the Duke–Harvard Collaborative Coronary Artery Disease Data Bank [24]. This survey also included a mixture of totally asymptomatic and partially asymptomatic patients with angiographically documented coronary artery disease. Thirty-two had prior infarctions. The 44 patients were matched with 127 symptomatic patients from the same data bank. The computerized matching process was based on five variables that reflected coronary anatomy and left ventricular function. Originally we had hoped to match each of the 44 asymptomatic patients with three symptomatic patients to ensure a large enough data base, but this was not always possible; hence, the final figure for the control group was 127 rather than 132. In addition to the five variables noted earlier, we also compared the frequency of other variables once the groups were selected by the computer. This was to insure that the results of the survival analysis were not influenced by descriptors that were not selected to be matched by the computer. This comparison is depicted in Table 1; there were

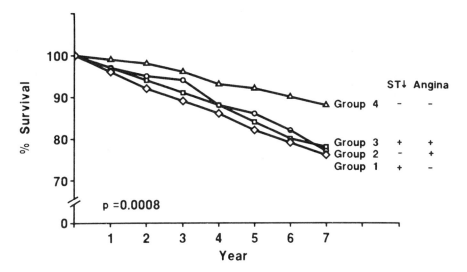

Figure 10   Cumulative survival for patients in groups 1 through 4. The 7-year survival was similar to patients in groups 1 (the silent ischemia group), 2, and 3. Group 4 patients (with neither angina nor ST depression) had a substantially better 7-year survival. (From Weiner DA, Ryan TJ, McCabe CH, Luk S, Chaitman BR, Sheffield LT, Tristani F, Fisher LD. Am J Cardiol 1987; 59:725.)

no significant differences between the two groups. Mean follow-up time was 3 ½ years. There was an 81% survival rate for the total asymptomatic group at years (yearly mortality 2.7%), compared with a 62% survival rate for the symptomatic group (yearly mortality 5.4%). The worst prognosis was in the subgroup with three-vessel disease (4.7% vs. 8.7% in the symptomatic group (Fig. 12). Two of the four patients in the symptomatic group who died had anginal symptoms at least 6 months before their death; development of anginal symptoms eventually was reported in 30% of the patients by the end of the 4-year follow-up.

In addition to these studies, there are numerous reports describing prognosis in patients who have sustained an *acute* myocardial infarction. Short-term survival statistics based on the postinfarction exercise studies indicate that exercise-induced ST segment depression markedly increases the 1-year mortality. In some of these studies, prognosis in those patients who were asymptomatic and had positive exercise tests denoting active, though silent, myocardial ischemia could be gleaned from the raw data. For example, in the classic study by Theroux et al. [25], 210 patients who had no overt heart failure and had been

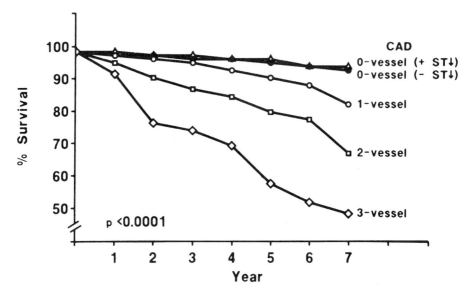

Figure 11 Seven-year survival rates for group 1 patients in Figure 7 based on the severity of coronary artery disease (CAD); a separate group of 282 patients without CAD who had ischemic ST segment depression (+ST↓) without angina during exercise testing; and a control group of 1117 patients without CAD and without either ischemic ST depression (–ST↓) or angina during exercise testing. (From Weiner DA, Ryan TJ, McCabe CH, Luk S, Chaitman BR, Sheffield LT, Tristani F, Fisher LD. Am J Cardiol 1987; 59:725.)

free of chest pain for at least 4 days were exercised 1 day before discharge from the hospital. The 1-year mortality rate was 2.1% (3 of 146) in patients without ischemic ST changes during exercise and 27% (17 of 64) in those with such changes ($p < 0.001$). The authors reported that angina in the presence of ST segment depression had no effect on these statistics. Thus, 10 of 37 patients with ST depression on the exercise test but without angina died, compared with 7 of 27 with both exercise-induced ST depression and angina. DeBelder et al. [26] studied 262 patients 7 days after infarction; 104 had a positive exercise test and 67 had silent ischemia. In the first year after the infarction, these latter patients had 12 times as high a cardiac mortality rate compared to negative responders (and twice as high a rate as patients with angina and ST depression). These figures are similar to those reported by Theroux et al. [25]. Gibson and Beller [27] have reported that postinfarction patients with painless exercise ST

Table 1 Clinical and Angiographic Findings in Study Patients with and Without Anginal Symptoms

	Without anginal symptoms (*n* = 44)	With anginal symptoms (*n* = 127)
Mean age	47.6	49.0
Male sex	41 (93%)	107 (84%)
Diabetes	2 (4%)	8 (6%)
Hypertension	13 (29%)	27 (21%)
Diagnostic Q waves in electrocardiogram	23 (53%)	76 (60%)
Positive exercise test	17/31 (55%)	48/96 (50%)
Two-vessel disease	13 (30%)	38 (30%)
Three-vessel disease	18 (40%)	51 (40%)
Left main coronary arterial stenosis	0	0
Left anterior descending arterial stenosis	36 (82%)	91 (72%)
Totally occluded vessels	12 (27%)	34 (27%)
Abnormal left ventricular contraction pattern	32 (73%)	95 (75%)
Left ventricular end-diastolic pressure > 18 mmHg	8 (18%)	18 (14%)
Arteriovenous oxygen difference > 5.5 volumes percent	9 (21%)	23 (18%)

Source: Cohn PF, Harris P, Barry WH, Rosati RA, Rosenbaum P, Waternaux C. Am J Cardiol 1981; 47:233.

depression at the highest risk for further cardiac events are those with abnormal exercise thallium-201 scintigrams. The use of dobutamine stress echocardiography after an uncomplicated myocardial infarction was reported by Bigi et al. in 1998 [28]. Patients who experienced abnormalities—with or without angina—were at increased risk for future cardiac events.

The resting ECG itself has also been used as a prognostic indicator after a myocardial infarction. Two separate studies [29,30] have shown that persistent recurrent ischemia (defined as ST segment depression) was associated with subsequent infarction or death.

The number of Holter studies in postinfarction patients has increased dramatically in the past several years. In 1988, Gottlieb et al. [31] reported that in postinfarction patients who were not suitable for exercise testing, silent

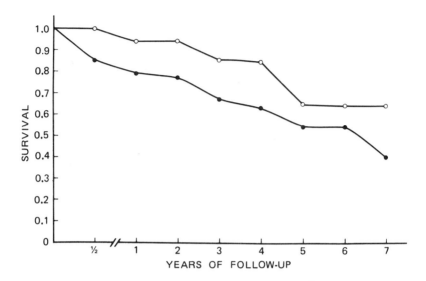

Figure 12 Survival curves for 17 patients (○) with three-vessel coronary artery disease but without angina symptoms, compared to 49 patients (●) with three-vessel disease and anginal symptoms, in the Duke–Harvard Coronary Artery Disease (CAD) Data Bank.

ischemia on Holter monitoring was a significant predictor of 1-year mortality. That same year, Tzivoni et al. [32] compared the value of Holter monitoring vs. exercise testing as risk prognosticators. The subsequent cardiac event rate was significantly higher in those patients with *both* abnormal Holter reports and abnormal exercise tests. Ouyang et al. [33] also evaluated postinfarction patients with Holter monitoring during their hospital stay. Silent ischemia occurred frequently and identified a group of patients at risk for adverse in-hospital clinical outcomes (Table 2). Since these reports a number of other studies have been published. The studies by Quintana et al. [34] and Gill et al. [35] confirm earlier studies on the adverse prognosis seen with transient ischemic episodes (Fig. 13), while Jereczek et al. [36] found risk stratification only when Holter monitoring was combined with exercise test results. Stevenson et al. found Holter monitoring useful for identifying patients at increased risk after thrombolysis for acute infarcts [37], while Currie and Saltissi reported that there was no relation between transient myocardial ischemia and ventricular arrhythmias [38]. ST segment elevation after an acute myocardial infarction has also been adversely linked to long-term prognosis [39]. Perhaps the most

Table 2 Clinical Ischemic Events During Hospital Stay

	ST changes ($n = 27$)	No ST changes ($n = 32$)	p value
Death (%)	1 (4)	1 (3)	NS
Recurrent MI (%)	0 (0)	0 (0)	NS
Pulmonary edema (%)	5 (19)	1 (3)	0.06
Angina after AMI (%)	11 (41)	6 (19)	0.06
At least 1 ischemic outcome (%)	14 (52)	7 (22)	<0.02

AMI = acute myocardial infarction; NS = not significant.
Source: Ouyang P, Chandra NC, Gottlieb SO. Am J Cardiol 1990; 65:267.

interesting of these studies is that of Ruberman et al. [40], who conducted a case-control analysis of 261 deaths during the Beta Blocker Heart Attack Trial. They found an "independent contribution to mortality by the presence of ST-segment depression of more than one minute's duration when other relative variables were taken into account." This study also has implications for the effects of medical therapy on prognosis and will be discussed further in Chapter 15. Other prognostic studies involving results of medical and surgical therapy are also discussed in Chapters 15 and 16.

III. PROGNOSIS IN PATIENTS WITH BOTH SYMPTOMATIC AND ASYMPTOMATIC ISCHEMIC EPISODES

Several studies have investigated the prognosis of patients with *chronic angina* who have a positive exercise test without pain. (Usually a painful but positive test remains so with repeat testing some months later [41].) Presumably, these individuals have both symptomatic and silent ischemic episodes during daily activities. Several studies have evaluated prognosis after exercise testing in patients with chronic angina. Falcone et al. [42] followed 269 patients with painful ischemia during exercise and 204 patients with painless ischemia. Survival curves were similar regardless of the presence or absence of pain during the test (Fig. 14). Callahan et al. [43] reported similar results, as did Dagenais et al. [44]. By contrast, Mark et al. [45] found ST depression without angina to have the same prognostic importance as a *negative* exercise test. Studies using radionuclide techniques have not supported the results of Mark et al. For example, Assey et al. [46] found a worse prognosis in silent compared to painful ischemia in their series of 55 patients studied with exercise thallium tests (Table

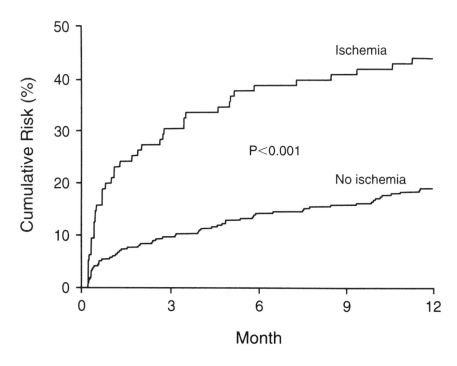

Figure 13   Cumulative risk of death, nonfatal myocardial infraction, or hospitalization for unstable angina, according to the presence or absence of ischemia on ambulatory ECG monitoring in 406 patients with myocardial infarction. (Reproduced with permission from Gill JB, Cairns JA, Roberts RS, Tech M, Sealy BJ, Fallen EF, Tomlinson CW, Gent M. N Engl J Med 1996; 334:65–70.)

3). Other reports citing exercise thallium scintigraphy [47] or exercise radionuclide ventriculography [48] have shown silent ischemia to carry the same adverse prognosis as painful ischemia.

There is now a considerable amount of data concerning prognosis in stable angina patients who have undergone long-term ambulatory ECG monitoring. These reports show that Holter evidence of ischemia adds important incremental data to that obtained from clinical history and/or exercise testing

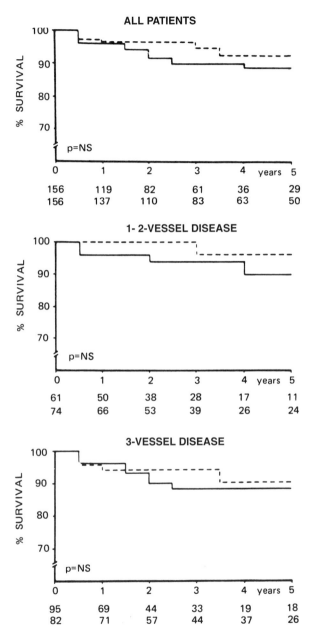

Figure 14   Survival curves of medically treated patients with (Group I) (*dashed lines*) or without (Group II) (*solid lines*) angina during stress testing. No statistically significant difference was found between the two groups, even when patients were classified according to the number of disease. (From Falcone C, DeServi S, Poma E, Campana C, Scire A, Montemartini C, Specchia G. J Am Coll Cardiol 1987; 9:295.)

Table 3 Cardiac Events of Study Population During Follow-Up

Event	Group I (n = 27)	Group II (n = 28)	p value
Acute MI	6 (22%)	1 (4%)	0.05
Death	3 (11%)	0 (0%)	NS
Hospitalization for unstable angina	13 (48%)	16 (57%)	NS

MI = myocardial infarction; NS = not significantly different.
Source: Assey ME, Waters GL, Hendrix GH, Carabello BA, Usher BW, Spann JF, Jr. Am J Cardiol 1987; 59:497.

[49–51]. For example, Deedwania and Carbajal [50] found that silent ischemia occurs frequently (even in medically treated patients) and identifies a subset of patients at high risk for cardiac death (Fig. 15). Not all groups find a positive correlation between Holter findings and prognosis. Mulcahy et al. reported in 1997 [52] that transient ischemia in ambulatory monitoring in 221 low-risk stable angina patients did not help assess long-term (over 4 year) prognosis. In an accompanying editorial, Ambrose and Fuster [53] point out the problems of trying to predict future coronary events when the lesions that cause these events are not severe enough to be identified using conventional ischemia detection methods.

Additional Holter data are also available in patients with unstable angina. Gottlieb et al. studied 70 patients with this syndrome; 37 had Holter ECG evidence of silent ischemia, 33 did not. Thirty-day [54] and 2 year [55] follow-up showed a significant pattern of adverse events associated with silent ischemia (Table 4), but not with negative Holter findings (Fig. 16). Similar findings were reported by Nademanee et al. [56], who also confirmed the importance of more than 60 min of ischemia/per 24 h of Holter monitoring (Fig. 17). Other studies have reported similar results [57], although some investigators have found exercise thallium scintigraphy to be more reliable than Holter monitoring [58].

Using a combination—or comparison—of the various noninvasive parameters to predict prognosis continues to be one of the most fruitful areas of research into silent ischemia. Rovai et al. [59] found that reversible ischemia at rest (detected by Holter monitoring) was a strong negative indicator of prognosis when compared to ischemia on effort (exercise tests). By contrast, Amanullah and Lindvall [60] found no advantage to Holter monitoring compared to thallium-201 myocardial perfusion imaging. In the ACIP study, Stone et al. [61] found that myocardial ischemia detected by both Holter monitoring and an

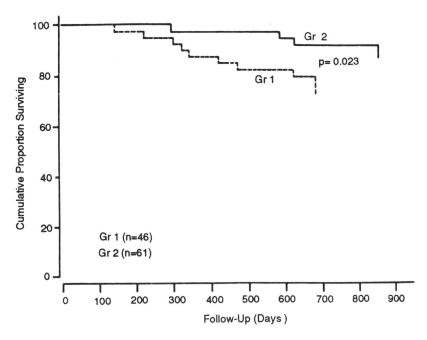

Figure 15 Graph showing Kaplan–Meier curves comparing cumulative proportion of patients surviving without cardiac death during mean follow-up of 2 years for 46 patients with silent ischemia (group 1) and 61 patients without ischemia (group 2) during ambulatory ECG monitoring ($p = 0.023$). (From Deedwania PC, Carbajal EV. Circulation 1990; 81:748. Reproduced with permission of American Heart Association.)

abnormal exercise test were each independently associated with an adverse outcome in patients subsequently managed with medical treatment. This kind of study leads to the intriguing question: What effect does therapy have on prognosis? Although this subject will be considered in more detail in subsequent chapters, it is worth noting at this time that Holter monitoring can be used to evaluate prognosis in such patients. For example, de Marchena et al. noted a high frequency of persistent silent myocardial ischemia in men with angina who were rendered pain-free by standard medical therapy [62] and this predicted a high cardiac event rate. Others have also looked into not only the problem of persistent ischemia despite treatment, but the additional adverse effects of interrupted treatment, especially beta-blockade [63].

Table 4   Two-Year Adverse Clinical Outcomes for Unstable Angina Patients with and Without Silent ST Segment Changes on Initial 48-h Holter Monitoring

Adverse clinical outcome	Group I: Silent ischemia ($n = 37$)	Group II: No silent ischemia ($n = 33$)	p value[a]
Cardiac death	2	0	<0.01
Nonfatal MI	8 (27%)	1 (3%)	
CABG or PTCA for symptoms	11 (30%)	5 (15%)	<0.05
Total	21 (57%)	6 (18%)	<0.001

[a] Derived from Kaplan–Meier analysis, Breslow test.
CAGB = coronary bypass surgery; MI = myocardial infarction; PTCA = percutaneous transluminal coronary angioplasty.
Source: Gottlieb SO, Weisfeldt ML, Ouyang P, Mellits ED, Gerstenblith G. J Am Coll Cardiol 1987; 10:756.

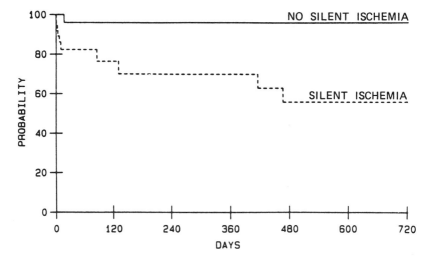

Figure 16   Kaplan–Meier curves illustrating the probability of *not* experiencing death or myocardial infarction over the 2-year follow-up period for the 37 patients with (Group I) and the 33 patients without (Group II) silent ischemic ST changes on initial Holter monitoring. The difference between the two groups is significant at the $p < 0.01$ level. (From Gottlieb SO, Weisfeldt ML, Ouyang P, Mellits ED, Gerstenblith G. J Am Coll Cardiol 1987; 10:756.)

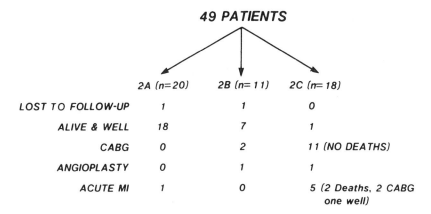

49 PATIENTS

	2A (n=20)	2B (n=11)	2C (n=18)
LOST TO FOLLOW-UP	1	1	0
ALIVE & WELL	18	7	1
CABG	0	2	11 (NO DEATHS)
ANGIOPLASTY	0	1	1
ACUTE MI	1	0	5 (2 Deaths, 2 CABG one well)

Figure 17   Flow diagram demonstrating the clinical outcome of 49 patients with unstable angina relative to the presence and duration of transient myocardial ischemia (TMI) in patients with unstable angina. CABG = coronary artery bypass surgery; MI = myocardial infarction.   Patients were subgrouped as follows: 2A = no transient myocardial ischemia; 2B and 2C = transient myocardial ischemia <60 min/24 h and >60 min/24 h, respectively. (From Nadamanee K, Intarachot V, Josephson MA, Rieders D, Mody FV, Singh BN. J Am Coll Cardiol 1987; 19:1.)

IV.   PROGNOSIS FOR NONCARDIAC SURGERY

It is becoming increasing clear that not only exercise testing (with or without thallium scintigraphy) but also Holter monitoring can be used to assess perioperative risk of cardiovascular morbidity and mortality in patients undergoing a variety of noncardiac surgical procedures. Most of the ischemia found by these tests is silent. Eagle et al. [64] have reviewed the value of preoperative dipyridamole thallium imaging which continues to be popular in patients who cannot exercise because of peripheral vascular disease [65], although dipyridamole echocardiography can also be used for this purpose [66]. Studies comparing dipyridamole scintigraphy with Holter monitoring find each to be helpful. The latter procedure has grown in popularity, with both cardiologists and anesthesiologists [67–70]. Mangano et al. have published several studies attesting to its utility [68,69]. For example, they found that postoperative myocardial ischemia occurred in 41% of their Holter-monitored patients (Fig. 18) and was associated with a significant increase in the risk of an adverse cardiovascular event. Others have reported similar results [70]. How preoperative medication can improve prognosis is discussed in Chapter 15.

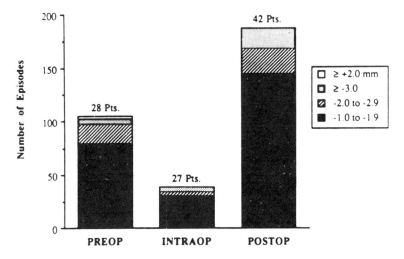

Figure 18   Incidence and severity of ischemia during the preoperative (PREOP), intra-operative (INTRAOP), and postoperative (POSTOP) periods. Shown are the total number of episodes per period and the number of patients (Pts.) with ischemia during each period. The severity of ischemia is shown as the number of episodes with an ST change from baseline of ≥+2 mm (elevation) and ≥–1 to –1.9, ≥–2 to –2.9, and ≥–3 (depression). The ST change was calculated by subtracting the baseline ST level from the maximal ST level. (From Mangano DT, Hollenberg M, Febert G, Meyer ML, London MJ, Tubau JF, Krupski WC, the Study of Perioperative Ischemia (SPI) Research Group. J Am Coll Cardiol 1991; 17:843. Reproduced with permission.)

V.   PROGNOSIS FOLLOWING CORONARY REVASCULARIZATION

The exercise test has been used to predict prognosis after both coronary angioplasty [71] and coronary bypass surgery [72]. Now the Holter monitor is being employed for the same purpose [73]. Although the results with angioplasty are encouraging, it is not clear that either the exercise test or Holter monitor results can reliably predict adverse events following coronary artery surgery.

VI.   CONCLUSIONS

In general, prognosis in totally asymptomatic individuals with silent myocardial ischemia appears good, the exception being those with three-vessel disease. Similarly, patients who are asymptomatic after an infarction contain a subgroup of individuals with three-vessel disease who have far from a benign prognosis. Mortality in this group averages 6%. The adverse effect that the presence of frequent silent ischemic episodes has on the prognosis of patients with chronic angina is now well documented, and with few exceptions exercise test data indicate prognosis is similar with exercise-induced ST depression whether angina is present or not. Holter data in both stable and unstable angina indicate that continuing ischemia, which is usually silent ischemia, has an adverse effect on cardiovascular morbidity and mortality [74], though there are those who would differ with these conclusions.

REFERENCES

1. Froelicher VF, Thompson AJ, Longo MR, Triebwasser J, Lancaster MC. Value of exercise testing for screening asymptomatic men for latent coronary heart disease. Prog Cardiovasc Dis 1976; 18:265.
2. Uhl GS, Froelicher V. Screening for asymptomatic coronary artery disease. J Am Coll Cardiol 1983; 1:946.
3. Uhl GS, Kay TN, Hickman JR, Jr. Comparison of exercise radionuclide angiography and thallium perfusion imaging in detecting coronary disease in asymptomatic men. J Cardiac Rehabil 1982; 2:118.
4. Hickman JR, Jr., Uhl GS, Cook RL, Engel PJ, Hopkirk A. A natural history study of asymptomatic coronary disease (abstr). Am J Cardiol 1980; 45:422.
5. Langou RA, Huang EK, Kelley MJ, Cohen LD. Predictive accuracy of coronary artery calcification and abnormal exercise test for coronary artery disease in asymptomatic men. Circulation 1980; 62:1196.
6. Erikssen J, Thaulow E. Follow-up of patients with asymptomatic myocardial ischemia. In: Rutishauser W, Roskamm H, eds. Silent Myocardial Ischemia. Berlin: Springer-Verlag, 1984:156–164.
7. Erikssen J, Mundal R. The patient with coronary disease without infarction: Can a high risk group be identified? Ann NY Acad Sci 1982; 382:483.
8. Thaulow E, Erikssen J, Sandvik L, Erikssen G, Jorgensen L, Cohn PF. Initial clinical presentation of cardiac disease in asymptomatic men with silent myocardial ischemia and angiographically documented coronary artery disease (the Oslo Ischemia Study). Am J Cardiol 1993; 72:629–633.
9. Fleg, JL, Gerstenblith G, Zonderman AB, Becker LC, Weisfeldt ML, Costa PT, Jr., Lakatta EG. Prevalence and prognostic significance of exercise-induced silent myocardial ischemia detected by thallium scintigraphy and electrocardiography in asymptomatic volunteers. Circulation 1990; 81:428.
10. Rywik TM, Zink RC, Gittings NS, Khan AA, Wright JG, O'Connor FC, Fleg JL. Independent prognostic significance of ischemic ST-segment response limited to recovery from treadmill exercise in asymptomatic subjects. Circulation 1998; 97:2117–2122.

11. Pinco J, O'Connor FC, Fleg JL. Does normalization of a previously ischemic exercise ECG in asymptomatic subjects predict a better prognosis than a persistently ischemic response? J Am Coll Cardiol 1999; 33 (suppl A):562A (abstr).

12. Detrano RC, Wong ND, Tang W, French WJ, Georgiou D, Young E, Brezden OS, Doherty TM, Narahara KA, Brundage BH. Prognostic significance of cardiac cinefluoroscopy for coronary calcific deposits in asymptomatic high risk subjects. J Am Cardiol 1994; 24:354–358.

13. Detrano RC, Wong ND, Doherty TM, Shavelle RM, Tang W, Ginzton LE, Budoff MJ, Narahara KA. Coronary calcium does not accurately predict near-term future coronary events in high-risk adults. Circulation 1999; 99:2633–2638.

14. Camp AD, Garvin PJ, Hoff J, Marsh J, Byers SL, Chaitman BR. Prognostic value of intravenous dipyridamole thallium imaging in patients with diabetes mellitus considered for renal transplantation. Am J Cardiol 1990; 65:1459.

15. Hedblad B, Moller SJ, Svensson K, Hanson BS, Isacsson S, Janzon L, Lindell SE, Steen B, Johansson BW. Increased mortality in men with ST segment depression during 24-h ambulatory long-term ECG recording: Results from prospective population study 'Men born in 1914,' from Malmo, Sweden. Eur Heart J 1989; 10:149.

16. Hedblad B, Janzon L, Johansson BW, Juul-Moller S. Survival and incidence of myocardial infarction in men with ambulatory ECG-detected frequent and complex ventricular arrhythmias. Eur Heart J 1997; 18:1787–1795.

17. Fleg JL, Kennedy HL. Prognostic significance of Holter monitoring in apparently healthy older subjects (abstr). J Am Coll Cardiol 1991; 17:330A.

18. Cohn PF. Prognosis in exercise-induced silent myocardial ischemia and implications for screening asymptomatic populations. Prog Cardiovasc Dis 1992; 34:399.

19. Murabito JM, Evans JC, Anderson KM, Levy D. Prognosis following the initial presentation of coronary heart disease: The Framingham Heart Study (abstr). Circulation, 1991; 84(suppl II):334.

20. Kent KM, Rosing DR, Ewes CJ, Lipson L, Bonow R, Epstein SE. Prognosis of asymptomatic or mildly symptomatic patients with coronary artery disease. Am J Cardiol 1982; 49:1823.

21. Bonow RO, Kent KM, Rosing DR, Lan KKG, Lakatos E, Borer JS, Bacharach SL, Green MV, Epstein SE. Exercise-induced ischemia in mildly symptomatic patients with coronary artery disease and preserved left ventricular function: Identification of subgroups at risk of death during medical therapy. N Engl J Med 1984; 311:1339.

22. Bonow RO, Bacharach SL, Green MV, LaFreniere RL, Epstein SE. Prognostic implications of symptomatic versus asymptomatic (silent) myocardial ischemia induced by exercise in mildly symptomatic and in asymptomatic patients with angiographically documented coronary artery disease. Am J Cardiol 1987; 60: 778.

23. Weiner DA, Ryan TJ, McCabe CH, Luk S, Chaitman BR, Sheffield LT, Tristani F, Fisher LD. Significance of silent myocardial ischemia during exercise testing in patients with coronary artery disease. Am J Cardiol 1987; 59:725.

24. Cohn PF, Harris P, Barry WH, Rosati R, Rosenbaum P, Waternaux C. Prognostic importance of anginal symptoms in angiographically defined coronary artery disease. Am J Cardiol 1981; 47:233.

25. Theroux P, Waters DD, Halphen C, Debaisieux JC, Mizgala HF. Prognostic value of exercise testing soon after myocardial infarction. N Engl J Med 1979; 301:341.

26. deBelder M, Skehan D, Pumphrey C, Khan B, Evans S, Rothman M, Mills P. Identification of a high risk subgroup of patients with silent ischaemia after myocardial infarction: A group for early therapeutic revascularisation? Br Heart J 1990; 63:145.

27. Gibson RS, Beller GA. Prevalence and clinical significance of painless ST segment depression during early post infarction exercise testing. Circulation 1987; 75(suppl II):II-36.

28. Bigi R, Galati A, Curti G, Coletta C, Ricci R, Fedeli F, Occhi G, Ceci V, Fiorentini C. Different clinical and prognostic significance of painful and silent myocardial ischemia detected by exercise electrocardiography and dobutamine stress echocardiography after uncomplicated myocardial infarction. Am J Cardiol 1998; 81:75–78.

29. Krone RJ, Greenberg G, Dwyer EM, Kleiger RE, Boden WE, and the Multicenter Diltiazem Postinfarction Trial Research Group. Long-term prognostic significance of ST segment depression during acute myocardial infarction. J Am Coll Cardiol 1993; 22:361–367.

30. Silva P, Galli M, Campolo L, for the IRES (Ischemia Residua) Study Group. Prognostic significance of early ischemia after acute myocardial infarction in low-risk patients. Am J Cardiol 1993; 71:1142–1147.

31. Gottlieb SO, Gottlieb SH, Achuff SC, Baumgardner R, Mellits ED, Weisfeldt ML, Gerstenblith G. Silent ischemia on Holter monitoring predicts mortality in high-risk postinfarction patients. J A M A 1988; 259:1030.

32. Tzivoni D, Gavish A, Zin D, Gottlieb S, Moriel M, Keren A, Banai S, Stern S. Prognostic significance of ischemic episodes in patients with previous myocardial infarction. Am J Cardiol 1988; 62:661.

33. Ouyang P, Chandra NC, Gottlieb SO. Frequency and importance of silent myocardial ischemia identified with ambulatory electrocardiographic monitoring in the early in-hospital period after acute myocardial infarction. Am J Cardiol 1990; 65:267.

34. Quintana M, Lindvall K, Carlens P, Bevegard S, Brolund F. ST-segment depression on ambulatory electrocardiography in the early in-hospital period after acute myocardial infarction predicts early and late mortality: a short-term and a 3-year follow-up study. Clin Cardiol 1995; 18:392–400.

35. Gill JB, Cairns JA, Roberts RS, Tech M, Constantini L, Sealey BJ, Fallen EF, Tomlinson CW, Gent M. Prognostic importance of myocardial ischemia detected by ambulatory monitoring early after acute myocardial infarction. N Engl J Med 1996; 334:65–70.

36. Jereczek M, Andresen D, Schroder J, Voller H, Bruggemann T, Deutschmann C,

Schroder R. Prognostic value of ischemia during Holter monitoring and exercise testing after acute myocardial infarction. Am J Cardiol 1993; 72:8–13.

37. Stevenson R, Ranjadayalan K, Wilkinson P, Marchant B, Timmis AD. Assessment of Holter ST monitoring for risk stratification in patients with acute myocardial infarction treated by thrombolysis. Br Heart J 1993; 70:233–240.

38. Currie P, Saltissi S. Transient myocardial ischaemia after acute myocardial infarction does not induce ventricular arrhythmias. Br Heart J 1993; 69:303–307 (1993).

39. Mickley H, Nielsen JR, Berning J, Junker A, Moller M. Characteristics and prognostic importance of ST-segment elevation on Holter monitoring early after acute myocardial infarction. Am J Cardiol 1995; 76:537–542.

40. Ruberman W, Crow R, Rosenberg CR, Rautaharju PM, Shore RE, Pasternack BS. Intermittent ST depression and mortality after myocardial infarction. Circulation 1992; 85:1440.

41. Weisz G, Stern S, Tzivoni D. Is a silent or painful treadmill test predictive of a silent or painful treadmill test repeated one year later? Circulation 1987; 76 (suppl IV):361.

42. Falcone C, deServi S, Poma E, Campana C, Scire A, Montemartini C, Specchia G. Clinical significance of exercise-induced silent myocardial ischemia in patients with coronary artery disease. J Am Coll Cardiol 1987; 9:295.

43. Callaham PR, Froelicher VF, Klein J, Risch M, Dubach P, Friis R. Exercise-induced silent ischemia: Age, diabetes mellitus, previous myocardial infarction and prognosis. J Am Coll Cardiol 1989; 14:1175.

44. Dagenais G, Rouleau JR, Hochart P, Magrina J, Cantin B, Dumesnil JG. Survival with apinless strongly positive exercise electrocardiogram. Am J Cardiol 1988; 62:892.

45. Mark DB, Hlatky MA, Califf RM, Morris JJ, Jr., Sisson SD, McCants CB, Lee KL, Harrell FE, Jr., Pryor DB. Painless exercise ST deviation on the treadmill: Long-term prognosis. J Am Coll Cardiol 1989; 14:885.

46. Assay ME, Walters GL, Hendrix GH, Crabello BA, Usher BW, Spann JF, Jr. Incidence of acute myocardial infarction in patients with exercise-induced silent myocardial ischemia. Am J Cardiol 1987; 59:497.

47. Heller LI, Tresgallo M, Sciacca RR, Blood DK, Seldin DW, Johnson LL. Prognostic significance of silent myocardial ischemia on a thallium stress test. Am J Cardiol 1990; 65:718.

48. Breitenbucher A, Pfisterer M, Hoffmann A, Burckhardt D. Long-term follow-up of patients with silent ischemia during exercise radionuclide angiography. J Am Coll Cardiol 1990; 15:999.

49. Tzivoni D, Weisz G, Gavish A, Zin D, Keren A, Stern S. Comparison of mortality and myocardial infarction rates in stable angina pectoris with and without ischemic episodes during daily activities. Am J Cardiol 1989; 63:273.

50. Deedwania PC, Carbajal EV. Silent ischemia during daily life is an independent predictor of mortality in stable angina. Circulation 1990; 81:748.

51. Yeung AC, Barry J, Orav J, Bonassin E, Raby KE, Selwyn AP. Effects of asymp-

tomatic ischemia on long-term prognosis in chronic stable coronary disease. Circulation 1991; 83:1598.

52. Mulcahy D, Husain S, Azlos G, Rehman A, Andrews NP, Schenke WH, Geller NL, Quyyumi A. Ischemia during ambulatory monitoring as a prognostic indicator in patients with stable coronary artery disease. JAMA 1997;

53. Ambrose JA, Fuster V. Can we predict future acute coronary events in patients with stable coronary artery disease? JAMA 1997; 277:343–344.

54. Gottlieb SO, Weisfeldt ML, Ouyang P, Mellits ED, Gerstenblith G. Silent ischemia as a marker for early unfavorable outcomes in patients with unstable angina. N Engl J Med 1986; 314:1214.

55. Gottlieb SO, Weisfeldt ML, Ouyang P, Mellits ED, Gerstenblith G. Silent ischemia predicts infarction and death during 2 year follow-up of unstable angina. J Am Coll Cardiol 1987; 19:756.

56. Nademanee K, Interachot V, Josephson MA, Rieders D, Mody V, Singh BN. Prognostic significance of silent myocardial ischemia in patients with unstable angina. J Am Coll Cardiol 1987; 19:1.

57. Wilcox I, Freedman B, Kelly DT, Harris PJ. Clinical significance of silent ischemia in unstable angina pectoris. Am J Cardiol 1990; 65:1313.

58. Marmur JD, Freeman MR, Langer A, Armstrong PW. Prognosis in medically stabilized unstable angina: Early Holter ST-segment monitoring compared with predischarge exercise thallium tomography. Ann Intern Med 1990; 113:575.

59. Rovai D, Landi P, Michelassi C, Severi S, L'Abbate A. Clinical features and prognostic implications of myocardial ischemia at rest in patients with exertional angina pectoris. Am J Cardiol 1994; 74:433–477.

60. Amanullah AM, Lindvall K. Prevalence and significance of transient predominantly asymptomatic—myocardial ischemia on Holter monitoring in unstable angina pectoris, and correlation with exercise test and thallium-201 myocardial perfusion imaging. Am J Cardiol 1993; 72:144–148.

61. Stone PH, Chaitman BR, Forman S, Andrews TC, Bittner V, Bourassa MG, Goldberg AD, MacCallum G, Ouyang P, Pepine CJ, Pratt CM, Sharaf B, Steingart R, Knatterud GL, Sopko G, Conti R for the ACIP Investigators. Prognostic significance of myocardial ischemia detected by ambulatory electrocardiography, exercise treadmill testing, and electrocardiogram at rest to predict cardiac events by one year [the Asymptomatic Cardiac Ischemia Pilot (ACIP) study]. Am J Cardiol 1997; 80:1395–1401.

62. de Marchena E, Asch J, Martinez J, Wozniak P, Posada JD, Pittaluga J, Breuer G, Chakko S, Kessler KM, Myerburg RJ. Usefulness of persistent silent myocardial ischemia in predicting a high cardiac event rate in men with medically controlled, stable angina pectoris. Am J Cardiol 1994; 73:390–392.

63. Madjlessi-Simon T, Mary-Krause M, Fillette F, Lechat P, Jaillon P. Persistent transient myocardial ischemia despite beta-adrenergic blockade predicts a higher risk of adverse cardiac events in patients with coronary artery disease. J Am Coll Cardiol 1996; 27:1586–1591.

64. Eagle KA, Coley CM, Newell JB, Brester DC, Darling RC, Strauss HW, Guiney TE, Boucher CA. Combining clinical and thallium data optimizes preoperative assessment of cardiac risk before major vascular surgery. Ann Intern Med 1989; 110:859.

65. Urbinati S, DiPasquale G, Andreoli A, Lusa AM, Ruffini M, Lanzino G, Pinelli G. Frequency and prognostic significance of silent coronary artery disease in patients with cerebral ischemia undergoing carotid endarterectomy. Am J Cardiol 1992; 69:1166.

66. Tischler MD, Lee RT, Lee TH, Creager MA, Lord C, Hirsch AT, Raby K. Dipyridamole echocardiography versus ambulatory ischemia monitoring in the assessment of perioperative risk (abstr). J Am Coll Cardiol 1991; 17:264A.

67. Ouyang P, Gerstenblith G, Furman WR, Golueke PJ, Gottlieb SO. Frequency and significance of early postoperative silent myocardial ischemia in patients having peripheral vascular surgery. Am J Cardiol 1989; 64:1113.

68. Mangano DT, Browner WS, Hollenberg M, London MJ, Tubau JF, Tateo IM, and the Study of Perioperative Ischemia Research Group. Association of perioperative myocardial ischemia with cardiac morbidity and mortality in men undergoing noncardiac surgery. N Engl J Med 1990; 323:1781.

69. Mangano DT, Hollenberg M, Fegert G, Meyer ML, London MJ, Tubau JF, Krupski WC, and the Study of Perioperative Ischemia (SPI) Research Group. Perioperative myocardial ischemia in patients undergoing noncardiac surgery. J Am Coll Cardiol 1991; 17:843.

70. Aronow WS, Ahn C, Mercando AD, Epstein S. Prognostic significance of silent ischemia in elderly patients with peripheral arterial disease with and without previous myocardial infarction. Am J Cardiol 1992; 69:137.

71. Deligonul U, Vandormael MG, Younis LT, Chaitman BR. Prognostic significance of silent myocardial ischemia detected by early treadmill exercise after coronary angioplasty. Am J Cardiol 1989; 64:1.

72. Dubach P, Froelicher V, Klein J, Detrano R. Use of the exercise test to predict prognosis after coronary artery bypass grafting. Am J Cardiol 1989; 63:530.

73. Kennedy HL, Seiler SM, Sprague MK, Homan SM, Whitlock JA, Kern MJ, Vandormael MG, Barner HB, Codd JE, Willman VL. Relation of silent myocardial ischemia after coronary artery bypass grafting to angiographic completeness of revascularization and long-term prognosis. Am J Cardiol 1990; 65:14.

74. Reis SE, Gottlieb SO. Prognostic implications of transient asymptomatic myocardial ischemia as detected by ambulatory electrocardiographic monitoring. Prog Cardiovasc Dis 1992; 35:77.

13
Relation of Silent Myocardial Ischemia to Sudden Death, Silent Myocardial Infarction, and Ischemic Cardiomyopathy

In addition to the overall prognostic picture provided in Chapter 12, there are three potential complications of silent myocardial ischemia that warrant special comment: sudden death, silent myocardial infarction, and ischemic cardiomyopathy.

I. SILENT MYOCARDIAL ISCHEMIA, VENTRICULAR ARRHYTHMIAS, AND SUDDEN DEATH

Sudden death is defined as death occurring within 1 to 24 h of collapse in a person with or without prior overt cardiac disease in whom there is no other probable cause of death. In witnessed deaths (in-hospital or out-of-hospital) the most common arrhythmia is ventricular fibrillation [1].

Sudden death represents a major source of cardiovascular mortality in the United States. It has been estimated that some 300,000 persons die in this manner every year [2]. Most have coronary artery disease and many have not had *any* prior clinical evidence of heart disease.

The Framingham study has analyzed the risk factors for this phenomenon in 5209 persons and found that the "classical" risk factors of coronary artery disease appear to be risk factors for sudden death as well, especially in men [2]. Pathological studies at necropsy have revealed several differences between those patients who were previously asymptomatic compared to those patients who had histories of angina pectoris and/or a clinical acute myocardial infarction [3]. In one study, peak age was 41 to 60 (Fig. 1) and men predominated. There was a higher frequency of left main disease and a lower frequency of one-vessel disease in the symptomatic group. Quantitative analysis showed

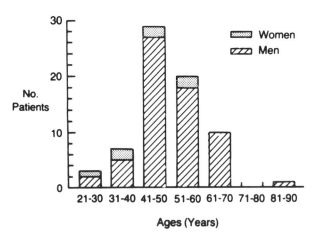

Figure 1   Age distribution in 70 patients with sudden coronary death. (From Warnes CA, Roberts WC. Am J Cardiol 1984; 54:65.)

a significantly higher mean percent of severely narrowed segments in the symptomatic group and less minimal narrowing (Fig. 2).

The degree of vascular pathology notwithstanding, the intriguing question is whether patients with silent myocardial ischemia are as likely—or more likely—to develop sudden death than their symptomatic counterparts. In the absence of an effective anginal warning system [4], will individuals at high risk because of severe coronary stenoses continue to exert themselves until catastrophic events (sudden death or myocardial infarction) occur?

It is obvious that the widespread and extensive coronary atherosclerosis present at autopsy in individuals dying suddenly and unexpectedly did not occur overnight (although complete occlusion due to a thrombus—when present—is presumably a sudden event). Few studies have addressed the issue of whether the population with asymptomatic coronary artery disease forms the pool from which a certain number of persons will surface each year as victims of sudden death or nonfatal myocardial infarctions. Evidence from a study performed at the Hennepin County Medical Center in Minnesota [5] provides some tentative conclusions in this regard. These investigators studied 15 persons who were successfully resuscitated from ventricular fibrillation that took place outside the hospital. Nine of the 15 had no prior history of heart disease. During bicycle exercise testing in the catheterization laboratory, nearly all the patients developed silent myocardial ischemia on their ECGs. Ventriculography also showed painless wall motion abnormalities (Fig. 3). The severity of left ventricular dysfunction was similar in asymptomatic compared to the previously symptomatic patients. Thus, one could speculate that silent ischemia may have occurred prior to the episode of ventricular fibrillation and may play a role in the genesis of sudden death in some individuals. Norris et al. [6] found that 25% of 43 out-of-hospital survivors of ventricular fibrillation had silent ischemia on subsequent Holter monitoring, and Myerburg et al. [7] induced silent ischemia and ventricular tachycardia with ergonovine in five survivors of cardiac arrest who had evidence of coronary spasm, but Peters et al. [8] could not duplicate these findings.

Conversely, ventricular arrhythmias have been reported with varying frequency in patients with silent ischemia who are undergoing Holter monitoring. Stern et al. [9] found ventricular arrhythmias in 32 of the 75 patients with silent ischemia that they studied, whereas Hausmann et al. [10] found only 10 of their 87 patients had silent ischemic episodes associated with ventricular arrhythmias. Complex ventricular ectopic activity was not common in any of these studies. In postinfarction patients, Camacho et al. [11] could not find a clearcut relationship between asymptomatic ST depression and ventricular arrhythmias. In hypertensive subjects with abnormal thallium exercise tests, Szlachcic

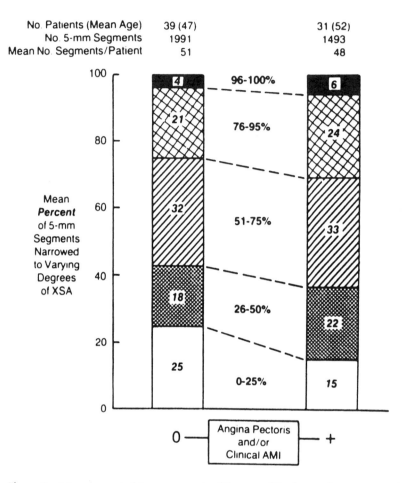

Figure 2 Mean percent of 5-mm segments of the sum of the four major coronary arteries narrowed to varying degrees in cross-sectional area (XSA) in 70 patients with sudden coronary death: comparison of 39 patients without and 31 patients with a clinical acute myocardial infarction (AMI) or angina or both. (From Warnes CA, Roberts WC. Am J Cardiol 1984; 54:65.)

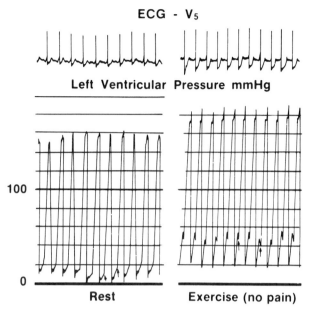

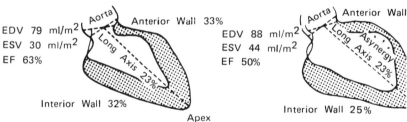

Left Ventriculogram

Figure 3 Simultaneous recording of chest lead V_5, left ventricular pressure, and ventriculogram during exercise indicating electrocardiographic (ECG), hemodynamic, and left ventriculographic evidence of painless myocardial ischemia in an asymptomatic patient with out-of-hospital ventricular fibrillation (patient 3). Note the increase in end-diastolic pressure from rest to exercise (arrows). EDV = end-diastolic volume; EF = ejection fraction; ESV = end-systolic volume. (From Sharma B, Asinger R, Francis GS, Hodges M, Wyeth RP. Am J Cardiol 1987; 59:740.)

et al. [12] reported a 24% incidence of ventricular tachycardia if left ventricular hypertrophy was also present.

Looking at this subject from yet another point of view, there are also studies in which Holter records of patients dying during the monitoring period are reviewed for evidence of silent ischemia. Hohnloser et al. report striking evidence of this phenomenon in two patients [13]. Dubner et al. [14] also found it in two patients and Santinelli et al. in one [15]. In the largest series of patients studied to date, Pepine et al. [16] found that 34% of 35 cases of sudden death had new ST abnormalities preceding the cardiac arrest (Fig. 4). Further evidence suggesting a relationship between ventricular arrhythmias and silent ischemia has been reported by Goseki et al. [17]. Their study showed heart rate variability—a measure of autonomic nervous system activity—to be impaired in the last 10 min before the ischemic events. Pozzati et al. found similar autonomic dysfunction to occur even sooner—5 min before ischemic sudden death (Fig. 5) [18]. A circadian pattern has also been noted in these episodes by Goseki et al. and confirmed by Peckova et al. [19], when cardiac arrest occurs. This circadian variation can be abolished by beta-blockers [20] in a similar manner to ischemic events. We concur with Pepine et al. [16], who concluded that "ischemia may be found more often than previously anticipated in patients with sudden cardiac death." Despite these reports, the arrhythmogenic potential of silent ischemia—or any ischemic event for that matter—is still controversial [21,22]. Mehta et al. [23] have recently summarized the controversy as to whether acute ischemia versus scar/substrate is related to sudden cardiac death and note that Holter monitoring is merely one of the clinical investigations used to document ischemia-related events. Nonetheless, in Erikssen's study in Norway [24], 5 of 50 totally asymptomatic persons died suddenly and unexpectedly. Interestingly, five others developed silent myocardial infarctions prior to death.

In the U.S. Air Force study, Hickman et al. [25] recorded two cases of sudden death (for an annual rate of 4.4/1000), while Feruglio [26] reported rates of 10/1000 in one series and 12/1000 in another series. This compares to rates of 2.9/1000 in epidemiological studies using positive exercise tests without angiographic confirmation. By contrast, rates of 20 to 27/1000 for stable angina patients and 40 to 60/1000 for those with unstable angina have been reported (Table 1).

What implications do these data have in relation to vigorous exercise in asymptomatic individuals who may have latent coronary artery disease? There are several reports of exertion-related sudden death in which silent ischemia appears causally related. Hong et al. [27] documented this association in three patients, and Hoberg et al. [28] postulated that "silent ischemia-related ventricular arrhythmias could be the missing link between the increased risk of car-

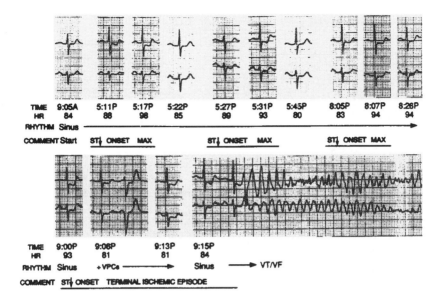

Figure 4   Example of a patient with multiple ischemic episodes terminating in ventricular tachycardia (VT)/fibrillation (VF). The ambulatory electrocadiographic recorder was applied at 9:05 A.M. when the patient was in sinus rhythm. The ST segment remained isoelectric until 5:11 P.M. and reached a maximum (MAX) of 2.0 mm 6 min later in lead V5 (top tracing) as R-wave amplitude and heart rate (HR) increased. This initial ischemic episode subsided slowly over the next 5 min. A second ischemic episode was recorded at 5:27 P.M. with a similar pattern of increasing R-wave amplitude and ST segment depression. Another ischemic episode was recorded at 8:05 P.M., and a fourth and terminal ischemic episode was recorded at 9 P.M. During this episode, ST segment depression reached 2.0 mm and at 9:06 P.M. was associated with ventricular premature contractions (VPCs) occurring late in the cycle. At 9:15 P.M. a ventricular premature contraction occurred during the T wave followed by ventricular tachycardia/fibrillation. (From Pepine CJ, Morganroth J, McDonald JT, Gottlieb SO. Am J Cardiol 1991; 68:785. Reproduced with permission.)

diac arrest and lack of premonitoring symptoms in cardiac rehabilitation programs." They based this conclusion on their studies of strenuous physical exercise in patients with coronary artery disease who wore Holter monitors during the training periods. We know there is a small risk of sudden death in persons participating in vigorous sports. Northcote and Ballantyne reviewed the literature and found 109 such instances of which 80 (73%) were attributed to coronary artery disease found at autopsy [29]. They felt medical screening, includ-

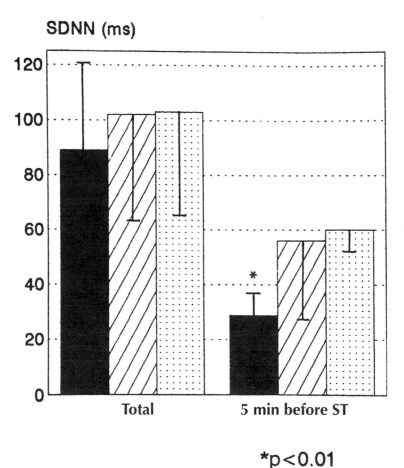

SDNN (ms)

*p<0.01

Figure 5 Values for the standard deviation of normal RR intervals (SDNN) are reported for control subjects (hatched bars, 24 ischemic episodes in 20 patients) and patients with ischemic sudden death (solid bars, 8 fatal episodes in 8 patients; dotted bars, 7 nonfatal episodes in 4 of the 8 patients). At left, values refer to overall recording; at right, values refer to those obtained 5 min before ST shift. The SDNN is significantly reduced at the onset of fatal ischemic episodes when compared with either that recorded in nonfatal episodes or before ST shifts in control subjects. (Reproduced with permission from Pozzati A, Pancaldi LG, Di Pasquale G, Pinelli G, Bugiardini R. J Am Coll Cardiol 1996; 27:847–852.)

Table 1 Incidence of SD in Coronary Artery Disease

Patient category		Annual incidence (per 1000)
Symptomatic	Stable effort angina	20–27
	Unstable angina	40–60
	Acute myocardial infarction	≥20%
	Previous infarction	50
Asymptomatic	No previous acute myocardial infarction	4.4 [16]
		2.9 [17]
		10 [8,18]
	Previous myocardial infarction	12 [24]

SD = sudden death.
Numbers in brackets indicate references in original article.
Source: Geruglio GA. In: Rutishauser W, Roskamm H, eds. *Silent Myocardial Ischemia.* Berlin: Springer-Verlag, 1984.

ing exercise testing, might be helpful in identifying some of the individuals at highest risk. They have been particularly interested in squash playing in the United Kingdom and in 1986 reported on 60 deaths occurring between 1976 and 1984 [30]. Only 22 of the persons had known medical conditions possibly related to heart disease, yet 51/60 had autopsy-proven coronary artery disease. Proximal symptoms were present in some, but not all, of the patients without known heart disease (Madsen [31] has observed that about 20% of sudden death victims have neither prodromes nor overt heart disease). In contrast to the British experience, Malinow et al. found only one case of sudden death in a 10-year retrospective analysis of YMCA sports facilities in the United States [32]. Therefore, they felt it was not important to screen such persons. Siscovick et al. [33] interviewed the wives of 133 men without known prior heart disease who had suffered a cardiac arrest. They concluded that those persons who engaged in low levels of habitual physical activity had a greater risk of sudden death during vigorous exercise compared to more physically active men. Whether exercise or Holter ECG screening prior to performing vigorous activity would have detected latent coronary artery disease in these individuals is unclear [34]. However, a report on coronary patients who were engaged in swimming as part of their rehabilitation training suggests that Holter monitoring during this activity could detect patients at risk for ischemic sudden death [35] (Fig. 6).

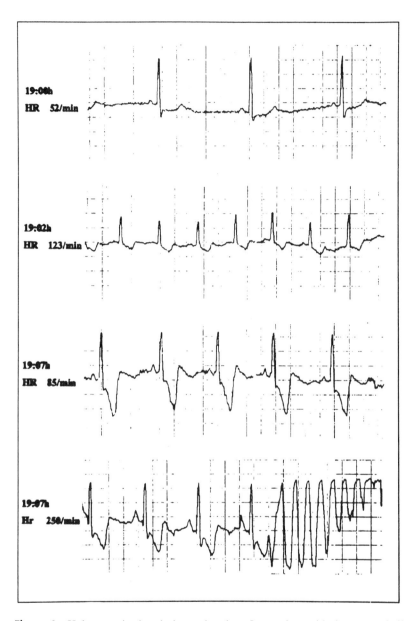

Figure 6 Holter monitoring during swimming. One patient with documented silent ischemia considerably exceeded his recommended heart rate (HR) while wearing a Holter monitor during a swimming session. Immediately after he stopped swimming in order to rest, he suddenly became unconscious, and electrocardiographic tracings revealed increasing ST segment depression that degenerated into ventricular fibrillation. (Reproduced with permission from Niebauer J, Hambrecht R, Hauerk, Marburger C, Schoppenthau M, Kalberer B, Schlierf G, Kubler W, Schuler G. Am J Cardiol 1994; 74:651–656.)

II. SILENT MYOCARDIAL ISCHEMIA AND SILENT MYOCARDIAL INFARCTION

It is tempting to speculate that if myocardial infarction occurs—rather than sudden death—it is more likely to be silent in this group of individuals. Are there any data to support this conjecture? Only in Erikksen's study [24], where 6 of 50 asymptomatic patients with angiographically confirmed disease developed silent infarctions, five of whom died. Whether patients with both silent ischemia and angina tend to develop silent infarctions is also unclear, though one could speculate that this circumstance must be common, since 20 to 25% of all infarctions are unrecognized.

III. SILENT MYOCARDIAL ISCHEMIA AND ISCHEMIC CARDIOMYOPATHY

Ischemia of the myocardium can cause diffuse fibrosis with the resultant clinical syndrome being indistinguishable from that of a primary congestive cardiomyopathy. It has generally been assumed that these cases preresent "burned out" postinfarction patients who no longer have ischemic foci. A history of angina is usually, but not invariably, present. However, in many cases there has been neither an anginal history nor a history of a symptomatic infarction. Pantely and Bristow [36] speculate that "repeated episodes of silent ischemia, though brief, or silent infarction, though small, may result in congestive ischemic cardiomyopathy" in such patients. Presumably the mechanism would be similar to that of the "stunned" or "hibernating" myocardium described in Chapter 4. Raper et al. [37] in their small series of patients with severe painless ischemia offer dramatic evidence of how a painless episode can lead to marked left ventricular dysfunction, including pulmonary edema. Another etiology for the left ventricular dysfunction, myocarditis, has recently been suggested by Frustaci et al. [38].

Survival in patients with this syndrome—as in all types of cardiomyopathy—is directly related to the degree of left ventricular dysfunction.

IV. CONCLUSIONS

It is intriguing to speculate that silent myocardial ischemia can lead to sudden death, silent infarcts, or even ischemic cardiomyopathy. There is evidence to confirm this sequence in some patients, but the numbers are too small to permit sweeping generalizations [39].

REFERENCES

1. Goldstein S, Friedman L, Hutchinson R, Canner P, Romhilt D, Schlant R, Sobrino R, Verter J, Wasserman A, and the Aspirin Myocardial Infarction Study Research Group. Timing, mechanism and clinical setting of witnessed deaths in post-myocardial infarction patients. J Am Coll Cardiol 1984; 3:111.

2. Schatzkin A, Cupples LA, Heeren T, Morelock S, Mucatel M, Kannel WB. The epidemiology of sudden unexpected death: Risk factors for men and women in the Framingham Heart Study. Am Heart J 1984; 107:1300.

3. Warnes CA, Roberts WC. Sudden coronary death: Relation of amount and distribution of coronary narrowing at necropsy to previous symptoms of myocardial ischemia, left ventricular scarring and heart weight. Am J Cardiol 1984; 54:65.

4. Cohn PF. Silent myocardial ischemia in patients with a defective anginal warning system. Am J Cardiol 1980; 45:697.

5. Sharma B, Asinger R, Francis GS, Hodges M, Wyeth RP. Demonstration of exercise-induced painless myocardial ischemia in survivors of out-of-hospital ventricular fibrillation. Am J Cardiol 1987; 59:740.

6. Norris B, Callahan DB, Emery M, Cobb LA. Silent ischemia in survivors of out-of-hospital ventricular fibrillation (abstr). J Am Coll Cardiol 1988; 11:96A.

7. Myerburg RJ, Kessler KM, Mallon SM, Cox MM, deMarchena E, Interian A, Jr., Castellanos A. Life-threatening ventricular arrhythmias in patients with silent myocardial ischemia due to coronary artery spasm. N Engl J Med 1992; 326:1451.

8. Peters PHJ, Wever EJD, Hauer RNW, de Medina EOR. Low prevalence of coronary artery spasm in patients with normal coronary angiograms and unexplained ventricular fibrillation. Eur Heart J 1998; 19:1070–1074.

9. Stern S, Banai S, Keren A, Tzivoni D. Ventricular ectopic activity during myocardial ischemic episodes in ambulatory patients. Am J Cardiol 1990; 65:412.

10. Hausmann D, Nikutta P, Trappe H-J, Daniel WG, Wenzlaff P, Lichtlen PR. Incidence of ventricular arrhythmias during transient myocardial ischemia in patients with stable coronary artery disease. J Am Coll Cardiol 1990; 16:49.

11. Camacho AM, Guindo J, Bayes-de-Luna A. Usefulness of silent subendocardial ischemia detected by ST-segment depression in postmyocardial infarction patients as a predictor of ventricular arrhythmias. Am J Cardiol 1992; 69:1243.

12. Szlachcic J, Tubau JF, O'Kelly B, Ammon S, Daiss K, Massie BM. What is the role of silent coronary artery disease and left ventricular hypertrophy in the genesis of ventricular arrhythmias in men with essential hypertension? J Am Coll Cardiol 1992; 19:803.

13. Hohnloser SH, Kasper W, Zehender M, Geibel A, Meinertz T, Just H. Silent myocardial ischemia as a predisposing factor for ventricular fibrillation. Am J Cardiol 1988; 61:461.

14. Dubner SJ, Pinski S, Palma S, Elencwajg B, Tronge JE. Ambulatory electrocardiographic findings in out-of-hospital cardiac arrest secondary to coronary artery disease. Am J Cardiol 1989; 64:801.

15. Santinelli V, Oppo I, Materazzi C, Rabuano A, Piscitelli MM, Basile F, Palma M, Giunta A. Causal relation between silent myocardial ischemia and sudden death. Am Heart J 1994; 128:816–20.

16. Pepine CJ, Morganroth J, McDonald JT, Gottlieb SO. Sudden death during ambulatory electrocardiographic monitoring. Am J Cardiol 1991; 68:785.

17. Goseki Y, Matsubara T, Takahashi N, Takeuchi T, Ibukiyama C. Heart rate variability before the occurrence of silent myocardial ischemia during ambulatory monitoring. Am J Cardiol 1994; 73:845–849.

18. Pozzati A, Pancaldi LG, Di Pasquale G, Pinelli G, Bugiardini R. Transient sympathovagal imbalance triggers "ischemic" sudden death in patients undergoing electrocardiographic Holter monitoring. J Am Coll Cardiol 1996; 27:847–852.

19. Peckova M, Fahrenbruch CE, Cobb LA, Hallstrom AP. Circadian variations in the occurrence of cardiac arrests initial and repeat episodes. Circulation 1998; 98:31–39.

20. Aronow WS, Ahn C, Mercando AD, Epstein S. Circadian variation of sudden cardiac death or fatal myocardial infarction is abolished by propranolol in patients with heart disease and complex ventricular arrhythmias. Am J Cardiol 1994; 74:19–21.

21. Mathes P, Reinke A, Michel D. Arrhythmogenic potential of silent myocardial ischemia after myocardial infarction. In: von Arnim T, Maseri A, eds. Silent Ischemia: Current Concepts and Management. Darmstad: Steinkopff, 1987; 56–61.

22. Gomes JA, Alexopoulos D, Winters S, Fuster V, Suh K. The role of silent ischemia, the arrhythmic substrate and the genesis of sudden cardiac death. J Am Coll Cardiol 1989; 14:1618.

23. Mehta D, Curwin J, Gomes A, Fuster V. Sudden death in coronary artery disease. Circulation 1997; 96:3215–3223.

24. Thaulow E, Erikssen J, Sandik L, Erikssen G, Jorgensen L, Cohn PF. "Warning" signs and symptoms in 50 asymptomatic men with silent myocardial ischemia and angiographically documented coronary artery disease followed for 15 years (abstr). Circulation 1991; 84 (suppl II):II-650.

25. Hickman JR, Jr., Uhl GS, Cook RL, Engel PJ, Hopkirk A. A natural study of asymptomatic coronary disease (abstr). Am J Cardiol 1980; 45:422.

26. Feruglio GA. Sudden death in patients with asymptomatic coronary heart disease. In: Rutishauser W, Roskamm H, eds. Silent Myocardial Ischemia. Berlin: Springer-Verlag, 1984; 144–150.

27. Hong RA, Bhandari AK, McKay CR, Au PK, Rahimtoola SH. Life-threatening ventricular tachycardia and fibrillation induced by painless myocardial ischemia during exercise testing. JAMA 1987; 257:1937.

28. Hoberg E, Schuler G, Kunze B, Obermoser A-L, Hauer K, Mautner HP, Schlierf G, Kubler W. Silent myocardial ischemia as a potential link between lack of pre-

monitoring symptoms and increased risk of cardiac arrest during physical stress. Am J Cardiol 1990; 65:583.

29. Northcote RJ, Ballantyne D. Sudden cardiac death in sports. Br Med J 1983; 287:1357.

30. Northcote RJ, Flannigan C, Ballantyne D. Sudden death and vigorous exercise—A study of 60 deaths associated with squash. Br Heart J 1986; 55:198.

31. Madsen JK. Ischaemic heart disease and prodromes of sudden cardiac death: Is it possible to identify high risk groups for sudden cardiac death? Br Heart J 1985; 54:27.

32. Malinow MR, McGarry DL, Kuehl KS. Is exercise testing indicated for asymptomatic active people? J Cardiac Rehabil 1984; 4:376.

33. Siscovick DS, Weiss NS, Fletcher RH, Lasky T. Relation between vigorous exercise and primary cardiac arrest. N Engl J Med 1984; 311:874.

34. Cohn PF. Silent myocardial ischemia: Clinical significance and relation to sudden cardiac death. Chest 1986; 90:597.

35. Niebauer J, Hambrecht R, Hauer K, Marburger C, Schoppenthau M, Kalberer B, Schlierf G, Kubler W, Schuler G. Identification of patients at risk during swimming by Holter monitoring. Am J Cardiol 1994; 74:651–656.

36. Pantely GA, Bristow JD. Ischemic cardiomyopathy. Prog Cardiovasc Dis 1984; 27:95.

37. Raper AJ, Hastillo A, Paulsen WJ. The syndrome of sudden severe painless myocardial ischemia. Am Heart J 1984; 107:813.

38. Frustaci A, Chimenti C, Maseri A. Global biventricular dysfunction in patients with asymptomatic coronary artery disease may be caused by myocarditis. Circulation 1999; 99:1295–1299.

39. Stern S, Tzivoni D. Ventricular arrhythmias, sudden death, and silent myocardial ischemia. Prog Cardiovasc Dis 1992; 35:19.

14

Prognosis After Silent Myocardial Infarction and Myocardial Infarction Without Preceding Angina

Cardiologists have long appreciated that the natural history of coronary artery disease is complex because of the numerous "subsets" of patients with or without angina, with or without infarctions, etc. [1]. Unfortunately, data on prognosis following silent infarctions are sparse. The greatest source of data concerning this subset of patients has been the Framingham study.

I. SILENT MYOCARDIAL INFARCTION

The Framingham survey was begun in 1948. A standard, thorough, cardiovascular examination was done biennially to detect newly developed cardiovascu-

253

lar disease. In addition, data on cardiovascular endpoints was also obtained by daily surveillance of hospital admission records at Framingham Union Hospital.

As discussed in Chapter 5, the myocardial infarctions were designated as "unrecognized" and then further subdivided into atypical or silent, depending on whether the patients—in retrospect—could identify any complaints as having possibly been compatible with an acute myocardial infarction. (About half of the 108 infarctions were of the truly silent type.) As reported in the 20-year follow-up, the 3-year mortality rates for both unrecognized and recognized myocardial infarctions were similar [2]. (In the Israeli study of Medalie and Goldbourt [3], the mortality following unrecognized myocardial infarctions was markedly lower than after recognized myocardial infarctions—unlike the Framingham experience.)

In their most recent report (26-year follow-up), the Framingham investigators have updated their results [4,5]. As before, there are no data available on prognosis in the immediate convalescent period since, by definition, these patients are not identified until the next routine ECG is performed. However, in those who survived the initial period, the mortality statistics are sobering. As depicted in Figure 1, unrecognized infarctions are as potentially lethal as the symptomatic kind. After 10 years, 45% of patients with unrecognized and 39%

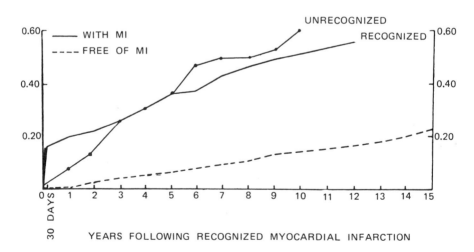

Figure 1 Death following recognized and unrecognized myocardial infarctions (MI) in men of all ages in the Framingham study. ——— = with MI; ---- = free of MI. (From Kannel WB, Abbott RD. In: Rutishauser W, Roskamm H, eds. Silent Myocardial Ischemia. Berlin: Springer-Verlag, 1984: 131–137.)

of those with recognized infarctions were dead. Sudden deaths occurred with equal frequency, and at about nine times the rate seen in the general population. Although less prone to angina (18% vs. 59%) (Table 1), patients with unrecognized infarctions develop congestive heart failure just as often (Table 2). Reinfarction is also common (3%/year in men and 10%/year in women). About 50% of the recurrences are fatal. In the elderly population in the Framingham study, patients with recognized and unrecognized infarctions also had similar mortality rates [6] Sigurdsson et al. [7] in the Reykjavik study also reported similar mortality rates (Fig. 2). By contrast, Yano and MacLean in the Honolulu Heart Program found unrecognized infarctions to carry a *worse* prognosis than recognized infarctions [8].

Silent infarction can also be followed by silent ischemia either on the exercise test, Holter monitoring, or both [9], as well as by other manifestations of coronary disease [7].

Table 1 Proportion of ECG-Documented Myocardial Infarctions (MI) Followed by Angina Pectoris (AP) in Subjects Aged 30 to 62 Years on Entry. Framingham Study, 22-Year Follow-Up

	Number with MI	Followed by AP	
		n	%
Unrecognized	98	18	18
Recognized	190	113	59
Total	288	114	45

Eighty-nine patients had prior angina pectoris or died and were eliminated from consideration.
Source: Kannel WB, Abbott RD. In: Rutishauser W, Roskamm H, eds. Silent Myocardial Ischemia. Berlin: Springer-Verlag, 1984:131–137.

Table 2 Proportion of ECG-Documented Myocardial Infarctions Followed by Cardiac Failure in Subjects 30 to 62 Years of Age at Entry. Framingham Study, 22-Year Follow-Up

	Number	Followed by cardiac failure	
		n	%
Unrecognized	100	21	21
Recognized	221	55	25
Total	321	76	24

Source: Kannel WB, Abbott RD. In: Rutishauser W, Roskamm H, eds. Silent Myocardial Ischemia. Berlin: Springer-Verlag, 1984:131–137.

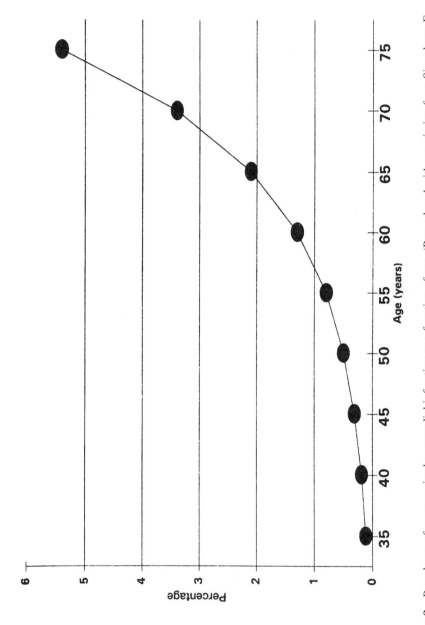

Figure 2 Prevalence of unrecognized myocardial infarction as a function of age. (Reproduced with permission from Sigurdsson E, Thorgeirsson G, Sigvaldson H, Sigfusson N. Ann Intern Med 1995; 122:956–1002.)

II. MYOCARDIAL INFARCTION WITHOUT PRECEDING ANGINA

In patients who survive an acute myocardial infarction, about half did not have angina pectoris before the infarction [10–12]. As noted previously in Chapter 5, there is a high association of one-vessel disease (82%) in such patients [13]. One would suspect that prognosis might, therefore, be better in this type of patient and indeed Midwall et al. [13] reported a lower frequency of postinfarction angina. Mortality figures were not available in this study, but they were in the study by Pierard et al. [12]: 3-year mortality was 16% (angina) vs. 7% (no angina). This was similar to what Harper et al. [10] had reported in their series; hospital mortality was 12% in patients without preceding angina compared to 20% in patients with chronic stable angina. Long-term mortality statistics were also not available in this study. Behar et al. [14] found that preexisting angina identified a group at higher risk of death both during hospitalization and up to 5 years after discharge (Table 3). Barbash et al. [15] reported similar findings in another recent study of patients receiving thrombolytic therapy for acute infarctions. A study by Matsuda et al. [16] suggests that postinfarction left ventricular function is better in patients with angina and an occluded left anterior descending coronary artery compared to those with a similar lesion but without angina. No ready explanation for this finding is available, though the authors suggest better developed collaterals may be involved. Cortina et al. [17] reported similar findings. A protective effort on LV function before the acute myocardial infarction (due to preinfarction angina) was reported by Azai et al. [18] and a similar effect on infarct size by Kloner et al.

Table 3 In-Hospital and Long-Term Mortality Rates in Patients with and Without Angina Pectoris Before a First AMI

Mortality	Angina pectoris ($n = 1801$)		No angina pectoris ($n = 2365$)		p value
	No.	%	No.	%	
In hospital	284	16	276	12	0.0001
After discharge (yr)					
1	124 ·	8	130	6	0.05
5	401	26	407	19	0.001

Source: Behar S, Reicher-Reiss H, Abinader E, Agmon J, Friedman Y, Barzilai J, Kaplinsky E, Kauli N, Kishou Y, Palant A, Peled B, Rbinovich B, Reisin L, Schlesinger Z, Zahavi I, Ziou M, Goldbourt U. Am Heart J 1992; 123:1481.

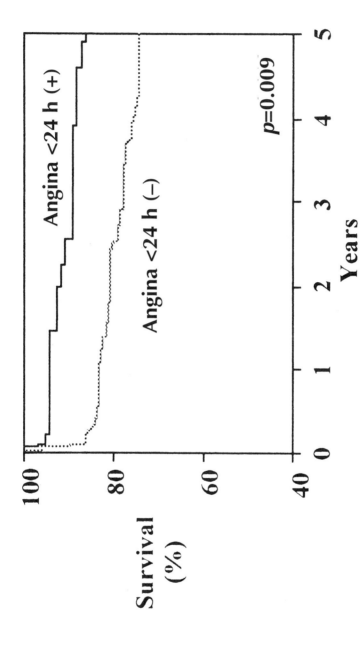

Figure 3 Five-year survival curves for patients with [angina <24 h (+)] versus those without [angina <24 h (−)] prodromal angina in the 24 h before infarction. (Reproduced with permission from Ishihara M, Sato H, Tateishi H, Kawagoe T, Shimatani Y, Kurishu S, Sakai K, Ueda K. J Am Coll Cardiol 1997; 30:970–975.)

[19] as well as reduced incidence of cardiac rupture, cardiogenic shock, and/or congestive heart failure by Kobayashi et al. [20]. Ischemic preconditioning may be the common basis for all three reports as well as another report that angina before the myocardial infarction is associated with favorable in-hospital and postdischarge survival rates (Fig. 3) [21].

III. CONCLUSIONS

Silent myocardial infarctions are as potentially lethal as the symptomatic kind. When a symptomatic infarction occurs, there are conflicting reports as to whether or not prognosis is better if the patient did or did not have angina preceding the infarction.

REFERENCES

1. Goldman GJ, Pichard AD. The natural history of coronary artery disease: Does medical therapy improve the prognosis? Prog Cardiovasc Dis 1983; 25:513.
2. Kannel WB, Sorlie P, McNamara PM. Prognosis after initial myocardial infarction: The Framingham study. Am J Cardiol 1979; 44:53.
3. Medalie JH, Goldbourt MA. Unrecognized myocardial infarction: Five-year incidence, mortality and risk factors. Ann Intern Med 1976; 84:526.
4. Kannel WB, Abbott RD. Incidence and prognosis of unrecognized myocardial infarction: Based on 26 years follow-up in the Framingham study. In: Rutishauser W, Roskamm H, eds. Silent Myocardial Ischemia. Berlin: Springer-Verlag, 1984:131–137.
5. Kannel WB, Abbott RD. Incidence and prognosis of unrecognized myocardial infarction. An update on the Framingham study. N Engl J Med 1984; 311:1144.
6. Vokonas PS, Kannel WB, Cupples LA. Incidence and prognosis of unrecognized myocardial infarction in the elderly, The Framingham study (abstr). J Am Coll Cardiol 1988; 11:51A.
7. Sigurdsson E, Thorgeirsson G, Sigvaldason H, Sigfusson N. Unrecognized myocardial infarction: epidemiology, clinical characteristics, and the prognostic role of angina pectoris. Ann Intern Med 1995; 122:956–1002.
8. Yano K, MacLean CJ. The incidence and prognosis of unrecognized myocardial infarction in the Honolulu, Hawaii, Heart Program. Arch Intern Med 1989; 149:1528.
9. Cohn PF, Sodums MT, Lawson WE, Vlay SC, Brown EJ, Jr. Frequent episodes of silent myocardial ischemia after apparently uncomplicated myocardial infarction. J Am Coll Cardiol 1986; 8:982.

10. Harper RW, Kennedy G, DeSanctis RW, Hutter AM, Jr. The incidence and pattern of angina prior to acute myocardial infarction: A study of 577 cases. Am Heart J 1979; 97:178.

11. Matsuda M, Matsuda Y, Ogawa H, Moritani K, Kusukawa R. Angina pectoris before and during acute myocardial infarction: Relation to degree of physical activity. Am J Cardiol 1985; 55:1255.

12. Pierard LA, Dubois C, Smeets J-P, Boland J, Carlier J, Kulbertus HE. Prognostic significance of angina pectoris before first acute myocardial infarction. Am J Cardiol 1988; 61:984.

13. Midwall J, Ambrose J, Pichard A, Abedin Z, Herman MV. Angina pectoris before and after myocardial infarction: angiographic correlations. Chest 1982; 81:681.

14. Behar S, Reicher-Reiss H, Abinader E, Agmon J, Friedman Y, Barzilai J, Kaplinsky E, Kauli N, Kishon Y, Palant A, Peled B, Rabinovich B, Reisin L, Schlesinger Z, Zahavi I, Zion M, Goldbourt U. The prognostic significance of angina pectoris preceding the occurrence of a first acute myocardial infarction in 4166 consecutive hospitalized patients. Am Heart J 1992; 123:1481.

15. Barbash GI, White HD, Modan M, Van de Werf F for the Investigators of the International Tissue Plasminogen Activator/Streptokinase Trial. Antecedent angina pectoris predicts worse outcome after myocardial infarction in patients receiving thrombolytic therapy: Experience gleaned from the International Tissue Plasminogen Activator/Streptokinase Mortality Trial. J Am Coll Cardiol 1992; 20: 36.

16. Matsuda Y, Ogawa H, Moritani K, Matsuda M, Naito H, Matsuzaki M, Ikee Y, Kusukawa R. Effects of the presence or absence of preceding angina pectoris on left ventricular function after acute myocardial infarction. Am Heart J 1984; 108:955.

17. Cortina A, Ambrose JA, Prieto-Granada J, Moris C, Simarro E, Holt J, Fuster V. Left ventricular function after myocardial infarction: Clinical and angiographic correlations. J Am Coll Cardiol 1985; 5:619.

18. Anzai T, Yoshikawa T, Asakura Y, Abe S, Meguro T, Akaishi M, Mitamura H, Handa S, Ogawa S. Effect on short-time prognosis and left ventricular function of angina pectoris prior to first Q-wave anterior wall acute myocardial infarction. Am J Cardiol 1994; 74:755–759.

19. Kloner RA, Shook T, Przyklenk K, Davis VG, Junio L, Matthews RV, Burstein S, Gibson CM, Poole WK, Cannon CP, McCabe CH, Braunwald E for the TIMI 4 Investigators. Previous angina alters in-hospital outcome in TIMI 4. Circulation 1995; 91:37–47.

20. Kobayashi Y, Miyazaki S, Itoh A, Daikoku S, Morii I, Matsumoto T, Goto Y, Nonogi H. Previous angina reduces in-hospital death in patients with acute myocardial infarction. Am J Cardiol 1998; 81:117–122.

21. Ishihara M, Sato H, Tateishi H, Kawagoe T, Shimatani Y, Kurishu S, Sakai K, Ueda K. Implications of prodromal angina pectoris in anterior wall acute myocardial infarciton: acute angiographic findings and long-term prognosis. J Am Coll Cardiol 1997; 30:970–975.

V

MANAGEMENT OF PATIENTS WITH ASYMPTOMATIC CORONARY ARTERY DISEASE

15

Medical Treatment of Asymptomatic Coronary Artery Disease

Having diagnosed patients as having silent ischemia, the physician must then decide on appropriate therapy—if he or she chooses to treat at all. Guidelines can be offered on the basis of the prognostic information provided in Part IV, as well as the results of trials reported in the 1980s [1–3], and newer multicenter studies whose results have recently become available and which will be discussed at length in subsequent sections of this chapter.

I.   MANAGEMENT OF PERSONS WHO ARE TOTALLY ASYMPTOMATIC

Perhaps no single area concerning asymptomatic coronary artery disease is as controversial as management [4]. Because the prognosis in persons in this category is generally favorable, the simplest approach is to (1) modify risk factors when they are present and (2) reduce physical activities so that myocardial ischemia does not develop. As we shall discuss in some detail later, the former approach now utilizes new cholesterol-lowering agents ("statins") and angiotensin-converting enzyme (ACE) inhibitors that can improve endothelial function, reduce myocardial ischemia, and dramatically inhibit the rate of subsequent coronary events [5]. The latter approach is to ward off possible damage to the patient with a defective angina warning system during strenuous exertion. It is the patients who demonstrate extensive ischemia that merit special concern [4]. These individuals are more likely to have multivessel disease with its correspondingly worse prognosis. As opposed to asymptomatic persons with single-vessel disease who may be in a "presymptomatic" stage and go on to angina or nonfatal infarction, asymptomatic individuals with triple-vessel or left main disease appear to be at higher risk for sudden death or massive infarctions. We believe every effort should be made to treat these latter patients with anti-ischemic agents. One endpoint could be improved exercise tolerance (i.e., prolonging the time at which ischemia develops). Another endpoint could be improved wall motion in ischemic zones. This can be documented in one of several ways. For example, in an early study from our laboratory [6], we treated 11 asymptomatic patients with silent myocardial ischemia (some of whom had prior infarctions) with propranolol or timolol and evaluated exercise ECGs and radionuclide ventriculograms before and after administration of the drugs. The beneficial results are depicted in Table 1. In the first study to show an improvement in event-free survival, Eme et al. [7] randomized 53 type-1 patients in Switzerland to either no treatment or a combination of anti-ischemic agents (Fig. 1). Another way to approach the asymptomatic patient with silent ischemia is to use Holter monitoring to document a reduction in ischemic activity (either frequency, duration, or both). Imperi et al. [8] used the beta-blocker metoprolol in a group of nine asymptomatic or minimally symptomatic patients. By titrating the metoprolol to an optimal dose (via

Table 1   Treatment of Silent Myocardial Ischemia with Beta-Adrenergic Blockade (BAB)

	Pre-BAB	Post-BAB	p value
Time to exercise-induced ST depression	207 s ± 75	348 s ± 89	$p < 0.05$
Maximum ST depression	1.41 mm ± 0.15	0.81 ± 0.20	$p < 0.05$
Change in regional exercise ejection fraction	–0.06 ± 0.01	–0.01 ± 0.01	$p < 0.01$

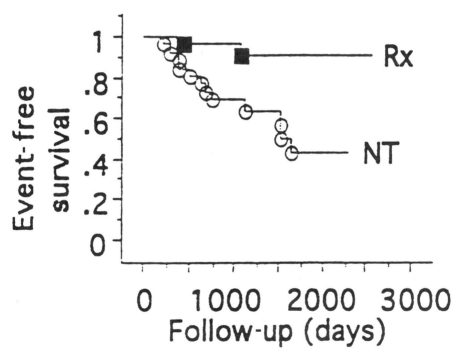

Figure 1   Event-free survival in 53 asymptomatic patients in the Swiss International Study on Silent Ischemia (SWISSI 1) randomized to either no therapy (NT) or medical therapy (RX). [Reproduced with permission from Eme P, Burckhardt D, Dubach P, Zuber M, Kowski W. J Am Coll Cardiol 1999; 33 (Suppl A): 340A.]

Table 2 Clinical, Angiographic, and Holter Findings Before and After Nifedipine in 12 Asymptomatic Patients

					Holter monitoring			
					Pretreatment		Nifedipine treatment	
		Narrowed CA			Ischemic episodes (n)	Duration of ischemic episodes (min)	Ischemic episodes (n)	Duration of ischemic episodes (min)
Pt	Right	LAD	LC	MI				
1	+	+	+	0	11	699	4	143
2	+	0	0	0	6	153	4	144
3	+	+	0	+(A)	4	15	1	2
4	0	+	+	+(A)	6	53	1	10
5	+	+	+	0	3	39	4	21
6	+	+	+	+(I)	17	120	5	59
7	+	0	0	0	4	14	1	2
8	+	+	0	0	8	40	0	0
9	+	+	+	0	6	37	6	55
10	0	+	0	0	4	197	7	177
11	+	+	+	+(A)	5	52	0	0
12	+	+	+	0	6	68	4	2

A = anterior; CA = coronary artery; I = inferior; LAD = left anterior descending coronary artery; LC = left circumflex coronary artery; MI = myocardial infarction.
Source: Cohn PF and Lawson WE. Am J Cardiol 1988; 61:908.

Holter monitoring), they were able to significantly reduce ischemic activity. We achieved similar results (Table 2) using the calcium blocker nifedipine in a standard dose, either 30 or 60 mg daily [9].

Although usually employed in symptomatic patients, percutaneous transluminal coronary angioplasty (PTCA) can be used in selected asymptomatic patients. Tuzcu et al. [10] reported excellent results in 34 patients, with 100% survival at the 3-year follow-up mark. In an even larger series of asymptomatic patients, Anderson et al. [11] reported their results in 114 individuals, 107 of whom had been initially detected by exercise testing. Again the results were excellent and are depicted in Figure 1.

Because psychological stress may exacerbate silent myocardial ischemia [11], psychological counseling may be important in these patients, especially since the implications of a potentially lethal, but silent, disease can be further anxiety-provoking and thus detrimental to the patient's emotional well-being

[13]. This is discussed further in the following section on postinfarction patients.

II. MANAGEMENT OF PATIENTS WHO ARE ASYMPTOMATIC FOLLOWING A MYOCARDIAL INFARCTION

There is now a general consensus concerning aggressive treatment of these patients. Even those who are skeptical of treating totally asymptomatic persons would treat postinfarction patients with silent ischemia. At present, medical treatment with beta-blockers is recommended for postinfarction patients in order to reduce short-term mortality and reinfarction [16]. Therefore, it is only logical that *all* patients with evidence of myocardial ischemia postinfarction should receive some form of medical treatment, whether or not they are symptomatic. That the absence of angina in postinfarction exercise studies is reliable evidence of silent ischemia rather than of "stoic endurance or denial of perceived symptoms"—was the conclusion of a 1996 study of psychological characteristics of 151 patients with exercise-induced silent ischemia [14]. A recent comparison of coronary angioplasty versus combination drug therapy (including beta-blockers) showed no difference in event-free survival in 201 type-2 Swiss patients but did show improved left ventricular function in the patients undergoing angioplasty. There are data suggesting that the mechanism of action by beta-blockers is not due only to a reduction in arrhythmias but in ischemia suppression per se. (The ischemia suppression hypothesis will be discussed further when the effect of therapy on prognosis is considered.) Data suggest, but do not prove, that the beta-blockers improve prognosis in postinfarction patients by reducing ischemia. Ruberman et al. [17] conducted a large case-control study using data from the previously completed Beta Blocker Heart Attack Trial (BHAT). There were 326 deaths during the BHAT follow-up period, and 261 of the patients had readable Holter tapes available for review. They were matched against appropriate controls from the BHAT registry who survived at least as long as the given case. The results are worth summarizing: The investigators found that ST depression on Holter monitoring was associated with increased mortality and that the more ischemic time on Holter monitoring, the greater the risk of subsequent death. Most importantly, in terms of medical management, the relative risk in the popranolol-treated group was significantly less than in the placebo-treated group (Table 3).

As discussed in Chapter 11, most physicians regard continuing evidence of ischemia as grounds for cardiac catheterization. Depending on the severity of the angiographic findings, some of these patients will be candidates for more aggressive medical management, coronary angioplasty, or coronary bypass

Table 3 Conditional Logistic Relative Risk Estimates for Mortality Caused by STD (Drug Effect Model)

Variable	RR	95% CL
Nongradient model		
STD (treated)	0.98	0.48–2.00
STD (placebo)	2.56	1.39–4.71
Gradient model		
STD (1–30 min, treated)	0.92	0.40–2.09
STD (> 30 min, treated)	1.15	0.35–3.71
STD (1–30 min, placebo)	1.91	0.92–3.96
STD (> 30 min, placebo)	4.33	1.60–11.71

STD, ST segment depression; RR, relative risk; CL, confidence limits. Deaths matched to controls on time, age, sex, and drug status. RR estimates adjusted for previous myocardial infarction (MI), history of angina, diastolic blood pressure, heart rate, cigarette smoking before MI, and presence of pulmonary edema.
Source: Ruberman W, Crow R, Rosenberg CR, Rautaharju PM, Shore RE, Pasternack BS. Circulation 1992; 85:1440.

surgery. Comparisons of medical versus surgical management (as in the CASS survey) will be discussed in Chapter 16.

Psychological reactions in these patients are also important, since many assume that once they have recovered from the acute infarction and are asymptomatic, they have little to worry about. When this assumption is corrected, the level of anxiety is raised. However, in a study of 15 patients [13] with asymptomatic coronary artery disease, most of whom had prior infarctions, we found that most patients felt their physicians had been supportive in explaining the problems to them. Because of trust in their physicians, patients often changed their lifestyles markedly in regard to exercise and diet. All agreed that public awareness of this disorder was unfortunately almost nonexistent.

III. MANAGEMENT OF PATIENTS WITH EPISODES OF BOTH SYMPTOMATIC AND ASYMPTOMATIC MYOCARDIAL ISCHEMIA

These patients are the ones that practitioners are most likely to encounter. In the past, there has been a tendency to discount the importance of the asymptomatic episodes and to treat "symptoms." With the report of several groups that asymptomatic episodes often greatly outnumber symptomatic episodes (as determined by Holter monitoring), there is a growing trend toward considering the asymptomatic episodes of equal importance to the symptomatic ones. Both can result in metabolic, hemodynamic and electrical abnormalities of myocardial function. As a result, a new approach to the treatment of myocardial ischemia is gaining acceptance. In this approach, the use of drugs, angioplasty, and surgery is used to reduce the *total ischemic burden* and not merely symptomatic episodes [1,18] especially since the greatest number of ischemic episodes per day appears to be in those patients with both symptomatic and painless ischemia [19].

Just as with type 1 and type 2 patients discussed earlier, choice of medications in type 3 patients depends on whether the ischemia is due to increased work of the heart, a vasospastic component, or both. In the former case, myocardial oxygen requirements are raised, usually because of increases in heart rate and blood pressure, two of the major factors regulating myocardial oxygen consumption. For these episodes, beta-blockers would appear to be reasonable agents.

Early studies suggested that many of the episodes did not appear to be associated with increased work of the heart. For example, Schang and Pepine [20] and then Cecchi et al. [21] reported that the ratio of asymptomatic episodes to symptomatic episodes recorded on Holter monitoring was greatest during nonstrenuous activities. The lack of increased heart rate or blood pressure preceding many episodes was noted by several investigators, as in the example in Figure 3, from the study of hospitalized patients by Chierchia et al. [22]. Ambulatory blood pressure records in out-of-hospital patients have shown similar results [23]. Furthermore, Deanfield et al. [24] demonstrated that in their patients the heart rate at the onset of ST segment depression was significantly lower after unprovoked ischemia than after exercise (Fig. 4). Peak heart rates showed the same trend. During silent myocardial ischemia due to mental stress, heart rate was also less than during exercise-induced ischemia. It seemed reasonable to conclude that for episodes of silent ischemia not associated with increased work of the heart, nitrates or calcium antagonists would provide the best approach to therapy. Schang and Pepine [20] were able to significantly reduce the frequency of asymptomatic episodes using hourly nitroglycerin tables (3.7 ± 0.02 episodes per monitoring period to 0.6 ± 0.02). Long-acting nitrates, either as ointment (Table 4) isosorbide dinitrate or isosorbite mononitrate (Table 5) preparations, have also proven efficacious, especially when intermittent dosing is used [25–29]. Johnson et al. [30] and Parodi et al. [31] reduced total ischemic episodes with verapamil. Frishman et al. did the same with diltiazem [32]. Theroux et al. [33] also used diltiazem with excellent effects (Fig. 5), as did Deedwania et al. with a longer acting preparation [34], while Tzivoni et al. [35] found only moderate benefits with nisoldipine. Most data on calcium antagonists have come from nifedipine studies, with mixed

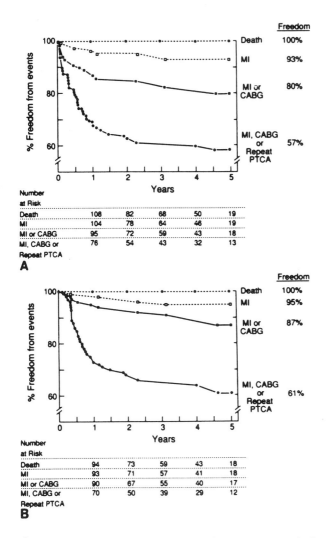

Figure 2 Event-free survival curves after coronary angioplasty for asymptomatic patients with coronary artery disease. (A) Event-free survival for entire group of 114 asymptomatic patients. (B) Event-free survival for group of 99 asymptomatic patients with successful angioplasty procedures. The tables below each graph show number of patients at risk for events at end of each year. CABG = coronary artery bypass graft surgery; MI = myocardial infarction; PTCA = percutaneous transluminal coronary angioplasty. (From Anderson HV, Talley JD, Black AJR, Roubin GS, Douglas JS, Jr., King SB, III. Am J Cardiol 1990; 65: 35. Reproduced with permission.)

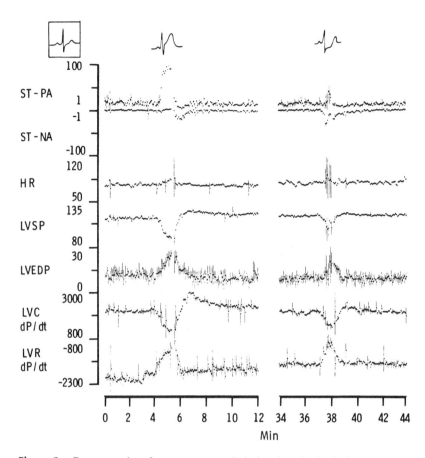

Figure 3 Computer plot of two asymptomatic ischemic episodes in the same patient. The averaged values of each derived variable are plotted with their standard deviation against time. The variables (top to bottom) were ST segment positive (PA) and negative areas (NA), heart rate (HR), left ventricular systolic (LVSP) and end-diastolic pressures (LVEDP) and left ventricular peak contraction (LVC) and relaxation (LVR) dP/dt. In the episode on the left, transient ST segment elevation (increase in ST segment positive area) was accompanied by an increase in left ventricular end-diastolic pressure, and decreases in both contract and relaxation dP/dt. Similar impairment of left ventricular function accompanied the asymptomatic episode of ST segment depression (increase in ST segment negative area) in the same electrocardiographic lead shown on the right. A vasospastic component is suggested by the lack of increase in the variables controlling myocardial oxygen demand (such as HR or LVSP) before either episode. (From Chierchia S, Lazzari M, Freedman B, Brunelli C, Maseri A. J Am Coll Cardiol 1983; 1:924.)

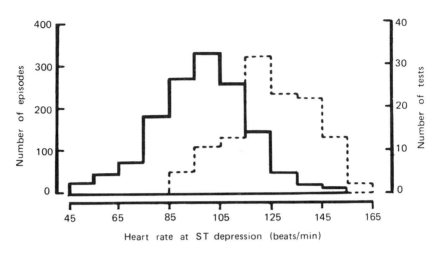

Figure 4   Distribution of heart rates at onset of ST depression during ambulatory monitoring (——) and during exercise testing (- - -). (From Deanfield JE, Selwyn AP, Krikler S, Morgan M. Lancet 1983; 2:753.)

results. In a small series of patients, Oakley et al. [36] used nifedipine with good results—though best results were observed when nifedipine and propranolol were combined. The combination of nifedipine and beta-blockers has also been used in the Nifedipine-Total Ischemia Awareness Program (TIAP) [37]. Nifedipine led to further and significant reduction in ischemic activity when added to either nitrates and/or beta-blockers. The beneficial effects of combination therapy were especially marked in the patients with the most total ischemic activity (Table 6). A new, long-acting nifedipine preparation was subsequently introduced and tested in another large multicenter study [38]. Again, the results were impressive, especially in combination with a beta-blocker. Others have reported lesser effects, especially when nifedipine is used as the

Table 4   Effect of Transdermal Nitroglycerin on Number and Duration of Ischemic Events in Eight Patients with Chronic Angina

	Prenitroglycerin (mean ± SEM)	Postnitroglycerin (mean ± SEM)
Silent ischemic episodes (no.)	5.3 ± 3.3	0.8 ± 1.2 ($p < 0.05$)
Depressed ST segment duration (min)	95.8 ± 87	17 ± 27.1 ($p = 0.05$)

Source: Adapted from Shell WE, Kivowitz CF, Rubins SB, See J. Am Heart J 1986; 212:222.

Table 5 Change in Silent Myocardial Ischemia per Week After Medication in 28 Patients

	Baseline phase (1)	Placebo phase (2)	IS-5-MN[a] phase (3)	Decreased (%)
No. of ischemic episodes	522	538	64	88
Duration of ischemia (min)	10,121	10,237	622	94
Integration (mm/min)	21,391	21,792	925	96
Total maximal ST segment (min)	1,001	1,037	142	86

[a] Isosorbide-5-mononitrate.
p Value: phases 1 and 2, >0.05; phases 1 and 3, <0.01; phases 2 and 3, <0.01.
Source: Fend J, Feng X-H, Schneeweiss A. Am J Cardiol 1990; 65:32J.

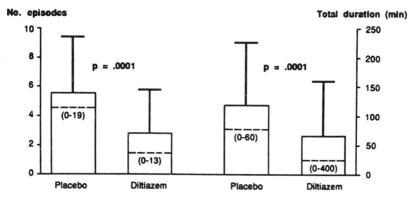

Figure 5 Total episodes and cumulative duration of ST depression during the double-blind crossover phase of the study. Diltiazem significantly reduced both the number of episodes and their total duration. Dashed lines within the bars show the median, and the numbers the ranges. (From Theroux P, Baird M, Juneau M, Warnica W, Klinke P, Kostuk W, Plugfelder P, Lavallee E, Chin C, Dempsey E, Grace M, Lalonde Y, Waters D. Circulation 1991; 84:15. Reproduced with permission of the American Heart Association.)

Table 6 Effect of Nifedipine on Number and Duration of Silent Ischemic Episodes in 38 Patients in the Total Ischemia Awareness Program (TIAP) with 60 Min or More of Ischemic Activity While Taking Nitrates and/or Beta-Blockers for Angina

	Pre-nifedipine (mean ± SEM)	Post-nifedipine (mean ± SEM)
ST segment changes without pain (no.)	5.7 ± 0.9	3.2 ± 0.6, $p < 0.001$
Depressed ST segment duration (min)	127 ± 13	68 ± 15, $p < 0.001$

sole anti-ischemic agent [39]. Newer calcium blockers have been reported to be very effective in reducing symptomatic and asymptomatic cardiac ischemic events. Perhaps the most thoroughly investigated of these agents is amlodipine. In the Circadian Anti-Ischemia Program in Europe (CAPE), 315 patients entered the active treatment phase and those patients receiving amlodipine showed a significant decrease in transient myocardial ischemia compared to placebo [40]. Similar results were reported from the United States [41]. This is in contrast to another study from Europe in which amlodipine was compared to diltiazem but neither was found to curtail the morning peak in ischemic events [42]. A newer calcium antagonist, mibefradil, created interest as an anti-ischemic agent but, unfortunately, a problem with unsafe side effects led the FDA to recommend its removal from the market in 1998.

Despite the previously cited observations concerning relatively low heart rates at the onset of most episodes of out-of-hospital ischemia and the lack of association with strenuous exercising, the sum of the data concerning treatment of ambulatory ischemia indicates that the beta-blockers are the most efficacious agents. Studies have involved metoprolol [43,44], propranolol [45], and atenolol [46].

The key to this seeming paradox is in the small, but significant, increase in heart rate preceding the ischemic event [47]. Thus, as shown in Figure 8 in Chapter 8, a resting heart rate of 75 bpm increases only to 90 bpm within 30 min, but this difference is important in increasing myocardial oxygen demand. By preventing this increase, beta-blockers can be a highly effective form of therapy, more so even than calcium blockers (Fig. 6), as demonstrated by Stone et al. [39], Anderson et al. [48], Hill et al. [49], Deedwania et al. [50], and Kawanishi et al. [51], though the latter again point out the value of combined therapy. In the last several years there have been a number of additional studies investigating the value of combination therapy, or comparing the beta-blockers to the calcium blockers. The larger multicenter studies will be considered subse-

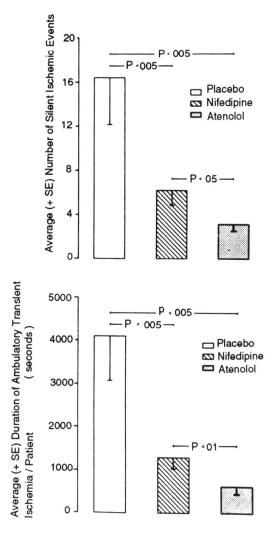

Figure 6 Comparison of anti-ischemic effects on the frequency (upper) and duration (lower) of ischemic episodes between the treatment groups. Compared with placebo, both atenolol (▢) and nifedipine (◩) significantly ($p < 0.005$) decreased the number of ischemic events during the monitoring period. However, atenolol was significantly better than nifedipine in reducing the frequency ($p < 0.05$) and duration ($p < 0.01$) of ischemic episodes. (From Deedwania PC, Carbajal EV, Nelson JR, Hait H. J Am Coll Cardiol 1991; 17:963. Reproduced with permission.)

quently when the effect of therapy on prognosis is discussed, but the conclusions of the smaller studies comparing amlodipine and atenolol alone or in combination [52,53], metoprolol and diltiazem [54], verapamil and amlodipine or atenolol [55], and bisoprolol and slow-release nifedipine [56] seemed to confirm the conclusions reached in earlier studies (i.e., combination regimens employing the beta-blockers appear superior in reducing ischemic episodes) (Fig. 7). Willich et al. [57] investigated the possibility that the effect of beta-blocking drugs on platelet aggregability was responsible for their abolition of the circadian variation (with a morning peak) in ischemic events. However, their study of 10 patients concluded that the "morning surge of transient ischemic events can be effectively blocked *without* changed platelet aggregability."

Studies using aspirin in silent ischemia have also been reported. Aspirin can reduce the number of ischemic events on Holter monitoring and be a protective agent against future infarctions [58]. Another study showed that the addition of heparin to aspirin in patients with unstable angina did not significantly reduce the number of transient ischemic episodes on the ECG nor reduce the incident of subsequent cardiac events [59]. This is in contrast to a study from Argentina evaluating aspirin plus low-molecular-weight heparin that did show a beneficial effect [60]. It is not only men who benefit from aspirin, but women as well [61].

Percutaneous transluminal coronary angioplasty represents a great advance in the treatment of myocardial ischemia, whether painful or silent. While we have commented earlier in the chapter on its usefulness in asymptomatic patients, it is obviously also of great value in patients with both silent and symptomatic episodes (Fig. 8). In addition, documentation of presistent but silent ischemia after angioplasty or stenting offers physicians an opportunity to diagnose restenosis before dangerous events occur [62,63]. Documentation of such ischemia does carry an unfavorable prognosis, however.

IV.   EFFECT OF MEDICAL THERAPY ON PROGNOSIS

Whether or not any therapies favorably affect the prognosis of patients with chronic myocardial ischemia is becoming clearer. In selected patients, both beta blockers and aspirin improve prognosis (in postinfarction patients, for example), but there is still no consensus that abolition of ischemic episodes per se has the same effect. Some data are available: Lim et al. [64] reported that patients who had their exercise-induced painless wall motion abnormalities abolished by medications did better at 9-month follow-up than patients in

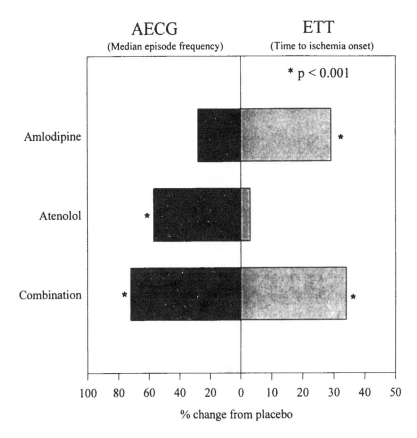

Figure 7 Relative efficacies of amlodipine, atenolol, and their combination on time-to-ischemia during treadmill exercise time versus episode frequency during ambulatory monitoring. Atenolol caused a greater reduction in ischemia during ambulatory monitoring, whereas amlodipine caused a greater delay in onset of ischemia during treadmill exercise. The combination was more effective than either drug alone in both settings. AECG = ambulatory electrocardiogram; ETT = exercise treadmill test. (Reproduced with permission from Davies RF, Habibi H, Klinke WP, Dessain P, Nadeau C, Phaneuf DC, Lepage F, Raman S, Herbert M, Foris K, Linden W, Buttars A. J Am Coll Cardiol 1995; 25:619–625.)

whom the abnormalities persisted (Fig. 9). Until recently, other evidence was less direct. In the BHAT study, for example, that we cited earlier in the chapter, patients on placebo had a much higher frequency of abnormal Holter recordings and a worse prognosis than those patients receiving propranolol. Some

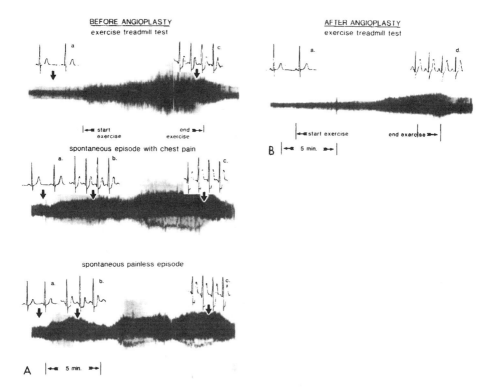

Figure 8 (A) Selected portions of the 24-h Holter compact analog record before angioplasty in a patient with an 80% stenosis in the proximal portion of the left anterior descending coronary artery. The *upper panel* was recorded during treadmill exercise test, the *middle panel* during a spontaneous episode of angina, and the *lower panel* during a spontaneous episode of ischemia without associated chest pain. The inserted printouts at a paper speed of 25 mm/s demonstrate the normal (a) QRST complex, (b) ST segment depression at the onset of ischemia, and (c) marked ST segment depression with T-wave augmentation. The ST segment depression and T-wave augmentation during spontaneous episodes of ischemia are similar to those induced during exercise. (B) After angioplasty, only (d) T-wave augmentation without ST segment depression occurred at 13.2 min of treadmill exercise. No spontaneous episodes were present on the Holter recording in this patient after angioplasty. (From Josephson MA, Nademanee K, Intarachot V, Lewis H, Singh BN. J Am Coll Cardiol 1987; 10:499.)

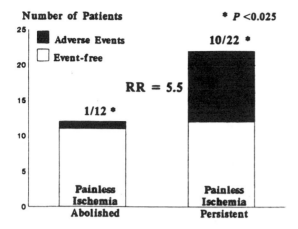

Figure 9   Relative risk (RR) of adverse cardiac events according to whether painless ischemia was abolished by or continued despite antiischemic therapy. (From Lim R, Dyke L, Dymond D S. Am J Cardiol 1992; 69 733. Reproduced with permission.)

resolution of this question has come from the results of multicenter trials in which patients are randomized to different treatment regimens (with ischemic episodes documented by exercise testing and Holter monitoring) and followed for subsequent development of cardiovascular events. The largest of these trials was sponsored by the National Institutes of Health (NIH) and directed by Conti: the Asymptomatic Cardiac Ischemia Pilot Study (ACIP). There is now a considerable amount of data available from this landmark study in which patients were randomized to either angina-guided medical therapy, ischemia-guided (Holter-driven) medical therapy, or revascularization (Fig. 10). The primary goal was to (1) compare the 12-week efficacy of the three treatment strategies in suppressing cardiac ischemia and (2) assess the feasibility of a larger prognosis trial in patients with asymptomatic ischemia [65]. Six-hundred-eighteen patients were enrolled in the pilot study with cardiac ischemia suppressed in 40 to 55% of patients at 12 week, (Fig. 11) using either low or moderate doses of a multidrug medical regimen (Table 7) or revascularization [66]. After 1 year of follow-up, revascularization was superior to both angina-guided and ischemia-guided medical strategies in suppressing ischemia and was also associated with a better clinical outcome [67] (Fig. 12). Within the revascularization arm, bypass surgery was superior to angioplasty in suppressing cardiac ischemia [68,69].

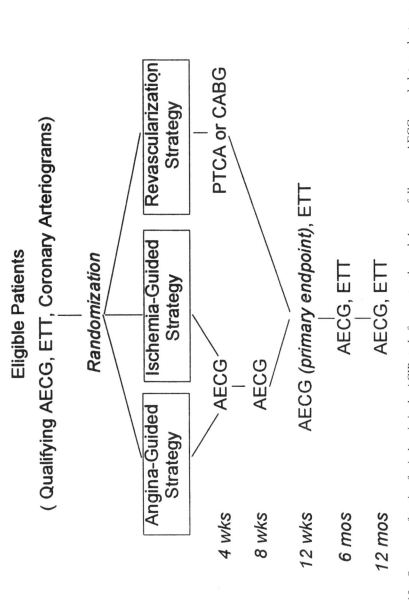

Figure 10 Sequence of testing for ischemia in the ACIP study from entry through 1-year follow-up. AECG = ambulatory electrocardiogram; CABG = coronary artery bypass graft surgery; ETT = treadmill exercise test (or equivalent); PTCA = percutaneous transluminal coronary angioplasty. (Reproduced with permission from Rodgers WJ, Bourassa MG, Andrews TC, Bertolet BD, Blumenthal RS, Chaitman BR, Forman SA, Geller NL, Goldberg AD, Habib GB, Masters RG, Moisa RB, Muellert Pearce DJ, Pepine CJ, Sopko G, Steingart RM, Stone PH, Knatterud GL, Conti R. J Am Coll Cardiol 1995; 26: 594–605.)

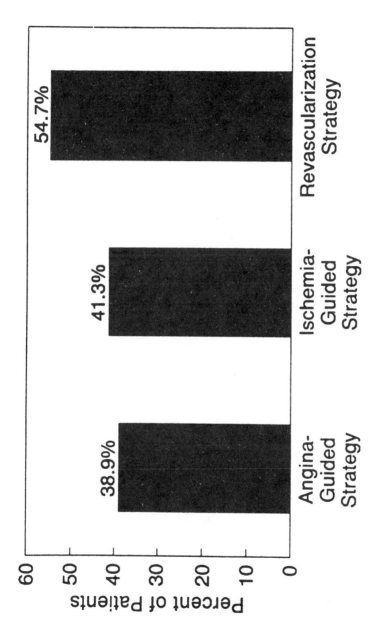

Figure 11   Percent of patients in the ACIP study ischemia-free on week 12 visit. Ambulatory electrocardiogram for each treatment strategy. (Reproduced with permission from Knatterud GL, Bourassa MG, Pepine CJ, Geller NL, Sopko G, Chaitman BR, Pratt C, Stone PH, Davies RF, Rogers WJ, Deanfield JE, Goldberg AD, Ouyang P, Mueller H, Sharaf B, Day P, Selwyn AP, Conti CR. J Am Coll Cardiol 1994; 24:11–20.)

Table 7   Medical Therapy Regimens in the ACIP Study

Regimen step	Atenolol/nifedipine regimen*	Diltiazem/isosorbide dinitrate regimen[a]
1	Atenolol, 50 mg qd (drug 1, dose 1)	Diltiazem SR, 60 mg bid (drug 1, dose 1)
2	Atenolol, 100 mg qd (drug 1, dose 2)	Diltiazem SR, 90 mg bid (drug 1, dose 2)
3	Atenolol, 100 mg qd (drug 1, dose 2), and nifedipine XL, 30 mg qd (drug 2, dose 1)	Diltiazem SR, 90 mg bid (drug 1, dose 2), and ISDN, 20 mg bid (drug 2, dose 1)
4	Atenolol, 100 mg qd (drug 1, dose 2), and nifedipine XL, 60 mg qd (drug 2, dose 2)	Diltiazem SR, 90 mg bid (drug 1, dose 2), and ISDN, 40 mg bid (drug 2, dose 2)

[a] Assigned randomly unless one regimen was indicated or contraindicated. Supply of unblinded medications was provided for each enrolled patient. A separate supply of blinded medications was provided for patients assigned to angina- or ischemia-guided strategies. Isosorbide dinitrate (ISDN) was to be given at 8 AM and 2 PM and diltiazem before the morning meal and at bedtime. bid = twice a day; qd = once a day; SR = slow release; XL = long acting.
Source: Knatterud GL, Bourassa MG, Pepine CJ, Geller NL, Sopko G, Chaitman BR, Pratt C, Stone PH, Davies RF, Rogers WJ, Deanfield JE, Goldberg AD, Ouyang P, Mueller H, Sharaf B, Day P, Selwyn AP, Conti CR. J Am Coll Cardiol 1994; 24:11–20.

Further analysis of patient characteristics [70], subgroup comparisons [71], and the relation between clinical, angiographic, and ischemic findings at baseline and follow-up at 1 year [72,73] have also been reported. At 2 years, the benefits of revascularization were still present [74]. Other trials of importance have also been completed, one in the United States using beta-blockers (the Atenolol Silent Ischemia Trial, or ASIST) [75] and one in Europe (the Total Ischemic Burden European Trial, or TIBET) [76]. In the ASIST trial, atenolol-treated patients with coronary disease and mild or no ischemia had fewer adverse events, fewer ischemic episodes, and shorter duration of ischemia [77] compared to placebo. At 1-year follow-up, the atenolol-treated patients also had fewer cardiac events (Table 8). The TIBET trial had a different protocol in that there was no placebo arm but rather treatment with atenolol, slow-release nifedipine, and a combination of the two drugs. The study showed no evidence of an association between ischemic events or hard and soft endpoints after 2 years of follow-up [78].

In another example of the value of beta-blockers, the use of atenolol to prevent perioperative ischemia in noncardiac surgical cases and improve the

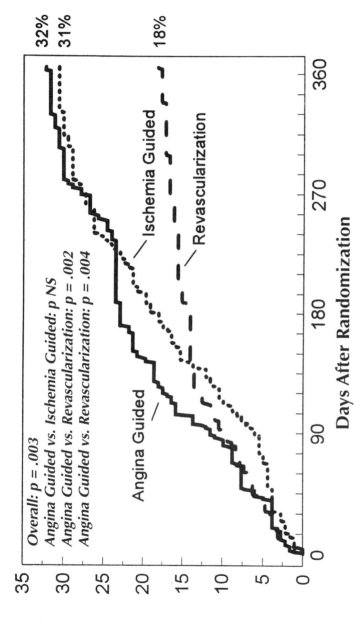

Figure 12 Death, myocardial infarction (MI), nonprotocol angioplasty (PTCA), bypass surgery (CABG), or hospital admission in the ACIP study. This composite secondary outcome was significantly less common among patients assigned to the revascularization strategy than among those assigned to the other two treatment strategies. (Reproduced with permission from Rodgers WJ, Bourassa MG, Andrews TC, Bertolet BD, Blumenthal RS, Chaitman BR, Forman SA, Geller NL, Goldberg AD, Habib GB, Masters RG, Moisa RB, Mueller H, Pearce DJ, Pepine CJ, Sopko G, Steingart RM, Stone PH, Knatterud GL, Conti R. J Am Coll Cardiol 1995; 26:594–605.)

Table 8 Outcomes During Treatment in the ASIST Trial

Outcomes at 1 year	Placebo ($n = 154$)	Atenolol ($n = 152$)	RR (95% CI)	p
Death or resuscitated VT/VF	4	1		
Nonfatal MI	3	2		
Hospitalized for unstable angina	6	4		
Death, VT/VF, MI, or hospitalization	13	7	0.55 (0.22 to 1.33)	0.175
Aggravation of angina	26	9	0.35 (0.17 to 0.72)	0.003
Revascularization	0	1		
Any adverse event	39	17	0.44 (0.26 to 0.75)	0.001

RR = relative risk; CI = confidence interval; VT = ventricular tachycardia; VF = ventricular fibrillation; and MI = myocardial infarction.
Source: Pepine CJ, Cohn PF, Deedwania PC. Circulation 1994; 90:762–768.

adverse prognosis commented on in Chapter 12 has been reported by Mangano et al., who found favorable results to last as long as 2 years after surgery [79] (Fig. 13).

In summary, while there is not yet enough evidence to *confirm* the hypothesis that suppressing myocardial ischemia per se favorably affects prognosis, all of these reports strongly suggest that is the case. Others argue, however, that ischemia is merely a marker for severe coronary lesions and the beta-blocker effect protects against ischemic triggers of morbid cardiac events.

V. ENDOTHELIAL DYSFUNCTION AND MYOCARDIAL ISCHEMIA

One of the more dramatic developments in the field of cardiology since the last edition of this book was published is the increasing realization that the pathogenesis of coronary artery disease may not be as clear-cut as once believed. The response-to-injury hypothesis for development of coronary atherosclerosis had endothelial denudation as the first step in this process, but endothelial dysfunction rather than denudation is now emphasized, raising the possibility of a chronic inflammatory state. The role of the vascular endothelium has come under intensive scrutiny because this structure is involved in the control of vascular tone and hemostasis by helping to regulate or influence (1) vascular remodeling; (2) fibrinolysis; (3) adhesion of activated platelets and leukocytes to the endothelium; and, therefore, (4) the intravascular inflammatory process.

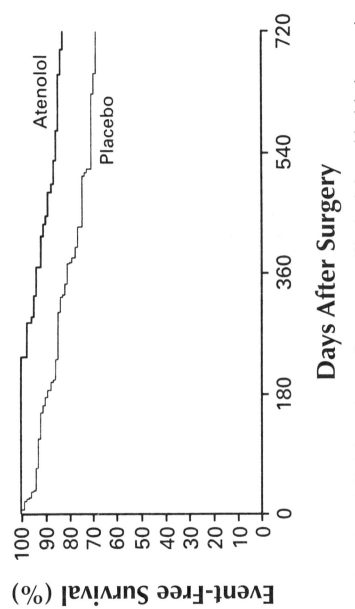

Figure 13   Event-free survival in the 2 years after noncardiac surgery among 192 patients in the atenolol and placebo groups who survived to hospital discharge. The outcome measure combined the following events: myocardial infarction, unstable angina, the need for coronary artery bypass surgery, and congestive heart failure. The rate of event-free survival at 6 months (180 days) was 100% in the atentolol group and 88% in the placebo group ($p < 0.001$); at 1 year (360 days), the rates were 92% and 78%, respectively; ($p = 0.003$); and at 2 years (720 days), 83% and 68% ($p = 0.008$). (Reproduced with permission from Mangano DT, Layug EL, Wallace A, Tateo I. N Engl J Med 1996; 335:1713–1763.)

One of the most exciting developments to emerge from research in endothelial dysfunction is that there are therapeutic interventions currently available that appear to limit or reverse endothelial dysfunction in humans. The ACE inhibitors and the statins are two such classes of drugs and there are some data suggesting that antibiotics may also be helpful.

The beneficial effects of ACE inhibitors on cardiovascular function are due to their blocking of the formation of angiotensin II, a potent vasoconstrictor. Because of the unexpected reduction in the number of ischemic events reported with the use of these drugs in the postinfarction studies of patients with impaired left ventricular function [80], their role as anti-ischemic agents has been—and continues to be—extensively evaluated. For example, a 1997 trial [81] demonstrated a reduction in ischemic events as early as 3 months after treatment. The Trial on Reversing Endothelial Dysfunction (TREND) [82] extended these findings to patients who did not have the severe left ventricular dysfunction reported in the earlier studies. A possible mechanism by which the ACE inhibitor quinapril improves vascular function was recently demonstrated by Koh et al. [83]. Quinapril increased nitric oxide bioavailability and, as a result, endothelial-dependent vasodilation improved. Protection against pacing-induced ischemia with ACE inhibitors has also been documented [84]. A study specifically designed to address effects on transient ischemia and subsequent clinical event rates is ongoing: The Quinapril Anti-Ischemia and Symptoms of Angina Reduction (QUASAR) study. The projected sample size is 450 patients with exercise tests and Holter monitoring used to document transient ischemia.

The other drugs that have excited investigators are the cholesterol-lowering agents commonly referred to as the statins. Originally it was thought that the improvement in prognosis seen with these drugs in both primary [85] and secondary prevention trials [86] was due to their ability to lower LDL cholesterol levels, but studies demonstrating positive effects on endothelial-mediated vasodilation suggested a dual mechanism of action: improving endothelial function as a well as lowering serum cholesterol levels. In 1996, Van Boven et al. [87] used ambulatory ECG monitoring in their pravastatin studies to confirm this impression, and in 1999, Andrews et al. reported similar results with lovastatin [88] (Fig. 14).

Because of elevations in acute-phase proteins and other systemic reponses to inflammation in some patients with coronary artery disease, the issue of intravascular inflammation due to bacteria is being vigorously pursued [89]. Two 1999 studies have suggested that antibiotic treatment directed against bacteria such as *Chlamdyia pneumoniae* can prevent and/or reduce cardiac events [90,91]. Large-scale trials (e.g., the Azithromycin Coronary Event Study) are now under way to provide more data for future decision making in

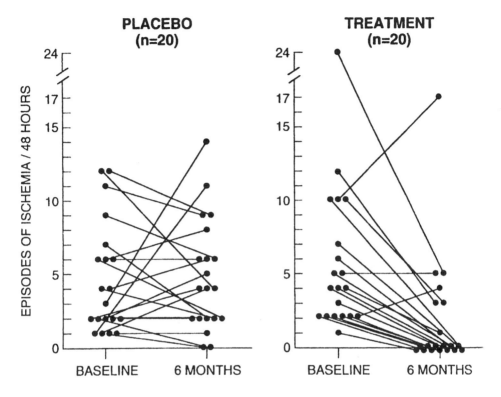

Figure 14   Patient-by-patient effect of cholesterol lowering (with lovastatin) over 6 months on the number of episodes of ischemic ST segment depression in patients with coronary disease. Two of 20 in the placebo group versus 13 of 20 in the treatment group show resolution of ischemia. (Reproduced with permission from Andrews TC, Roby K, Barry J, Naimi CL, Allred E, Ganz P, Selwyn AP. Circulation 1997; 95:324–328.)

this area. The concept of a bacterial role in coronary artery disease is provocative, but one must remember that reports of a causative relationship between *H. pylori* and peptic ulcers were also initially met with skepticism.

VI.   MANAGEMENT OF SILENT MYOCARDIAL INFARCTION

Recognition of these events invariably occurs too late for the usual treatment accorded patients with infarctions. However, patients at times may present with the acute *complications* of a silent infarction and require appropriate management. An example is the patient in pulmonary edema reported by Raper et al. [92].

VII. CONCLUSIONS

Medical management of silent myocardial ischemia involves modification of risk factors, use of drugs, and, in appropriate patients, angioplasty. In evaluating any therapy, however, the natural variability of ischemic events on Holter monitoring must be considered [93,94]. At the present time, beta-blockers appear to be the most efficacious medical therapy, but many of the ischemic episodes also respond to calcium antagonists and nitrates [95,96]. Combination therapy may offer the best approach, not only in abolishing ischemic episodes but in improving prognosis. Only long-term follow-up in studies like ACIP can establish this point in what may well turn out to be an inflammatory disease [97].

REFERENCES

1. Pepine CJ, Imperi GA, Hill JA. Therapeutic implications of silent myocardial ischemia during daily activity. Am J Cardiol 1987; 59:993.
2. Frishman WH, Teicher M. Antianginal drug therapy for silent myocardial ischemia. Am Heart J 1987; 114:140.
3. Mulcahy D, Fox K. Therapeutic implications of ischemia in the ambulatory setting. Prog Cardiovasc Dis 1992; 34:413.
4. Cohn PF, Brown EJ, Jr., Cohn JK. Detection and management of coronary artery disease in the asymptomatic population. Am Heart J 1984; 108:1064.
5. Pepine CJ. The effects of angiotensin-converting enzyme inhibition on endothelial dysfunction: potential role in myocardial ischemia. Am J Cardiol 1998; 82 (10A): 235–275.
6. Cohn PF, Brown EJ, Jr., Swinford R, Atkins HL. Effect of beta blockade on silent regional left ventricular wall motion abnormalities. Am J Cardiol 1986; 57:521.
7. Eme P, Burckhardt D, Dubach P, Zuber M, Kowski W. Antiischemic therapy improves event free survival in silent ischemia Type 1. Results of the Swiss Interventional Study on Silent Ischemia 1 (SWISSI 1). J Am Coll Cardiol 1999; 33 (suppl A):340A (abstr).
8. Imperi GA, Lambert CR, Coy K, Lopez L, Pepine CJ. Effects of titrated beta blockade (metoprolol) on silent myocardial ischemia in ambulatory patients with coronary artery disease. Am J Cardiol 1987; 60:519.

9. Cohn PF, Lawson WE. Effect of nifedipine on out-of-hospital silent myocardial ischemia in asymptomatic men with coronary artery disease. Am J Cardiol 1988; 61:908.

10. Tuzcu EM, Nisanci Y, Simpfendorger C, Dorosti K, Franco I, Hollman J, Whitlow P. Percutaneous transluminal coronary angioplasty in silent ischemia. Am Heart J 1990; 119:797.

11. Anderson HV, Talley JD, Black AJR, Roubin GS, Douglas JS, Jr., King SB, III. Usefulness of coronary angioplasty in asymptomatic patients. Am J Cardiol 1990; 65:35.

12. Freeman LJ, Nixon PGF, Sallbank P, Reaveley D. Psychological stress and silent myocardial ischemia. Am Heart J 1987; 114:477.

13. Cohn JK, Cohn PF. Patient reactions to the diagnosis of asymptomatic coronary artery disease: Implications for the primary physician and consultant cardiologist. J Am Coll Cardiol 1983; 1:956.

14. Freedland KE, Carney RM, Krone RJ, Case NB, Case RB. Psychological determinants of anginal pain perception during exercise testing of stable patients after recovery from acute myocardial infarction or unstable angina pectoris. Am J Cardiol 1996; 77:1–4.

15. Eme P, Burckhardt D, Pfisterer M, Dubach P, Zuber M, Klowski W. Effect of PTCA on outcome in patients with silent ischemia after myocardial infarction: results of the Swiss Interventional Study on Silent Ischemia Type II (SWISSI 11). J Am Coll Cardiol 1999; 33 (suppl A):38A.

16. Goldman L, Sia STB, Cook EF, Rutherford JD, Weinstein MC. Costs and effectiveness of routine therapy with long-term beta-adrenergic antagonists after acute myocardial infarction. N Engl J Med 1988; 319:152.

17. Ruberman W, Crow R, Rosenberg CR, Rautaharju PM, Shore RE, Pasternack BS. Intermittent ST depression and mortality after myocardial infarction. Circulation 1992; 85:1440.

18. Cohn PF. Time for a new approach to the management of patients with both symptomatic and asymptomatic episodes of myocardial ischemia. Am J Cardiol 1984; 54:1357.

19. Stern S, Gavish A, Weisz G, Benhorin J, Keren A, Tzivoni D. Characteristics of silent and symptomatic myocardial ischemia during daily activities. Am J Cardiol 1988; 61:1223.

20. Schang JJ, Jr., Pepine CJ. Transient asymptomatic ST-segment depression during daily activity. Am J Cardiol 1977; 39:396.

21. Cecchi AC, Dovellini EV, Marchi F, Pucci P, Santoro CM, Fazzini PF. Silent myocardial ischemia during ambulatory electrocardiographic monitoring in patients with effort angina. J Am Coll Cardiol 1983; 1:934.

22. Chierchia S, Lazzari M, Freedman B, Brunelli C, Maseri A. Impairment of myocardial perfusion and function during painless myocardial ischemia. J Am Coll Cardiol 1983; 1:924.

23. Crawford MH, Vittitoe J, O'Rourke RA. Ambulatory blood pressure recordings during silent ischemia episodes (abstr). Circulation 1987; 76 (suppl IV):79.

24. Deanfield JE, Shea M, Ribiero P, deLandsheere CM, Wilson RA, Horlock P, Selwyn AP. Transient ST segment depression as a marker of myocardial ischemia during daily life: A physiological validation in patients with angina and coronary disease. Am J Cardiol 1984; 54:1195.

25. Shell WE, Kovowitz CF, Rubins SB, See J. Mechanisms and therapy of silent myocardial ischemia: The effect of transdermal nitroglycerin. Am Heart J 1986; 212:222.

26. vonArnim T, Erath A. Nitrates and calcium antagonists for silent myocardial ischemia. Am J Cardiol 1988; 61:15E.

27. Dubiel JP, Moczurad KW, Bryniarski L. Efficacy of a single dose of slow-release isosorbide dinitrate in the treatment of silent or painful myocardial ischemia in stable angina pectoris. Am J Cardiol 1992; 69:1156.

28. Knuuti MJ, Wahl M, Wiklund I, Smith P, Alhainen L, Harkonen R, Puska P, Tzivoni D. Acute and long-term effects on myocardial ischemia of intermittent and continuous transdermal nitrate therapy in stable angina. Am J Cardiol 1992; 69:1525.

29. Feng J, Feng X, Schneeweiss A. Efficacy of isosorbide-5-mononitrate on painful and silent myocardial ischemia after myocardial infarction. Am J Cardiol 1990; 65:32J.

30. Johnson SM, Mauritson DR, Willerson JT, Hillis LD. A controlled trial of verapamil for Prinzmetal's variant angina. N Engl J Med 1981; 304:862.

31. Parodi O, Simonetii I, Michelassi C, Carpeggiani C, Biagini A, L'Abbate A, Maseri A. Comparison of verapamil and propranolol therapy for angina pectoris at rest: A randomized, multiple-crossover, controlled trial in the coronary care unit. Am J Cardiol 1986; 57:899.

32. Frishman W, Charlap S, Kimmel B, Teicher M, Cinnamon J, Allen L, Strom J. Diltiazem, nifedipine and their combination in patients with stable angina pectoris: Effects on angina, exercise tolerance and the ambulatory electrocardiographic ST segment. Circulation 1988; 77:774.

33. Theroux P, Baird M, Juneau M, Warnica W, Klinke P, Kostuk W, Pflugfelder P, Lavallee E, Chin C, Dempsey E, Grace M, Lalonde Y, Waters D. Effect of diltiazem on symptomatic and asymptomatic episodes of ST segment depression occurring during daily life and during exercise. Circulation 1991; 84:15.

34. Deedwania PC, Pool PE, Thadani U, Eff J, and the Dilacor XR Ambulatory Ischemia Study Group. Effect of morning versus evening dosing of diltiazem on myocardial ischemia detected by ambulatory electrocardiographic monitoring in chronic stable angina pectoris. Am J Cardiol 1997; 80:421–425.

35. Tzivoni D, Banai S, Botvin S, Zilberman A, Weiss TA, Gavish A, Medina A, Benhorin J, Rogel S, Caspi A, Stern S. Effects of nisoldipine on myocardial ischemia during exercise and during daily activity. Am J Cardiol 1991; 67:559.

36. Oakley GDG, Fox KM, Dargie HJ, Selwyn AP. Objective assessment of therapy in severe angina. Br Med J 1979; 1:1540.

37. Cohn PF, Vetrovec GW, Neso R, Gerber FR, and the Total Ischemia Awareness Program Investigators. The Nifedipine-Total Ischemia Awareness Program: A

national survey of painful and painless myocardial ischemia including results of antiischemic therapy. Am J Cardiol 1989; 63:534.

38. Parmley WW, Nesto RW, Singh BN, Deanfield J, Gottlieb SO, and the N-Cap Study Group. Attenuation of the circadian patterns of myocardial ischemia with nifedipine GITS in patients with chronic stable angina. J Am Coll Cardiol 1992; 19:1380.

39. Stone PH, Gibson RS, Glasser SP, DeWood MA, Parker JD, Kawanishi DT, Crawford MH, Messineo FC, Shook TL, Raby K, Curtis DG, Hoop RS, Young PM, Braunwald E, and the ASIS Study Group. Comparison of propranolol, diltiazem, and nifedipine in the treatment of ambulatory ischemia in patients with stable angina: Differential effects on ambulatory ischemia, exercise performance, and anginal symptoms. Circulation 1990; 82:1962.

40. Deanfield JE, Detry J M, Lichtlen PR, Magnani B, Sellier P, Thaulow E. Amlodipine reduces transient myocardial ischemia in patients with coronary artery disease: double-blind circadian anti-ischemia program in Europe (CAPE Trial). J Am Coll Cardiol 1994; 24:1460–1467.

41. Deedwania PC and the Amlodipine Study Group. Anti-ischemic effects of amlodipine in patients with stable angina pectoris and myocardial ischemia during daily life. Am J Cardiol 1999; 33:1117–1119.

43. Tzivoni D, Medina A, David D, Barzilai Y, Brunel P. Effect of metoprolol in reducing myocardial ischemic threshold during exercise and during daily activity. Am J Cardiol 1998; 81:775–777.

44. Tzivoni D, Medina A, David D, Barzilai Y, Gavish A, Shatboon D, Keren A, Brunel P. Comparison between metoprolol orally osmotic once daily and metoprolol two or three times daily in suppressing exercise-induced and daily myocardial ischemia. Am J Cardiol 1996; 78:1362–1368.

45. Kawanishi DT, Reid CL, Simsarian G, Amisola Y, Gonzales A, Rahimtoola SH. Effect of pharmacologic therapy on angina frequency, ST segment depression during ambulatory ECG monitoring, and treadmill performance in patients with chronic stable mild angina. Am Heart J 1998; 115:220.

46. Quyyumi AA, Crake T, Wright CM, Mockus LJ, Fox KM. Medical treatment of patients with severe exertional and rest angina: double blind comparison of beta blocker, calcium antagonist, and nitrate. Br Heart J 1987; 57:505.

47. Mcnachan JM, Weidinger FF, Barry J, Yeung A, Nable EG, Rocco NB, Selwyn AP. Relations between heart rate, ischemia, and drug therapy during daily life in patients with coronary artery disease. Circulation 1991; 83:1263.

48. Ardissino D, Savonitto S, Egstrup K, Marraccini P, Slavich G, Rosenfeld M, Feruglio GA, Roncarolo P, Glordano MP, Wahlqvist I, Rehnqvist N, Barberis P, Specchia G, L'Abbate A. Transient myocardial ischemia during daily life in rest and exertional angina pectoris and comparison of effectiveness of metoprolol versus nifedipine. Am J Cardiol 1991; 67:946.

49. Hill JA, Gonzalez JI, Kolb R, Pepine CJ. Effects of atenolol alone, nifedipine alone and their combination on ambulant myocardial ischemia. Am J Cardiol 1991; 67:671.

50. Deedwania PC, Carbajal EV, Nelson JR, Hait H. Anti-ischemic effects of atenolol versus nifedipine in patients with coronary artery disease and ambulatory silent ischemia. J Am Coll Cardiol 1991; 17:963.

51. Kawanishi DT, Reid CL, Morrison EC, Rahimtoola SH. Response of angina and ischemia to long-term treatment in patients with chronic stable angina: A double-blind randomized individualized dosing trial of nifedipine, propranolol and their combination. J Am Coll Cardiol 1992; 19:409.

52. Davies RF, Habibi H, Klinke WP, Dessain P, Nadeau C, Phaneuf DC, Lepage S, Raman S, Herbert M, Foris K, Linden W, Buttars A. Effect of amlodipine, atenolol and their combination on myocardial ischemia during treadmill exercise and ambulatory monitoring. J Am Cardiol 1995; 25:619–625.

53. Dunselman PHJM, van Kempen LHJ, Bouwens LHM, Holwerdo KJ, Herweijer AH, Bernink PJLM. Value of the addition of amlodipine to atenolol in patients with angina pectoris despite adequate beta blockade. Am J Cardiol 1998; 81:128–132.

54. Portegies MCM, Sijbring P, Gobel EJAM, Viersma JW, Lie KI. Efficacy of metoprolol and diltiazem in treating silent myocardial ischemia. Am J Cardiol 1994; 74:1095–1098.

55. Frishman WH, Glasser S, Stone P, Deedwania PC, Johnson M, Fakouhi TD. Comparison of controlled-onset, extended-release verapamil with amlodipine and amlodipine plus atenolol on exercise performance and ambulatory ischemia in patients with chronic stable angina pectoris. Am J Cardiol 1999; 83:507–514.

56. von Arnim T for the TIBBS Investigators. Medical treatment to reduce total ischemic burden: Total Ischemic Burden Bisoprolol Study (TIBBS), a multicenter trial comparing bisoprolol and nifedipine. J Am Coll Cardiol 1995; 25:231–238.

57. Willich SN, Pohjola-Sintonen S, Bhatia SJS, Shook TL, Tofler GH, Muller JE, Curtis DG, Williams GH, Stone PH. Suppression of silent ischemia by metoprolol without alteration of morning increase of platelet aggregability in patients with stable coronary artery disease. Circulation 1989; 79:557.

58. Nyman I, Larsson H, Wallentin L, the RISK Study Group in Southeast Sweden. Prevention of serious cardiac events by low-dose aspirin in patients with silent myocardial ischemia. Lancet 1992; 340:497.

59. Holdright D, Patel D, Cunningham D, Thomas R, Hubbard W, Hendry Gordon, Sutton G, Fox K. Comparison of the effect of heparin and aspirin versus aspirin alone on transient myocardial ischemia and in-hospital prognosis in patients with unstable angina. J Am Coll Cardiol 1994; 24:39–45.

60. Gurfinkel EP, Manos EJ, Mejail RI, Cerda MA, Duronto EA, Garcia CN, Daroca AM, Mautner B. Low molecular weight heparin versus heparin or aspirin in the treatment of unstable angina and silent ischemia. J Am Coll Cardiol 1995; 26:313–318.

61. Harpaz D, Benderly M, Goldbourt U, Kishon Y, Behar S for the Israeli BIP Study Group. Effect of aspirin on mortality in women with symptomatic or silent myocardial ischemia. Am J Cardiol 1996; 78:1215–1219.

62. Pirelli S, Danzi GB, Alberti A, Massa D, Piccalo G, Faletra F, Picano E, Campolo L, De Vita C. Comparison of usefulness of high-dose dipyridamole echocardiography and exercise electrocardiography for detection of asymptomatic restenosis after coronary angioplasty. Am J Cardiol 1991; 67:1335.

63. Kathiresan S, Jordan MK, Gimelli G, Lopez-Cuellar J, Madhi N, Jang I-K. Frequency of silent myocardial ischemia following coronary stenting. Am J Cardiol 1999; 84:930–932.

64. Lim R, Dyke L, Dymond DS. Effect of prognosis of abolition of exercise-induced painless myocardial ischemia by medical therapy. Am J Cardiol 1992; 69:733.

65. Pepine CJ, Geller NL, Knatterud GL, Bourassa MG, Chaitman BR, Davies RF, Day P, Deanfield JE, Goldberg AD, McMahon RP, Mueller H, Ouyang P, Pratt C, Proschan M, Rogers WJ, Selwyn AP, Sharaf B, Sopko G, Stone PH, Conti RC for the ACIP Investigators. The asymptomatic cardiac ischemia pilot (ACIP) study: design of a randomized clinical trial, baseline data and implications for a long-term trial. J Am Coll Cardiol 1994; 24:1–10.

66. Knatterud GL, Bourassa MG, Pepine CJ, Geller NL, Sopko G, Chaitman BR, Pratt C, Stone PH, Davies RF, Rogers WJ, Deanfield JE, Goldberg AD, Ouyang P, Mueller H, Sharaf B, Day P, Selwyn AP, Conti CR for the ACIP Investigators. Effects of treatment strategies to suppress ischemia in patients with coronary artery disease: 12-week results of asymptomatic cardiac ischemia (ACIP) study. J Am Coll Cardiol 1994; 24:11–20.

67. Rodgers WJ, Bourassa MG, Andrews TC, Bertolet BD, Blumenthal RS, Chaitman BR, Forman SA, Geller NL, Goldberg AD, Habib GB, Masters RG, Moisa RB, Mueller H, Pearce DJ, Pepine CJ, Sopko G, Steingart RM, Stone PH, Knatterud GL, Conti R for the ACIP Investigators. Asymptomatic cardiac ischemia pilot (ACIP) study: outcome at 1 year for patients with asymptomatic cardiac ischemia randomized to medical therapy or revascularization. J Am Coll Cardiol 1995; 26:594–605.

68. Bourassa MG, Pepine CJ, Forman SA, Rogers WJ, Dyrda I, Stone PH, Chaitman BR, Sharaf B, Mahmarian J, Davies RF, Knatterud GL, Terrin M, Sopko G, Conti CR for the ACIP Investigators. Asymptomatic cardiac ischemia pilot (ACIP) study: effects of coronary angioplasty and coronary artery bypass graft surgery on recurrent angina and ischemia. J Am Coll Cardiol 1995; 26:606–614.

69. Bourassa MG, Knatterud GL, Pepine CJ, Sopko G, Rogers WJ, Geller NL, Dyrda I, Forman SA, Chaitman BR, Sharaf B, Davies RF, Conti CR for the ACIP Investigators. Asymptomatic cardiac ischemia pilot (ACIP) study. Circulation 1995; 92 (suppl II):II-1-II-7.

70. Pepine CJ, Andrews T, Deanfield JE, Forman S, Geller N, Hill JA, Pratt C, Rogers WJ, Sopko G, Steingart R, Stone PH, Conti R for the ACIP Study Group. Relation of patient characteristics to cardiac ischemia during daily life activity (An Asymptomatic Cardiac Ischemia Pilot Data Bank Study). Am J Cardiol 1996; 77: 1267–1272.

71. Pratt CM, McMahon RP, Goldstein S, Pepine CJ, Andrews TC, Dyrda I, Frishman WH, Geller NL, Hill JA, Morgan NA, Stone PH, Knatterud GL, Sopko G, Conti R for the ACIP Investigators. Comparison of subgroups assigned to medical regimens used to suppress cardiac ischemia (the Asymptomatic Cardiac Ischemia Pilot [ACIP] Study). Am J Cardiol 1996; 77:1302–1309.

72. Pepine CJ, Sharaf B, Andrews TC, Forman S, Geller N, Knatterud G, Mahmarian J, Ouyang P, Rogers WJ, Sopko G, Steingart R, Stone PH, Conti CR for the ACIP Study Group. Relation between clinical, angiographic and ischemic findings at baseline and ischemia-related adverse outcomes at 1 year in the asymptomatic cardiac ischemia pilot study. J Am Coll Cardiol 1997; 29:1483–1489.

73. Conti CR, Geller NL, Knatterud GL, Forman SA, Pratt CM, Pepine CJ, Sopko G for the ACIP Investigators. Anginal status and prediction of cardiac events in patients enrolled in the asymptomatic cardiac ischemia pilot (ACIP) study. Am J Cardiol 1997; 79:889–892.

74. Davies RF, Goldberg AD, Forman S, Pepine CJ, Knatterud GL, Geller N, Sopko G, Pratt C, Deanfield J, Conti CR for the ACIP Investigators. Asymptomatic cardiac ischemia pilot (ACIP) study two-year follow-up. Circulation 1997; 95:2237–2043.

75. Pepine C, Cohn PF, Deedwania PC, Gibson R, Gottlieb S, Hill J. The prognostic and economic implications of a strategy to detect and treat asymptomatic ischemic: The Atenolol Silent Ischemia Trial (ASIST) Protocol. Clin Cardiol 1991; 14: 457.

76. Fox KM, Mulcahy D. Therapeutic rationale for the management of silent ischemia. Circulation 1990; 82 (suppl II):155.

77. Pepine CJ, Cohn PF, Deedwania PC. Effects of treatment on outcome in mildly symptomatic patients with ischemia during daily life: the Atenolol Silent Ischemia Study. Circulation 1994; 90:762–768.

78. Dargie HJ, Ford I, Fox KM on behalf of the TIBET study group. Total ischemic burden European trial (TIBET). Eur Heart J 1996; 17:104–112.

79. Mangano DT, Layug EL, Wallace A, Tateo I. Effect of atenolol on mortality and cardiovascular morbidity after noncardiac surgery. N Engl J Med 1996; 335: 1713–1763.

80. Yusuf S, Pepine CJ, Salem PH, Kostis SD, Benedict CM, Rousseau M, Bourassa M, Pitt B. Effect of enalapril on myocardial infarction and unstable angina in patients with low ejection fractions. Lancet 1992; 340:1173–1178.

81. van den Heuvel AFM, van Gilst WH, van Velduisen DJ, De Vries RJM, Dunselman PHJM, Kingma JH, for the Captopril and Thrombolysis Study (CATS) Investigators. Long-term anti-ischemic effects of angiotensin-converting enzyme inhibition in patients after myocardial infarction. J Am Coll Cardiol 1997; 30:400–405.

82. Mancini GBJ, Henry GC, Macaya C, O'Neill BJ, Pucillo AL, Carere RG, Wargovich TJ, Mudra H, Luscher TF, Klibaner MI, Haber HE, Uprichard ACG, Pepine CJ, Pitt B. Angiotensin-converting enzyme inhibition with quinapril improves

endothelial vasomotor dysfunction in patients with coronary artery disease: the TREND (Trial on Reversing Endothelial Dysfunction) study. Circulation 1996; 94:258–265.

83. Koh KK, Bui MN, Hathaway L, Csako G, Waclawiw MA, Panza JA, Cannon RO III. Mechanism by which quinapril improves vascular function in coronary artery disease. Am J Cardiol 1999; 83:327–331.

84. Bartels GL, van den Heuvel AFM, van Velduisen DJ, van der Ent M, Remme WJ. Acute anti-ischemic effects of perindoprilat in men with coronary artery disease and their relation with left ventricular function. Am J Cardiol 1999; 83:332–336.

85. West of Scotland Coronary Prevention Study. Influence of pravastatin and plasma lipids on clinical events in the West of Scotland Coronary Prevention Study (WOSCOPS). Circulation 1998; 97:1440–1445.

86. Pedersen TF, Olsson AG, Faergeman O, Kjekshus J, Wedel H, Berg K, Wihelmsen L, Haghfelt T, Thorgeirsson G, Kyorala K, Miettinen T, Christophersen B, Tobert JA, Musliner TA, Cook TJ for the Scandinavian Simvastatin Survival Study Group. Lipoprotein changes and reduction in the incidence of major coronary heart disease events in the Scandinavian Simvastatin Survival Study (4S). Circulation 1998; 97:1453–1460.

87. van Boven AJ, Jukema W, Zwinderman AH, Crijns HJGM, Lie KI, Bruschke AV G on behalf of the REGRESS Study Group. Reduction of transient myocardial ischemia with pravastatin in addition to the conventional treatment in patients with angina pectoris. Circulation 1996; 94:1503–1505.

88. Andrews TC, Raby K, Barry J, Naimi CL, Allred E, Ganz P, Selwyn AP. Effect of cholesterol reduction on myocardial ischemia in patients with coronary disease. Circulation 1997; 95:324–328.

89. Gabay C, Kushner I. Acute-phase proteins and other systemic responses to inflammation. N Engl J Med 1999; 340:448–454.

90. Meiser CR, Derby LE, Jick SS, Vasilakis C, Jick H. Antibiotics and risk of subsequent first-time acute myocardial infaraciton. JAMA 1999; 281:427–431.

91. Gurfinkel E, Bozovich G, Beckt E, Testat E, Liverllaras B, Mautner B for the ROXIS Study Group. Treatment with the antibiotic roxithromycin in patients with acute non-Q-wave coronary syndromes. Eur Heart J 1999; 20:121–127.

92. Raper AJ, Hastillo A, Paulsen WJ. The syndrome of sudden severe painless myocardial ischemia. Am Heart J 1984; 107:813.

93. Tzivoni D, Gavish A, Benhorin J, Banai S, Keren A, Stern S. Day-to-day variability of myocardial ischemic episodes in coronary artery disease. Am J Cardiol 1987; 60:1003.

94. Nabel EG, Barry J, Rocco MB, Campbell S, Mead K, Fenton T, Orav EJ, Selwyn AP. Variability of transient myocardial ischemia in ambulatory patients with coronary artery disease. Circulation 1988; 78:60.

95. Bertolet BD, Hill JA, Pepine CJ. Treatment strategies for daily life silent myocardial ischemia: A correlation with potential pathogenic mechanisms. Prog Cardiovasc Dis 1992; 35:97.

96. Mulcahy D, Fox K. Therapeutic implications of ischemia in the ambulatory setting. Prog Cardiovasc Dis 1992; 35:413.
97. Ross R. Atherosclerosis—an inflammatory disease. N Engl J Med 1999; 340: 115–126.

16

Surgical Treatment of Asymptomatic Coronary Artery Disease

Some investigators are adamantly against surgery in asymptomatic patients in general; others are in favor of it in very limited circumstances; yet others take a broader view. By necessity, prognosis—rather than relief of symptoms—is the key endpoint. Unfortunately, many of the surgical series have no medical controls and, therefore, do not provide enough "light," merely "heat." Furthermore, in most instances, there is no documentation that these asymptomatic patients demonstrate myocardial ischemia preoperatively. Because surgical patients who are totally asymptomatic are small in number, they are usually combined in follow-up reports with patients who are asymptomatic following a myocardial infarction. Specific surgical data on patients with angina who have frequent asymptomatic episodes is largely limited to the ACIP study cited in detail in Chapter 15 and commented on further later in this chapter. For these reasons, I have not used the same subheadings as in other chapters but rather discuss the findings in terms of nonrandomized versus randomized studies. The former are more numerous and will be discussed first.

I. NONRANDOMIZED STUDIES

Coronary bypass surgery in small numbers of asymptomatic patients has been performed at several hospitals (Table 1). Usually these patients are reported as part of a mixed series that includes asymptomatic and mildly symptomatic patients. The results involving the asymptomatic patients must then be dissected out from the main body of data. The study from the Seattle Heart Watch conducted by the University of Washington School of Medicine [1] is one such study. In this series, 114 patients were asymptomatic and 505 patients were mildly symptomatic. Prognosis was compared in medically and surgically treated patients. Even though the study was nonrandomized, it provides important data because the medically and surgically treated patients had similar baseline variables. The surgically treated patients had a lower mortality (via life-table analysis) than their medical counterparts, with the largest difference in survival seen in patients with triple-vessel disease and ejection fractions between 31 and 50% (Fig. 1). This is the only nonrandomized study with con-

Table 1 Surgical Therapy in Asymptomatic Patients with Coronary Artery Disease[a] (Nonrandomized Studies)

Reporting institution	No. of patients	Perioperative mortality	Mean follow-up (m.)	Late mortality
Cleveland Clinic	17	0	75	0
University of Washington	392	15 (3.8%)	65	NA
Peter Bent Brigham	20	0	34	1 (5%)
Montreal Heart Institute	55	0	69	4 (7.3%)

NA = not available.

[a] All studies include patients with prior myocardial infarction. University of Washington, Peter Bent Brigham, and Montreal Heart Institute studies also include patients with mild symptoms.

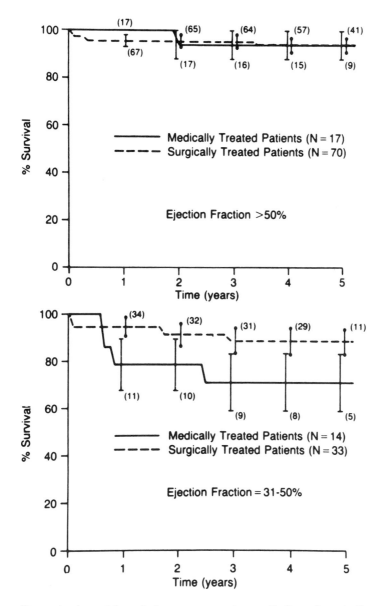

Figure 1 Actuarial survival curves comparing medically and surgically treated patients with three-vessel disease subgrouped according to ejection fraction. (From Hammermeister KE, DeRouen TA, Dodge HT. Circulation 1980; 62:98.)

trol patients; it suggests a beneficial effect of surgery on mortality in asymptomatic patients. Because prognosis in patients with normal ejection fractions and mild or no symptoms appeared excellent, the authors did not feel anything but an enormous sample size would be sufficient to test the hypothesis that surgical therapy improves survival in that type of patient. Furthermore, there were too few asymptomatic patients with left main lesions for the authors to make any definite statements about treatment for that type of lesion, but they did feel that on the basis of their study, they would recommend surgery in patients with triple-vessel disease and moderate impairment of left ventricular function.

In addition to this retrospective "matched" study from the University of Washington, there have also been several reports of surgical series without attempts to have control groups. Thus, Grondin et al. [2], at the Montreal Heart Institute, reported on 55 patients, 19 of whom were totally asymptomatic. Most patients had multivessel disease. There were four late deaths and seven late infarctions in the 69-month follow-up period, and despite the zero perioperative mortality, the authors questioned the value of this type of prophylactic surgery. Thurer et al. [3] operated on 17 patients at the Cleveland Clinic who were asymptomatic after an infarction. Sixteen of the seventeen remained asymptomatic. The Boston [4] experience was similar (Table 2). Twenty patients were studied, 14 of whom were totally asymptomatic. Six of these had sustained a prior myocardial infarction. This series was unique in that 16 patients had preoperative exercise tests, of which 14 demonstrated silent ischemia. The only death in this series occurred 5 years after surgery. There were 12 patients with both preoperative and postoperative exercise tests; in eight the test became completely normal, while in the other four, less of an ischemic response was observed compared to the preoperative test. Examples of these exercise tests are depicted in Figure 2. Schnellbacher et al. [5] recently reported that in a series of 22 surgically treated totally asymptomatic patients, all of them did well clinically and showed reduction or absence of ST depression on exercise tests. Fitzgibbon et al. [6] reported on a series of 723 consecutive patients operated on between 1971 and 1979. The authors separated the 118 patients who had no angina 3 years prior to the study from the 605 who had angina. No important differences in survival between the patients were noted.

II. RANDOMIZED STUDIES

The multicenter Coronary Artery Surgery Study (CASS) [7–10] has provided additional data both for and against surgical intervention. Unlike the Seattle report, this was a randomized study, but one with certain qualifying features.

Table 2 Clinical Data on Patients with Minimal or No Angina Pectoris Who Underwent CABG Surgery

Pt. no.	Age	MI	Angina pectoris	ETT Preop.	ETT Postop.	Diseased vessels (no.)	Grafts (no.)	Follow-up (mo)
1	49	+	−	0	0	2	2	80
2	54	−	−	+	−	LM	1	63
3	47	+	−	−	−	3	2	62 (1)
4	58	+	−	0	0	3	5	42
5	53	+	−	+	−	3	3	42
6	35	+	−	+	−	2	3	39
7	42	−	=	+	−	3	3	36
8	49	+	−	0	−	2	1	30
9	36	−	−	+	+	2	2	30
10	39	+	−	+	−	2	2	29
11	63	+	=	+	−	3	3	28
12	37	−	=	+	0	3	5	23
13	44	−	−	+	0	3	2	23
14	62	−	−	+	+	3	3	22
15	60	+	=	+	+	LM	3	22
16	43	+	=	−	0	2	3	21
17	55	−	=	+	−	LM	3	21
18	55	+	−	0	−	3	3	21
19	53	−	−	+	+	1	2	20
20	50	−	−	+	−	LM	2	19

CABG = coronary artery bypass graft; ETT = exercise tolerance test; + = positive or present; − = negative or absent; = = mild; 0 = not done; D = late death; LM = left main coronary; MI = prior myocardial infarction.
Source: Wynne J, Cohn LH, Collins JJ, Jr., Cohn PF. Circulation 1978; 58 (suppl I):1–92.

First, many patients had sustained myocardial infarctions. Second, they all had undergone coronary arteriography prior to randomization. Third, patients with left main lesions or ejection fractions less than 0.35 were excluded. Fourth, although only patients with no angina or mild angina (Class I and II NYHA) were included, many patients required medication to attain this pain-free or mild-pain classification. From the original 16,626 patients who underwent coronary arteriography at 15 sites from 1974 to 1979, 780 patients with stable ischemic heart disease were randomized to medical or surgical therapy; 390 patients were in each group. With only one exception, there were no statisti-

(a)

PREOPERATIVE

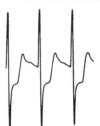

5-mm ST Depression
Heart Rate: 145 beats/min
Duration of Exercise: 4.5 min

POSTOPERATIVE

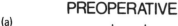
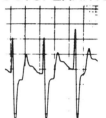

2-mm ST Depression
Heart Rate: 150 beats/min
Duration of Exercise: 10.5 min

(b)

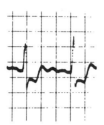

Positive 3-mm ST Depression
Heart Rate: 108 beats/min
Duration of Exercise: 7 min

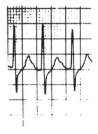

Negative
Heart Rate: 165 beats/min
Duration of Exercise: 10 min

Figure 2   Representative leads (V_4) from preoperative (left) and postoperative (right) exercise tolerance tests in two patients (a, b) demonstrating improvement after surgery. Improvement in degree of ST segment depression and duration of exercise was observed. [From Wynne J, Cohn LH, Collins JJ, Jr., Cohn PF. Circulation 1978; 58 (suppl 1): 1–92.]

cally significant differences in survival in patients receiving medical versus surgical therapy. The exception was the triple-vessel disease subgroup with <0.50 ejection fraction [8–10]. As discussed earlier in Chapter 12, the existence of high-risk patients within the three-vessel disease subgroup with normal left ventricular function can be verified only when additional tests besides the coronary angiogram and left ventriculogram are performed. For example, risk clarification is enhanced when the exercise test is employed. The best surgical candidates amongst patients with either normal or abnormal left ventricular function can now be identified. Patients with lesser degrees of ST depression and a greater duration of exercise are at low risk, whereas those with more severe indices are at high risk [10,11]. As seen in Figure 3, when these exercise parameters are related to left ventricular function (in the CASS Registry, a left ventricle score of under 9 is relatively normal, while 10 or above denotes increasing dysfunction), better risk stratification is obtained. Postoperative exercise

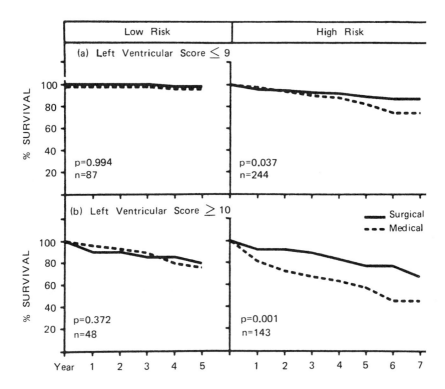

Figure 3 Cumulative survival rates in the surgical (solid line) and medical (dashed line) groups among patients with three-vessel coronary disease stratified by the left ventricular score according to the exercise risk classification. A lower risk subgroup comprised patients with less than 1 mm of ST segment depression and a final exercise stage of 3 or higher, whereas a higher risk subset consisted of patients with 1 mm or greater of ST segment depression and a final exercise stage of 1 or less. (From Weiner DA, Ryan TJ, McCabe CH, Chaitman BR, Sheffield LT, Fisher LD, Tristani T. Am J Cardiol 1987; 60:262.)

test results can also be used to predict prognosis. In the CASS survey, both silent and symptomatic ischemia on such tests adversely affected prognosis [12]. In 1999, the CASS investigators published their long-term (5-, 10-, and 15-year) survival rates [13]. Most striking were the benefits seen in those over age 75 at time of operation. The CASS Registry also included 53 asymptomatic patients with left main disease. Their outlook was significantly better when treated with bypass surgery compared to medical therapy [14]. Others have reported similar findings [15]. The CASS investigators updated their survival studies on left main disease [16] (Fig. 4) and left main equivalent disease [17] (see Fig. 5 for definition). The results remain impressive, with surgery prolonging life in most clinical and angiography subgroups.

A smaller randomized trial of medical versus surgical management was carried out at Green Lane Hospital in New Zealand [18]. One hundred patients who were asymptomatic after a myocardial infarction were followed for a mean period of 4.5 years. Annual mortality was 2% in both groups. These patients had at least two infarcts and had to survive at least 2 months postinfarction to be included in the randomization process. The patients—most with extensive coronary artery disease—again had a surprisingly low annual mortality and most were not on beta-blocking agents. This makes it difficult for surgical survival to be "better." Furthermore, of the four surgical deaths, one was from noncardiac causes and one died while awaiting surgery. This study has been criticized because of the 2-month lag before randomization began; it is in this period that most of the medical deaths occur. The most important new study dealing with surgical therapy is the ACIP trial described in Chapter 15 [19]. In that study, the revascularization arm consisted of either PTCA or CABG. In the initial 12-week and 1-year follow-up reports, revascularization had better results than medical therapy [20,21] and within the revascularization arm CABG was superior to PTCA (Figs. 6 and 7). (Interestingly, this latter finding is similar to what has been reported by others in regard to diabetics, who have a high incidence of silent ischemia [22].) The 2-year ACIP follow-up continued to show the superiority of revascularization over pharmacological therapy (Fig. 8) [23].

III. CONCLUSIONS

After reviewing these data, what is one to conclude? Should surgery be withheld from asymptomatic patients, as some argued early in the silent ischemia era [24]? Or is it indicated for prognostic reasons in selected instances such as patients with left main or triple-vessel disease, and left ventricular dysfunction,

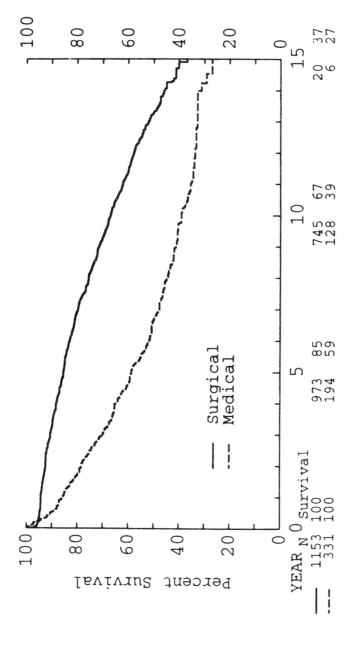

Figure 4 Graph showing 15-year cumulative survival estimates in 1484 Coronary Artery Surgery Study Registry patients with ≥50% left main coronary artery stenosis who were initially teated with coronary artery bypass graft surgery (1153 patients) and nonsurgical therapy (331 patients). The number of patients at risk for each follow-up interval is depicted next to the cumulative survival. (Reproduced with permission from Caracciolo EA, Davis KB, Sopko G, Kaiser GC, Corley SD, Schaff H, Taylor HA, Chaitman BR. Circulation 1995; 91:2325–2334.)

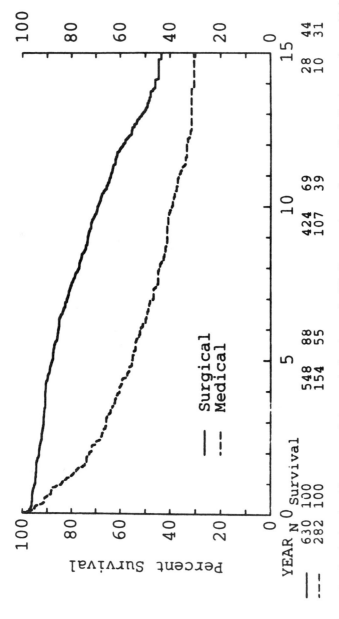

Figure 5 Graph showing 15-year cumulative survival estimates in 912 Coronary Artery Surgery Study Registry patients with left main equivalent disease, defined as combined stenoses of ≥70% in the proximal left anterior descending coronary artery before the first septal perforator and proximal circumflex coronary artery before the first obtuse marginal branch, who were initially treated with coronary artery bypass graft surgery (630 patients) and nonsurgical therapy (282 patients). The number of patients at risk for each follow-up interval is depicted next to the cumulative survival. (Reproduced with permission for Caracciolo EA, Davis KB, Sopko G, Kaiser GC, Corley SD, Schaff H, Taylor HA, Chaitma BR. Circulation 1995; 91:2335–2344.)

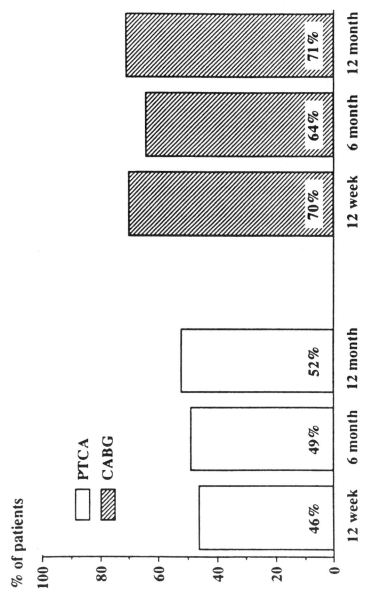

Figure 6 ACIP Study. Bar graph shows absence of ischemic episodes (or events) on 48-h AECG. The percentage of patients with no ischemic episodes was 46% after PTCA versus 70% after CABG ($p = 0.002$) at the 12-week visit; 49% versus 64%, respectively, ($p =$ NS) at the 6-month visit; and 52% versus 71%, respectively, ($p = 0.01$) at the 12-month visit. (Reproduced with permission from Bourassa MG, Pepine CJ, Forman SA, Rogers WJ, Dyrda I, Stone PH, Chaitman BR, Sharaf B, Mahmaria J, Davies RF, Knatterud GL, Terrin M, Sopko G, Conti CR. J Am Coll Cardiol 1995; 26:606–614.)

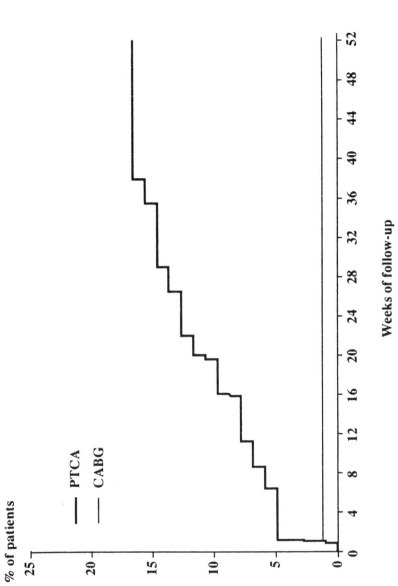

Figure 7 ACIP Study. Graph shows cumulative life-table event rates (death, myocardial infarction, repeat PTCA, or CABG). Seven PTCA patients versus one CABG patient had clinical events at the 12-week visit; the number of clinical events was 12 versus 1, respectively ($p = 0.004$) at the 6-month visit and 16 versus 1, respectively ($p < 0.001$, adjusted $p = 0.006$) at the 12-month visit. (Reproduced with permission from Bourassa MG, Pepine CJ, Forman SA, Rogers WJ, Dyrda I, Stone PH, Chaitman BR, Sharaf B, Mahmarian J, Davies RF, Knatterud GL, Terrin M, Sopko G, Conti CR. J Am Coll Cardiol 1995; 26:606–614.)

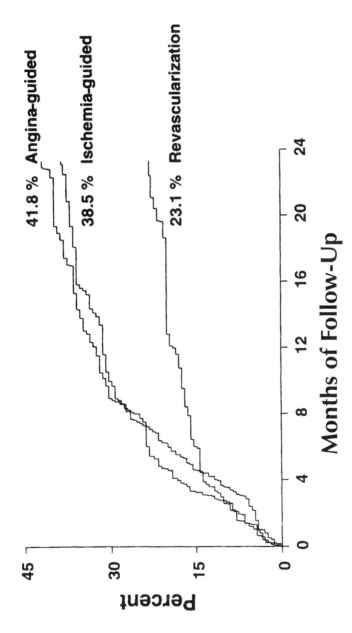

Figure 8 Two-year cumulative rates of death, MI, or cardiac hospitalization in the ACIP Study. Differences were significant between revascularization strategy and both angina-guided strategies ($p < 0.003$). The latter were not significantly different from each other ($p = 0.48$). (Reproduced with permission from Davies RF, Goldberg D, Forman S, Pepine CJ, Knatterud GL, Geller N, Sopko G, Pratt C, Deanfield J, Conti CR. Circulation 1997; 95:2037–2043.)

as others maintain [25,26] and the 1999 ACC/AHA guidelines seem to support [27]. In my view, it is the latter opinion that provides the best policy at present. Patients with less extensive disease can be managed with medical therapy and, at times, with angioplasty. It is of more than passing interest that patients who seem to benefit most from coronary artery surgery are those with active ischemia based on exercise test results, as initially reported by the European Coronary Artery Surgery Study in 1988, a finding still valid today [28]. This is dramatically depicted in Figure 9.

Survival figures are obviously the "hardest" endpoint, but evaluation of patients after surgery must also consider whether ischemia has been relieved. This is difficult to evaluate subjectively, but it can be done with objective tests of myocardial function such as exercise tests and ambulatory ECG monitoring. The latter represents an approach that may be especially useful in evaluating

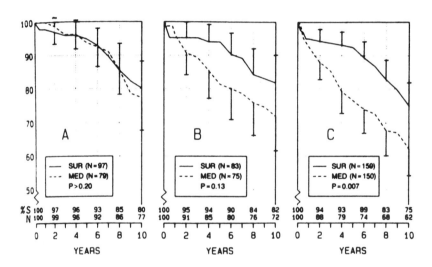

Figure 9   Ten-year cumulative survival rates and 95% confidence intervals for the surgically treated (SUR) and medically treated (MED) groups, stratified according to cardiovascular response to exercise graded by ST segment depression, maximal heart rate, and maximal workload. (A) Normal or slightly positive test result; (B) positive test result; and (C) markedly positive test result. N = number of patients; S = percentage surviving. (From Varnauskas E, and the European Coronary Surgery Study Group. N Engl J Med 1988; 319:332. Reproduced with permission.)

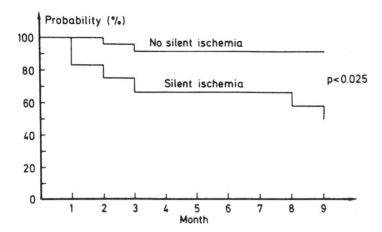

Figure 10 Kaplan–Meier curves of cumulative probabilities for cardiac events during a 9-month postoperative follow-up in 12 patients (group 1) with silent ischemia and 24 patients (group 2) without silent ischemia during ambulatory monitoring. (From Egstrup K. Am J Cardiol 1988; 61:248.)

patients with both symptomatic and asymptomatic episodes [29]. As with exercise testing, residual ischemic episodes without pain may be demonstrated. They are an adverse marker for future cardiac events (Fig. 10) [30,31]. Although the superiority of surgical procedures in patients with both angina and silent ischemia has been emphasized in the ACIP trial, we must remember this was only a 600-patient pilot study. The planned extension of this study in the next decade to include 6000 patients should provide more definitive data.

REFERENCES

1. Hammermeister KE, DeRouen TA, Dodge HT. Effect of coronary surgery on survival in asymptomatic and minimally symptomatic patients. Circulation 1980; 62:98.
2. Grondin CM, Kretz JG, Vouhe P, Tubau JF, Compeau L, Bourassa M G. Prophylactic coronary artery grafting in patients with few or no symptoms. Ann Thorac Surg 1978; 28:113.

3. Thurer RL, Lytle BW, Cosgrove DM, Loop FD. Asymptomatic coronary artery disease managed by myocardial revascularization: Results at 5 years. Circulation 1978; 61 (suppl 1):1–92.

4. Wynne J, Cohn LH, Collins JJ, Jr., Cohn PF. Myocardial revascularization in patients with multivessel coronary artery disease and minimal angina pectoris. Circulation 1978; 58 (suppl I):I–92.

5. Schnellbacher K, Droste KC, Roskamm H. Medical and surgical therapy of patients with asymptomatic ischemia. In: von Arnim T, Maseri A, eds. Silent Ischemia, Current Concepts in Detection and Management. Darmstad: Steinkopf, 1987:133.

6. Fitzgibbon GM, Buron JR, Keon WJ. Aortocoronary bypass surgery in "asymptomatic" patients with coronary artery disease. In: Rutishauser W, Roskamm H, eds. Silent Myocardial Ischemia. Berlin: Springer-Verlag, 1984: 180–193.

7. CASS Principal Investigators and Their Associates. Coronary Artery Surgery Study (CASS): A randomized trial of coronary artery bypass surgery: Survival data. Circulation 1983; 68:939.

8. Passamani E, Davis KB, Gillespie MJ, Killip T, and the CASS Principal Investigators and their associates. A randomized trial of coronary bypass surgery. Survival of patients with a low ejection fraction. N Engl J Med 1985; 312:1665.

9. Weiner DA, Ryan TJ, McCabe CH, Luk S, Chaitman BR, Sheffield LT, Fisher LD, Tristani FE. Comparison of coronary artery bypass surgery and medical therapy in patients with exercise-induced silent myocardial ischemia. J Am Coll Cardiol 1988; 12:595.

10. Weiner DA, Ryan TJ, McCabe CH, Chaitman BR, Sheffield LT, Fisher LD, Tristani F. Value of exercise testing in determining the risk classification and the response to coronary artery bypass grafting in three-vessel coronary artery disease: A report from the Coronary Artery Surgery Study (CASS) Registry. Am J Cardiol 1987; 60:262.

11. Weiner DA, Ryan TJ, McCabe CH, Ng G, Chaitman BR, Thomas Sheffield L, Tristani FE, Fisher LD. The role of exercise-induced silent myocardial ischemia in patients with abnormal left ventricular function: A report from the Coronary Artery Surgery Study (CASS) Registry. Am Heart J 1989; 118:649.

12. Weiner DA, Ryan TJ, Parson L, Fisher LD, Chaitman BR, Sheffield LT, Tristani FE. Prevalence and prognostic significance of silent and symptomatic ischemia after coronary artery bypass surgery: A report from the Coronary Artery Surgery Study (CASS) Randomized Population. J Am Coll Cardiol 1991; 18:343.

13. Myers WO, Blackstone EH, Davis K, Foster ED, Kaiser GC. CASS Registry—long term survival. J Am Coll Cardiol 1999; 33:488–498.

14. Taylor HA, Deumite J, Chaitman BR, Davis KB, Killip T, Rogers WJ. Asymptomatic left main coronary artery disease in the Coronary Artery Surgery Study (CASS) Registry. Circulation 1989; 79:1171.

15. Shawl FA, Chun PKC, Mutter ML, Slama RD, Donohue DJ, Zajtchuk R, Davia JE. Asymptomatic left main coronary artery disease and silent myocardial ischemia. Am Heart J 1989; 117:537.

16. Caracciolo EA, Davis KB, Sopko G, Kaiser GC, Corley SD, Schaff H, Taylor HA, Chaitman BR for the CASS Investigators. Comparison of surgical and medical group survival in patients with left main coronary artery disease. Circulation 1995; 91:2325–2334.

17. Caracciolo EA, Davis KB, Sopko G, Kaiser GC, Corley SD, Schaff H, Taylor HA, Chaitman BR. Comparison of surgical and medical group survival in patients with left main equivalent coronary artery disease. Circulation 1995; 91:2335–2344.

18. Norris RM, Agnes TM, Brandt PWT, Graham KJ, Jill DG, Kerr AR, Lowe JB, Roche AHG, Whitlock RML, Barrett-Boyes BG. Coronary surgery after a recurrent myocardial infarction: Progress of a trial comparing surgical with nonsurgical management for asymptomatic patients with advanced coronary disease. Circulation 1981; 63:785.

19. Pepine CJ, Sharaf B, Andrews TC, Forman S, Geller N, Knatterud G, Mahmarian J, Ouyang P, Rogers WJ, Sopko G, Steingart R, Stone PH, Conti R for the ACIP Study Group. Relation between clinical, angiographic, and ischemic findings at baseline and ischemia-related adverse outcomes at 1 year in the Asymptomatic Cardiac Ischemia Pilot Study. J Am Coll Cardiol 1997; 29:1483–1489.

20. Bourassa MG, Knatterud GL, Pepine CJ, Sopko G, Rogers WJ, Geller NL, Dyrda I, Forman SA, Chaitman BR, Sharaf B, Davies RF, Conti CR for the ACIP Investigators. Asymptomatic cardiac ischemia pilot (ACIP) study. Improvement in cardiac ischemia at 1 year after PTCA and CABG. Circulation 1995; 92 (suppl II):II-1–7.

21. Bourassa MG, Pepine CJ, Forman SA, Rogers WJ, Dyrda I, Stone PH, Chaitman BR, Sharaf B, Mahmarian J, Davies RF, Knatterud GL, Terrin M, Sopko G, Conti CR for the ACIP Investigators. Asymptomatic cardiac ischemia pilot (ACIP) study: effects of coronary angioplasty and coronary artery bypass graft surgery on recurrent angina and ischemia. J Am Coll Cardiol 1995; 26:606–614.

22. Detre KM, Guo P, Holubkov R, Califf RM, Sopko RJ, Rosen AD, Krone RJ, Frye RL, Feit F. Coronary revascularization in diabetic patients. Circulation 1999; 99:633–640.

23. Davies RF, Goldberg D, Forman S, Pepine CJ, Knatterud GL, Geller N, Sopko G, Pratt C, Deanfield J, Conti CR for the ACIP Investigators. Asymptomatic cardiac ischemia pilot (ACIP) study two-year follow-up. Circulation 1997; 95:2037–2043.

24. Selzer A, Cohn K. Asymptomatic coronary artery disease and coronary bypass surgery. Am J Cardiol 1977; 39:614.

25. Kent KM, Rosing DR, Ewels CJ, Kipson L, Bonow R, Epstein SE. Prognosis of asymptomatic or mildly symptomatic patients with coronary artery disease. Am J Cardiol 1982; 49:1823.

26. Epstein SE, Quyyumi AA, Bonow RO. Myocardial ischemia—Silent or symptomatic. N Engl J Med 1988; 318:1039.

27. Kirlin JW, Akins CW, Blackstone EH, Booth DC, Califf RM, Cohen LS, Hall RJ, Harrell F , Kouchoukos NT, McCallister BD, Naftel DC, Parker JO, Sheldon WC, Smith HC, Wechsler AS, Williams JF. Guidelines and indications for coronary artery bypass graft surgery. A report of the American College of Cardiology/ American Heart Association Task Force on assessment of diagnostic and thera-

peutic cardiovascular procedures (Committee to revise the 1991 guidelines for Coronary Artery Bypass Graft Surgery). J Am Coll Cardiol 1999; 34:1263–1342.

28.   Varnauskas E, and the European Coronary Surgery Study Group. Twelve-year follow-up of survival in the randomized European Coronary Surgery Group. N Engl J Med 1988; 319:332.

29.   Ribeiro P, Shea M, Deanfield JE, Oakley CM, Sapsford R, Jones T, Walesby R, and Selwyn AP. Different mechanisms for the relief of angina after coronary bypass surgery: Physiological versus anatomical assessment. Br Heart J 1984; 52:502.

30.   Egstrup K, Asymptomatic myocardial ischemia as a predictor of cardiac events after coronary artery bypass grafting for stable angina pectoris. Am J Cardiol 1988; 61:248.

31.   Pimentel CX, Paranandi SN, Goodhart DM, Sapp SK, Lytle BW, Simpfendorfer CC. Clinical markers, management, and long-term follow-up of early ischemia after coronary artery bypass grafting. Am J Cardiol 1995; 76:967–970.

VI

FUTURE DIRECTIONS

17

Silent Myocardial Ischemia and Silent Myocardial Infarction

What Issues Remain to Be Resolved?

Since the first edition of this book in 1986, there has been a considerable increase in the amount of information available to physicians concerning silent coronary artery disease. Some of the issues raised in the first edition have been clarified, others have not, and new issues have emerged. The 1986 workshop sponsored by the National Institutes of Health (NIH) helped to focus attention on many of the problems that were considered in the two subsequent editions in 1989 and 1993.

I. SILENT MYOCARDIAL ISCHEMIA

Present lines of investigation still include studies of the pathophysiologic mechanisms of silent myocardial ischemia. The work of Droste and Roskamm [1] on pain thresholds seems confirmed by the work of Glazier et al. [2]. Thus, there appears to be an alteration in the somatic pain mechanisms in some individuals. The basis of a neurological or humoral abnormality still remains unclear, but the role of adenosine as a chemical mediator has gained increased prominence [3]. If there is an alteration in somatic or cardiac pain perception, is this alteration found only in individuals with type 1 or type 2 silent ischemia? Do anginal patients with episodes of silent ischemia (type 3 patients) have a different pathophysiological mechanism (i.e., less myocardium at jeopardy)? The coronary balloon angioplasty data seem to suggest this is *not* the case in the type 3 patient, but better techniques to quantitate the amount of ischemic myocardium—during both symptomatic and asymptomatic episodes—will be necessary to arrive at a consensus. The widespread use of angioplasty now offers a safe way of producing transient transmural ischemia in an "approved" manner and has led to even more data for comparisons of symptomatic versus asymptomatic episodes. As far as the triggering mechanism that actually precipitates the ischemic event, exciting new research into endothelial dysfunction and inflammation [4] may be able to resolve this issue—for both painful and painless episodes.

Estimates of the prevalence of the various types of silent myocardial ischemia are more reliable now that more centers report data in type 2 and type 3 patients. While it will be difficult logistically and financially for one center in the United States to duplicate Erikssen's Norwegian study [5], it would certainly be interesting to see the results of this kind of diagnostic approach in type 1 persons in a multicentered study in the United States. But the cost of this kind of study still argues against its feasibility, as do the financial and ethical questions of confirmatory coronary angiography. The use of ultrafast CT scanning may change this perspective, however [6]. It is much simpler to obtain hard data on the prevalence of silent ischemia in asymptomatic *postinfarction* patients. The frequency of exercise testing (and Holter monitor studies) in this subgroup make it a fertile source of information and several groups have begun multicenter collaborations. Similarly, Holter monitoring in angina patients has provided reliable figures on the prevalence of type 3 silent ischemia. The ASIST [7], TIBET [8] and ACIP [9,10] surveys discussed in Chapters 15 and 16 have provided additional prevalence figures in treated populations.

Management decisions will require more than prevalence and natural history data. They will require different intervention arms to evaluate the effect of different therapies. The most comprehensive of these strategies is the ACIP study [9,10] with its "Holter-driven" approach to therapy, although both ASIST [7] and TIBET [8] also employ comparison drug regimens. These studies have helped to answer the key question: Can therapy—especially pharmacological therapy—favorably alter prognosis in patients with active ischemia? Finally, what happens to the subgroup of totally asymptomatic patients with left main and/or three-vessel disease? Are they truly as susceptible to sudden death and nonfatal infarcts as suggested by the Norwegian data [5], or are they always warned by symptoms and their course more benign [11]? How should they be treated? Medically? Surgically? Answers to these questions will be difficult to ascertain because of the small numbers of patients available for study, but guidelines can be established based on the results of the multicenter studies in patients with varying degrees of silent *and* painless ischemia cited above, as well as the ongoing SWISSI trial in type 1 and type 2 patients [12,13].

II. SILENT MYOCARDIAL INFARCTION AND SUDDEN CARDIAC DEATH

We have made important strides in documenting the prevalence of silent myocardial infarction; the Framingham Study [14] and the more recent Reykjavik study [15] are good examples of this kind of prospective investigation. Again, as in silent myocardial ischemia, we are not sure why nondiabetic individuals do not experience pain with their infarcts. Even though these are "softer" data (because physicians in general do not observe the infarct as we do the transient episodes of silent ischemia), there is still much that can be learned about these patients. Are they also experiencing episodes of silent ischemia? What is the incidence of recurrent silent infarctions? These questions remain unclear. With widespread Holter monitoring, we should be documenting many more of these infarctions and their arrhythmic complications as they occur, which leads us to the last and perhaps most important issue.

What is the relationship of silent ischemia and infarctions to sudden cardiac death? Some evidence from Erikssen's study [5] supports this link, but more data are necessary. There are many aspects of sudden cardiac death that remain to be unraveled, but one aspect of this syndrome is particularly fascinating. Are these individuals experiencing silent ischemia prior to their demise? The landmark study by Sharma et al. [16] suggests that this is so. To take survivors of cardiac death and systematically test them for silent ischemia requires a concerted effort from several centers and, by definition, we can only investigate survivors. Is this somehow a skewed population? This is one question we may never be able to answer, but, even in an era of declining mortality from cardiovascular disease, the public health consequences remain enormous.

REFERENCES

1. Droste C, Roskamm H. Experimental pain measurements in patients with asymptomatic myocardial ischemia. J Am Coll Cardiol 1983; 1:940.
2. Glazier JJ, Chierchia S, Brown MJ, Maseri A. Importance of generalized defective perception of painful stimuli as a cause of silent myocardial ischemia in chronic stable angina pectoris. Am J Cardiol 1986; 58:667.
3. Crea F, Gaspardone A. New look to an old symptom: angina pectoris. Circulation 1997; 96:3766–3773.
4. Ross R. Atherosclerosis—an inflammatory disease. N Engl J Med 1999; 340: 115–126.
5. Thaulow E, Erikssen J, Sandvik L, Erikssen G, Jorgensen L, Cohn PF. Initial clinical presentation of cardiac disease in asymptomatic men with silent myocardial ischemia and angiographically documented coronary artery disease (The Oslo Ischemia Study). Am J Cardiol 1993; 72:629–633.
6. Rumberger JA, Behrenbeck T, Breen JF, Sheedy P F. Coronary calcification by electron beam computed tomography and obstructive coronary artery disease: A model for costs and effectiveness of diagnosis as compared with conventional cardiac testing methods. J Am Cardiol 1999; 33:453–463.
7. Pepine CJ, Cohn PF, Deedwania PC, et al. Effects of treatment on outcome in mildly symptomatic patients with ischemia during daily life: the Atenolol Silent Ischemia Study. Circulation 1994; 90:792–798.
8. Dargie HJ, Ford I, Fox KM on behalf of the TIBET study group. Total ischemic burden European trial (TIBET). Eur Heart J 1996; 17:104–112.
9. Rodgers WJ, Bourassa MG, Andrews TC, Bertolet BD, Blumenthal RS, Chaitman BR, Forman SA, Geller NL, Goldberg AD, Habib GB, Masters RG, Moisa RB, Mueller H, Pearce DJ, Pepine CJ, Sopko G, Steingart RM, Stone PH, Knatterud GL, Conti R for the ACIP Investigators. Asymptomatic cardiac ischemia pilot (ACIP) study: outcome at 1 year for patients with asymptomatic cardiac ischemia randomized to medical therapy or revascularization. J Am Coll Cardiol 1995; 26:594–605.
10. Davies RF, Goldberg AD, Forman S, Pepine CJ, Knatterud GL, Geller N, Sopko G, Pratt C, Deanfield J, Conti C R for the ACIP Investigators. Asymptomatic cardiac ischemia pilot (ACIP) study two-year follow-up. Circulation 1997; 95:2037–2043.
11. Epstein SE, Quyyumi AA, Bonow RA, Myocardial ischemia—Silent or symptomatic. N Engl J Med 1988; 318:1039.
12. Eme P, Burckhardt D, Dubach P, Zuber M, Kowski W. Antiischemic therapy improves event free survival in silent ischemia Type 1. Results of the Swiss Inter-

ventional Study on Silent Ischemia 1 (SWISSI 1). J Am Coll Cardiol 1999; 33(suppl A):340A (abstr.)

13. Eme P, Burckhardt D, Pfisterer M, Dubach P, Zuber M, Klowski W. Effect of PTCA on outcome in patients with silent ischemia after myocardial infarction: results of the Swiss Interventional Study on Silent Ischemia Type II (SWISSI 11). J Am Coll Cardiol 1999; 33:(suppl A) 38A.

14. Kannel WB, Abbott RD. Incidence and prognosis of unrecognized myocardial infarction: An update on the Framingham Study. N Engl J Med 1984; 311:1144.

15. Sigurdsson E, Thorgeirsson G, Sigvaldason H, Sigfusson N. Unrecognized myocardial infarction: epidemiology, clinical characteristics, and the prognostic role of angina pectoris. Ann Intern Med 1995; 112:96–102.

16. Sharma B, Asinger R, Francis GS, Hodges M, Wyeth RP. Demonstration of exercise-induced ischemia without angina in survivors of out-of-hospital ventricular fibrillation. Am J Cardiol 1981; 59:740.

Index

Adenosine, 12
Ambulatory electrocardiographic
    (Holter) monitoring, 135–139,
    217, 223–228, 240–248
Amlodipine, 276, 278
Angina pectoris
    circulatory dynamics of, 58–61
    pathophysiology of, compared with
        silent myocardial ischemia,
        58–71
    prognosis of, compared with silent
        myocardial ischemia, 225–230
    treatment of, compared with silent
        myocardial ischemia, 270–278,
        300–313
    unstable, prognostic significance of
        painless episodes, 228
Angiotensin-converting enzyme
    inhibitors, 288

Apoprotein B, as marker for asympto-
    matic coronary artery disease,
    127
Arrhythmias
    exercise-induced, 166
    ventricular, as indicators of asympto-
        matic coronary artery disease,
        131, 240–248
Arteriography, coronary cardiac
    catheterization and (*see* Cardiac
        catheterization)
    findings of, in coronary artery
        patients with and without
        angina, 197–203, 217–230,
        241–242
    indications for, 195–197
Aspirin, 278
Asymptomatic Cardiac Ischemia Pilot
    study (ACIP), 281–284, 306

323